Dual Relationships and Psychotherapy

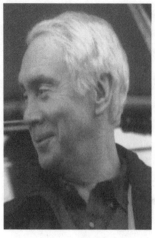

Arnold A. Lazarus, PhD, ABPP, is a Fellow of the Academy of Clinical Psychology and holds the rank of Distinguished Professor Emeritus of Psychology at Rutgers University. Previously, he served on the faculties of Stanford University, Temple University Medical School, and Yale University, where he was director of clinical training. A former president of several professional associations and societies, he has received many honors and awards for his contributions to clinical theory and therapy. These include the Distinguished Service Award from the American Board of Professional Psychology, the prestigious Cummings PSYCHE Award, and two Lifetime Achievement Awards (California Psychological Association and the Association for Advancement of Behavior Therapy). With 18 books and more than 250 professional and scientific articles to his credit, Dr. Lazarus is widely recognized as an international authority on effective and efficient psychotherapy.

His interest in examining the impact of licensing boards and ethics committees was spawned circa 1993 when two of his colleagues were severely censured by state licensing boards for transcending minor boundaries.

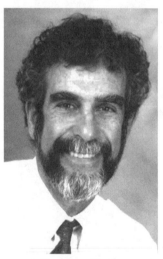

Ofer Zur, PhD, is a licensed psychologist, forensic consultant, and a pioneer of the managed-care-free private practice movement. In his nationwide workshops he has taught about ethics, private practice, burnout, and consulting to thousands of psychotherapists. He also presented the first course ever on dual relationships and how they can increase clinical effectiveness. For many years he taught courses on ethics, research, psychology of gender, and psychology of war at graduate schools, such as the California School of Professional Psychology (CSPP, Alameda, CA) and the California School of Integral Studies (CSIS, San Francisco, CA), where he also served as the associate program director. He has written dozens of articles in professional journals on topics, such as dual relationships, effective therapy, private practice development, therapists' families, burnout, victims, gender roles, and the psychology of peace and war. His 1999 article "The Managed Care Free Private Practice Kit" was given the Best Feature Article Award by the Division of Independent Practice (42) of APA.

Dual Relationships and Psychotherapy

Arnold A. Lazarus, PhD, ABPP
Ofer Zur, PhD
Editors

 Springer Publishing Company

Springer Publishing Company, Inc.
536 Broadway
New York, NY 10012-3955

Acquisitions Editor: Sheri W. Sussman
Production Editor: Sara Yoo
Cover design by Joanne Honigman

01 02 03 04 05 / 5 4 3 2 1

Library of Congress Cataloging-in-Publication Data

Dual relationships and psychotherapy / Arnold A. Lazarus, Ofer Zur, editors.
    p. cm.
    Includes bibliographical references and index.
    ISBN 0-8261-4899-9
    1. Psychotherapist and patient.   2. Therapeutic alliance.
I. Lazarus, Arnold A.   II. Zur, Ofer.
    RC480.8
    616.89'14—dc21   2002022549
                                               CIP

Printed in the United States of America by Sheridan Books.

Contents

v

Part 2: The Ethics of Dual Relationships

Part 3: Boundaries

Part 4: Laws, Boards, Ethics, and Other Forensic Matters

Part 5: Dual Relationships in Special Populations

Part 6: Dual Relationships in University Counseling Centers

Contributors

Jeffrey E. Barnett, PsyD, is a licensed psychologist in independent practice in Arnold, Maryland. He is also a core adjunct associate professor in the psychology department of Loyola College of Maryland. Dr. Barnett is a frequent presenter and author specializing in ethics, legal, and professional practice issues in psychology. Much of his work has focused on a practical and nondogmatic approach to ethical standards and professional practice, to include in the areas of boundary issues and multiple relationships. He is also a past president of the Maryland Psychological Association and is president-elect of the American Psychological Association's division of State and Provincial Psychological Associations. Dr. Barnett has received the Outstanding Professional Contributions award from each of these organizations. He presently represents Maryland on the American Psychological Association's Council of Representatives and is a Fellow of APA.

Nicholas A. Cummings, PhD, ScD, is Distinguished Professor, University of Nevada, Reno; president, Foundation for Behavioral Health; board chair, University Alliance for Behavioral Care, Inc.; and board chair, The Nicholas & Dorothy Cummings Foundation, Inc. He is also a former president of the American Psychological Association. He is the founding CEO, American Biodyne (MedCo/Merck, then Merit, and now Magellan Behavioral Care) and founder of the four campuses of the California School of Professional Psychology. In addition, Dr. Cummings has been the chief psychologist (retired), Kaiser Permanente. He is the founder of the National Academies of Practice and of American Managed Behavioral Healthcare Association, as well as the National Council of Professional Schools of Psychology. Dr. Cummings is the former executive director of the Mental Research Institute, Palo Alto. He is the author of more than 400 refereed journal articles and book chapters, and author of 18 books.

Patrick DeLeon, PhD, JD, ABPP, MPH, the past president of the American Psychological Association, has been awarded three honorary doctorates and is affiliated with the University of Hawaii, having served on the faculties of George Mason University, The George Washington University, and Widener University. He is a diplomate in clinical psychology and in forensic psychology. Dr. DeLeon is a member of numerous professional associations and societies, and he has served on many boards and advisory committees. He has been a staff member for U.S. Senator Inouye since 1973 and now is Chief-of-Staff. Dr. DeLeon is the recipient of numerous distinguished awards and citations, and he is the author of hundreds of articles.

Tana Dineen, PhD, RPsych (BC), CPsych (Ontario), is a Canadian psychologist with membership in both the American and the Canadian Psychological Associations. Through her wide-ranging career, beginning with research in the early 1970s that demonstrated how the belief systems of individual clinicians influence their diagnostic and treatment decisions, Dr. Dineen has become progressively more concerned about the role mental health professionals are playing in people's lives and in society. In 1993 she closed her clinical practice in Toronto, Ontario, and moved to Victoria, B.C., where she researched and wrote the book *Manufacturing Victims: What the Psychology Industry Is Doing to People.*

Bruce W. Ebert, PhD, JD, ABPP, obtained his PhD in clinical psychology from California School of Professional Psychology in 1979. In 1990 he was awarded his juris doctor degree from McGeorge School of Law. Dr. Ebert teaches law and ethics at the Professional School of Psychology and a course called "The Psychologist and the Law" at John F. Kennedy University. For more than 8 years Dr. Ebert served as a member of the Board of Psychology of California, including five terms as president. He was also a member of the California Psychological Association ethics committee. Dr. Ebert was recently elected Fellow of the Association of State and Provincial Psychology Boards. His latest writings include a book on dual/multiple role relationships and conflict of interest for mental health professionals. He is currently writing a book on ethical dilemmas in forensic practice.

Allen Fay, MD, is associate clinical professor of psychiatry at the Mt. Sinai School of Medicine and has a part-time private practice in New

York City. He is a graduate of New York Medical College and did his residency training at the Mount Sinai Hospital in New York. He is the author of *Making It as a Couple, Making Things Better by Making Them Worse, The Invisible Diet*, and coauthor of *I Can If I Want To* and *Don't Believe It for a Minute.* He has also published professional and scientific chapters and articles in books and journals.

John L. Fleer, PhD, JD, is the senior partner in the Walnut Creek, California, law firm Fleer, Daugherty & Raub. He is a litigation attorney with 20 years of practice who specializes in the defense of mental health professionals and institutions in civil lawsuits and disciplinary proceedings. Prior to becoming a lawyer, Dr. Fleer completed formal training as a clinical psychologist. He has written and lectured on professional ethics, suicide, involuntary treatment, sexual misconduct, and litigation techniques.

Marjorie Goldin, DSW, has practiced psychotherapy since 1973 when she completed her training at the Columbia University School of Social Work, later earning her doctorate from Adelphi University. She has served as staff and supervisor at several social service agencies, maintained a private practice, and taught on the college and postgraduate level. Currently she is a social worker with Sachem public schools, counseling children. Dr. Goldin is a past president and founding member of the Long Island chapter of the American Association for Marriage and Family Therapy.

Steve Gonzalez, PsyD, is a commissioned officer and clinical psychologist in the United States Navy. He earned his bachelor's degree from Tufts University in 1995 and his doctorate degree in clinical psychology from Nova Southeastern University in 2000. He is currently in his third year of active duty military service and is stationed at Marine Corps Base Camp LeJeune in North Carolina. His primary duties involve clinical and forensic evaluations, psychological/psychometric assessment, and consultation/liaison services. Additional duties include leading the Critical Incident Stress Management Team and providing terrorist/hostage negotiation training. He is published in the area of hostage negotiation.

Miriam Greenspan, MEd, LMHC, is a psychotherapist and consultant in private practice. For the past 27 years, she has been a workshop leader and public speaker with an international reputation in the area of women's psychology and psychotherapy. Her first book, *A New Ap-*

proach to Women and Therapy, was a landmark work in this field. She is currently working on the book *Healing Through the Dark Emotions: Turning Grief, Fear, Anger and Despair to Gratitude, Joy, Courage and Faith.*

Debra Guthmann, EdD, is the director of Pupil Personnel Services at the California School for the Deaf, Fremont. She is the former director and current project director for the Minnesota Chemical Dependency Program for Deaf and Hard of Hearing Individuals. Dr. Guthmann has made more than 100 national and international presentations and written numerous articles and several book chapters focusing on ethical issues, substance abuse, and treatment models to use with the deaf and hard of hearing. She is on the adjunct faculty at San Francisco State University, is the president for the National Association on Alcohol, Drugs and Disability, and is treasurer of the American Deafness and Rehabilitation Association.

Rafael S. Harris, Jr., PsyD, is a licensed clinical psychologist within Appalachian State University's Counseling and Psychological Services Center. His professional concentration has been the practice of psychology within university counseling center environments. Dr. Harris's therapeutic foundation lies within the existential-humanistic schools of thought, but he intervenes with a variety of ethical means depending on the particular client; thus, his emphasis on client-driven therapy in which the focus is to ascertain and implement the client's theory of change. Dr. Harris's interests within the field include positive psychology, substance abuse treatment, groups, couples therapy, psychotherapy process and outcome, and the demystification of the psychotherapist.

Scott M. Hyman, MS, is a doctoral student of clinical psychology at Nova Southeastern University. He works as a researcher in the Trauma Resolution and Integration Program and is a therapist in the Adolescent Drug Abuse Prevention and Treatment Program and Student Counseling Center of the university. His research interests include traumatic memory recall of childhood sexual abuse survivors and the mediating role of social support in the development of post traumatic stress disorder.

Miriam Iosupovici, MSW, recently retired from Psychological and Counseling Services, University of California at San Diego where she worked with a university population for more than 20 years. Much of her career was devoted to developing group treatment models and group therapy training programs. Her interests have focused extensively on intervention for sexual abuse recovery in groups with male and female survivors, graduate student populations, integrating relational therapy and Ericksonian treatment models, and supervision. Intensive postgraduate training with Miriam Polster and Erving Polster (Gestalt Training Center, San Diego) and Michael Yapko have significantly contributed to her treatment orientation. She maintains a private practice in San Diego, California.

Roberto Kertész, MD, PhD, studied at the Buenos Aires National University. He is a psychiatrist, doctor of medicine, former assistant professor of psychiatry, and professor of organizational psychology at National University of La Plata. He is the rector of University of Flores and director of the Private Institute of Medical Psychology. Dr. Kertész is the former president of the Latin American Transactional Analysis Association and former executive secretary/treasurer of the International College of Psychosomatic Medicine. He introduced transactional analysis, stress management, multimodal therapy, and other developments to Latin America, Spain, and Hungary. He translated and edited in Spanish *The Practice of Multimodal Therapy* and *Marital Myths,* by A. Lazarus. Dr. Kertész is the author/coauthor of 12 books, including *Buddhist Wisdom and Self-Actualization,* and he has published more than 100 papers in Spanish and English.

Clifford N. Lazarus, PhD, received his PhD in clinical psychology from Rutgers University in 1989. He is a licensed psychologist currently in full-time practice in Princeton, New Jersey, where he directs Comprehensive Psychological Services. From 1989 to 1994, Dr. Lazarus was the associate director of Princeton Biomedical Research, Private Association, a leading facility dedicated to evaluating new generation psychiatric medications for pharmaceutical companies and the Food and Drug Administration. Dr. Lazarus has published numerous professional papers, articles, and book chapters, and he has coauthored two popular books: *Don't Believe It for a Minute—Forty Toxic Ideas That Are Driving You Crazy* and *The 60-Second Shrink—101 Strategies for Staying Sane in a Crazy World.* In addition to his clinical, research, and scholarly activities, Dr. Lazarus is noted for his seminars, workshops, and lectures on effective psychological treatment, and for integrating psychopharmacology with psychosocial therapy.

Russell C. Llewellyn, ThM, PhD, received his degrees from Dallas Theological Seminary and Graduate School of Psychology, Fuller Theological Seminary, respectively. He is a clinical psychologist in full-time private practice and founder as pastor of Central Peninsula Church and as psychologist of Center for the Whole Person in San Carlos, California. He has served as a clinician since 1973. Dr. Llewellyn has contributed professionally as a supervisor and trainer of psychologists, facilitator of EMDR training, presenter of papers in the areas of self-esteem and humility, the use of prayer in psychotherapy, and he has served as president of the Christian Association for Psychological Studies, Western Region. He specializes in the integration of Christian faith and prayer into psychotherapy, self-esteem, and dissociative identity disorder.

Equilla Luke, PhD, is director of Psychological Counseling Services at California State University, Sacramento. She is the former clinical director of Psychological and Counseling Services at the University of California, San Diego. Dr. Luke is a member of Divisions 17 and 45 of American Psychological Association and is a licensed psychologist. Her professional interests include supervision, group psychotherapy, dynamics of intercultural relationships, and gender issues.

Simon Shimshon Rubin, PhD, is professor and chairman of the Clinical Psychology Program at the University of Haifa in Israel. Professor Rubin is affiliated with the university's International Center for Health, Ethics, and Law; has served as director of the Postgraduate Psychotherapy Program; and has chaired the university-wide ethics committee. Alongside his academic and research interests, Professor Rubin maintains an active practice as a clinician and as a consultant to individuals and institutions. Professor Rubin has been a visiting professor at the Northwestern and Harvard University Medical Schools, director of the Ministry of Health's Haifa Child, Adolescent and Family Clinic, and senior clinical psychologist at Michael Reese Medical Center in Chicago. Professor Rubin has lectured and published extensively on ethics, bereavement, and training in psychotherapy.

Katherine A. Sandberg, LADC, is the former program manager of the Minnesota Chemical Dependency Program for Deaf and Hard of Hearing Individuals. The program provides chemical dependency education, assessment, treatment, and training related to the deaf and hard of hearing. She has also presented at conferences and training sessions and published articles related to substance abuse and deafness. Ms. Sandberg is a licensed alcohol and drug counselor and a licensed teacher of deaf students. Ms. Sandberg is currently the coordinator of the Rice County Family Services Collaborative.

T. Richard Saunders, PhD, ABPP, has been in independent practice since 1976. He is a Fellow of APA Divisions 12 (Clinical), 29 (Psychotherapy), 31 (State Psychological Association Affairs), and 42 (Independent Practice). He has served on the APA council and is a former president of the Maryland Psychological Association. Currently, Dr. Saunders is associate editor of the journal *Psychotherapy*, having previously edited *The Independent Practitioner*, bulletin of the Division of Independent Practice. He has been elected to the boards of Divisions 29 and 42, and he received the Distinguished Professional Contribution Award of Division 42 in 1999. Dr. Saunders's main specific professional interests are in child maltreatment and child custody, as well as disability and some personal injury matters. Since 1999, he has served on the Division 42 Task Force on the APA Ethics Revision, where he advocated self-regulation of the profession, in the context of protecting the legal and civil rights of both the public and psychologists in adjudication.

Alan W. Scheflin, BA, JD, LLM, MA, is a professor of law at Santa Clara University School of Law. He holds a BA with High Honors in philosophy, a JD with Honors, an LLM, and an MA in counseling psychology. Professor Scheflin has authored six books and more than 50 articles, book chapters, and book reviews. He has delivered more than 100 invited addresses and workshops at the major American mental health professional organizations and at many international meetings. He has appeared frequently as an expert in court on issues of brainwashing, mind control, suggestion, hypnosis, and memory. Since 1991, Professor Scheflin has received numerous distinguished awards. Most recently (2001) he was given the American Psychological Association, Division 30, Distinguished Contribution to Professional Hypnosis Award, and the American Board of Psychological Hypnosis, Professional Recognition Award.

James Lawrence Thomas, PhD, is a clinical psychologist and neuropsychologist, on the faculty of NYU Medical Center for the last 20 years, with seven books to his credit, including *Do You Have Attention Deficit Disorder?* He has specialized in diagnosing and treating adult ADD, LD, and mild head injury for more than 2 decades, and has postdoctoral certificates in group therapy, cognitive therapy, relationship therapy, and neuropsychology. Dr. Thomas has degrees from Yale, UC Berkeley, and CUNY (Clinical Psychology, 1980) and is currently president of the Neuropsychology Division of the New York State Psychological Association. He is on the board of directors of the International Dyslexia

Association and was awarded the Distinguished Service Award by the New York State Psychological Association in June of 2000.

Karl Tomm, MD, is a professor in the department of psychiatry, Faculty of Medicine, at the University of Calgary where he founded the Family Therapy Program in 1973. He is highly regarded in the field of family therapy of his work commenting upon, explicating, and elaborating on new developments in the continuing evolution of theoretical frameworks and patterns of therapeutic practice. His articles have appeared in the *Journal of Marriage and Family Therapy* and *Family Process* as well as in numerous other publications. He has devoted much time to the application of systems theory and second order cybernetics to systemic therapy. Dr. Tomm has also served on the AAMFT board of directors.

Lenore E. A. Walker, EdD, ABPP, is a psychologist in the independent practice of clinical and forensic psychology and professor of psychology at Nova Southeastern University's Center for Psychological Studies where she coordinates the forensic psychology concentration. She was a founder and first president of the Feminist Therapy Institute and is current executive director of the Domestic Violence Institute and frequently lectures around the world. She has served on the APA Council of Representatives and board of directors and is currently president of the APA Division 46 on Media Psychology and president-elect of APA Division 42, Independent Practice of Psychology where she also served as chair of the Task Force on Revisions of the Ethics Code. She is author of 12 books including *The Battered Woman* (1979), *The Battered Woman Syndrome: Second Edition* (2000), and *Abused Women and Survivor Therapy* (1994).

Martin H. Williams, PhD, testifies nationwide and internationally in psychotherapy malpractice cases, as well as in litigation in which emotional damage or competency to practice are at issue. He continues to participate in the revision of the Ethics Code of the American Psychological Association and has served as the official observer of Psychologists in Independent Practice, Division 42 of the American Psychological Association, to the Ethics Code Task Force (the group that is drafting the revision to be adopted in August of 2002). Dr. Williams earned his doctorate in psychology from the University of California, Berkeley, in 1975. He is in clinical practice at the Kaiser Permanente Medical Center in Santa Clara, California, and has offices in Redwood Estates and Los Angeles, California. Dr. Williams often conducts continuing education seminars on the subject of ethics and risk management.

Barbara A. Yutrzenka, PhD, is currently a professor of psychology and directs the Clinical Psychology Training Program at the University of South Dakota. Prior to her faculty appointment in 1984, she served 3 years as the director of the Emergency Services Unit at Henrico Mental Health Center in Glen Allen, Virginia. Dr. Yutrzenka has been honored for her teaching and student involvement and is the author and coauthor of more than 75 professional presentations and publications. She is a past member of the South Dakota Governor's Mental Health Advisory Board and currently serves on the executive boards of the South Dakota Psychological Association and the Council of University Directors of Clinical Psychology. Her current teaching and research interests are in the areas of training and supervision and professional issues and ethics. Specific research interests include peer reporting, ethical decision-making, and nonsexual dual relationships in academic, rural, and ethnic minority communities.

Foreword: Meaningful Change Always Takes Time

Patrick H. DeLeon, PhD, JD, ABPP, MPH

One of the most interesting consequences of being personally involved, over a prolonged period of time, within the governance of the American Psychological Association (APA) is being exposed on a first-hand basis to the range of experiences and collective views of members who represent various elements of the discipline and profession of psychology. For more than a quarter of a century, I have been fortunate to have had this fantastic experience. It has been extraordinarily enriching, both professionally and personally. At times, I am simply amazed that as a national organization APA has done so well in fostering collegial discussions between such fundamentally disparate psychological communities. Science, Practice, Public Interest, and Education—they really do have entirely different ways of viewing the world and establishing priorities. Yet, we are still all one family. This sense of membership cohesion speaks very well for the quality of individuals who, year in and year out, volunteer to personally participate within the governance. I suspect that this is also the case for other professional, educational, and scientific organizations and personnel—psychiatrists, social workers, and counselors—a phenomenon that speaks well for the future of our nation. As one of the "learned professions," we have much to offer to one another and to society (DeLeon & Zimbardo, in press). My sincerest appreciation. Mahalo.

It has been my personal observation over the years that one of the areas in which we truly do not have one coherent and national voice has been that of ethics, and particularly what should be the appropriate role for APA, our state associations, and governmental licensing boards. During my tenure as APA president, the board of directors spent countless hours and retreat meeting time exploring in-depth the APA's historical approach to ethics adjudication, while also exploring a wide range of alternative options. Board members reported that they continually heard complaints from those in the field (e.g., the "grassroots"). It soon became evident to me that the various board members held very strong views on this matter. And, as I reflect upon the intensity of the discussions, I realize that throughout my service on the board over the past decade, this had always been true, regardless of the composition of the board. Ethical considerations, although superficially perhaps seemingly quite straightforward, are, in fact, clearly an area in which individual members bring intense personal experiences to the discussion and where social peer pressure per se has little impact. Board members needed considerable time to think through for themselves the various options and to test out among their colleagues what might be the resulting consequences of proposed modifications—in either the actual APA ethical standards or the historical role and functioning of the APA Ethics Committee. It also became evident that, over time, broad support steadily grew for what was essentially radical change. And, at the same time, a quite small but definitely vocal subset felt strongly that if any changes were to be adopted, they should essentially be in the opposite direction that a significant majority of the board was proposing. Again, one could see vastly different worlds and perspectives among the highest level of APA's governance officials.

As I reviewed the various public policy positions that are expressed in this book, which I personally consider to be highly reasonable, particularly regarding the complexity of "dual relationships," I could not help but think that they quite closely parallel the underlying thinking process of the vast majority of the APA board of directors, during my tenure. If so, they reflect a way of conceptualizing important policy issues that gives considerable weight to the practical realities of the practice environment of the 21st century and equally important, that reflect considerable confidence in the maturity, professionalism, and dedication of our profession's clinicians. One element is an appreciation for the extent to which professional guidelines (or standards) must be practically based, rather than purely abstract aspirations.

These arguments also reflect a philosophical orientation to providing health care (e.g., psychotherapy), which fundamentally grants considerable credence to the notion of the "educated consumer," the individual who will ultimately determine what the psychotherapeutic process (or in a larger sense, what the health care system) is all about. Yes, there may be an inherent power imbalance between the role of the therapist and that of the patient. However, if one truly appreciates that it is the patient (or client) who ultimately controls the existence, and the conditions of the therapeutic relationship, it then logically becomes the responsibility of both parties to jointly define (as coequals) the "correctness" of any dual relationship. As the authors in this book indicate, most, if not all, of the mental health disciplines have been addressing the complex issues surrounding dual relationships for a prolonged period of time.

As one reflects upon the chapters in this book that highlight the number of unusual circumstances that, at first glance, might seem to provide a practical justification for maintaining (and approving) dual relationships, one must wonder why so many colleagues have, for such a prolonged period of time, ever objected. I am referring to the discussions regarding the inherent isolation of rural America; possessing a disability such as blindness or deafness; or being of a particular cultural heritage, such as Native American. I still recall the discussion several years ago on the floor of the APA Council of Representatives regarding the ethical implications of bartering for services. Representatives from the rural states who were on the council explained to their colleagues (often from the larger cities) how this was commonplace where they resided and that it would continue to occur, notwithstanding any pronouncements from the national organization. Their persuasive arguments carried the day. Yet, at that time I began wondering—Why were we even having this discussion? If dual relationships were inherently bad, then they should be prohibited. If they were not inherently antitherapeutic (and highly respected senior colleagues clearly felt that they were not), then—Why were we even considering any prohibition? Didn't we institutionally trust the clinical competence and personal maturity of our practitioners?

One of the responsibilities one accepts when serving on the APA board of directors is to review those cases in which the Ethics Committee feels that significant sanctions, such as expulsion, are appropriate. From a decade of this experience, I know that a small, but significant number of our colleagues have acted in an inappropriate manner. From the reports we receive from the Insurance Trust, it is evident that this is a continuing reality. Nevertheless, I found myself steadily gravitating to the uncomfortable feeling that at the highest policy level within the association (e.g., at the board of directors) we could not ever find sufficient time to grapple with the underlying policy issues behind the actual "ethical standards." Individual cases were judged according to specific standards. But were the standards themselves appropriate? We did not seem to be acting in a manner that was truly responsive to our broader underlying charge. Somehow, I intuitively felt, we had lost sight of our unique responsibility as board members.

From a public policy perspective, I have always believed that it is important to constantly place what is before one in its proper perspective. The "slippery slope" argument discussed in this book is interesting and admittedly intriguing, but, as has been argued in several chapters, it has not been appropriately documented to my satisfaction. As is also described, when a national association promulgates standards (or guidelines), these are often given considerable weight by those outside of the specific profession, including those within our nation's judicial system. When one acts on behalf of all of psychology (and those who rely upon us) in proposing national standards, one must also act judiciously and with respect for the rights of all parties involved, including our practitioners. The alternative may seem at the time to be politically expedient; however, in my judgment, it does not reflect the actions of a mature profession, which is our societal obligation.

One of the refreshing challenges of this publication is the non-too-subtle reminder that psychology's clients are individual people, with all of the rights and responsibilities granted to them under our Constitution. As individuals, with their unique backgrounds and psychosocial environments, they are entitled to individualized treatment plans, after individualized assessments. It is not responsible behavior by any professional to attempt to categorize discussions surrounding dual relationships (or any other aspect of treatment for that matter) in an all-or-none fashion, or to propose blanket, uniform "solutions." Just as children are not little adults, psychodynamic-oriented therapy is not the same as providing biofeedback services. In my judgment, those who attempt to impose their vision of quality care upon others are not responsible professionals.

In many ways, the opinions expressed in this publication go directly to the challenges we collectively face as we enter the 21st century. Although the discipline of psychology dates back to the founding of Wundt's laboratory in 1879, we are, in fact, a very young profession. It was only back in 1977 that psychology became licensed or certified in all states and it was in 1988 that the APA Council of Representatives established our graduate student organization, the Committee for the

American Psychological Association of Graduate Students. Over the years, psychology has continued to be one of, if not the, most popular undergraduate majors. As we enter the 21st century, the APA membership numbers have grown to 155,000; with the American Psychological Association of Graduate Students possessing 59,700 members. These numbers suggest that within the public policy arena, psychology's collective voice will be heard. Accordingly, we must ensure that we act in a highly responsible manner. And in my judgment, this includes being willing to grapple with a number of our historical assumptions about the therapeutic process, our inherent responsibilities to clients, and the intelligent implementation of the open, flexible, and carefully thought out transactions underscored throughout this book. In so doing, we must affirmatively seek to develop a collaborative dialogue with colleagues in the other disciplines who also have a long history of providing high-quality care. The 21st century will be an era of unique challenges and unprecedented opportunities. Aloha.

REFERENCE

DeLeon, P. H., & Zimbardo, P. G. (in press). Presidential reflections—Past and future. *American Psychologist*.

Acknowledgments

Without the help of Azzia Zur and her eagle eye, editorial skills, tenacity, and patience, the compilation of this book would have been an arduous if not formidable task. Of course, true to the spirit of felicitous dual relationships, Azzia is Ofer Zur's (18-year-old) daughter. We also thank the geniuses who invented e-mails and fax machines and facilitated our frequent and rapid East–West Coast editorial communications. The process was indeed a 21st century experience and phenomenon.

Introduction

Arnold A. Lazarus, PhD, ABPP, and Ofer Zur, PhD

A dual relationship in psychotherapy refers to virtually any association outside the "boundaries" of the standard client-therapist relationship—for example, lunching, socializing, bartering, errand-running, or mutual business transactions (other than the fee-for-service). None of the codes of ethics of any major professional association states that nonsexual dual relationships are unethical. Nevertheless, many counselors and clinicians staunchly avoid entering into what have come to be called "multiple relationships," and lecturers who conduct risk-management seminars warn that therapists open themselves up to potentially serious negative consequences if they cross the threshold of professionalism into something less formal. Sexual activities are obviously and appropriately forbidden. It is also regarded as unethical to enter into a dual relationship that involves a conflict of interest, such as teachers or professors serving as therapists to students who will be graded by them, or employers entering into formal psychotherapeutic relationships with their employees. But the absolute ban on "dual relationships" so prevalent in most circles draws no distinction between "boundary violations" that can harm a client, and "boundary crossings" that produce no harm and often prove extremely helpful. Not all boundary crossings are dual relationships. It is important to note that some boundary crossings, such as hugging a grieving mother, flying with a client who suffers from a fear of flying, making home visits to a disabled client, or having lunch with an anorexic, do not necessarily constitute dual relationships. Other boundary crossings, such as socializing with clients, bartering, attending the same church or participating together in church projects and activities, working at an office at which the client is employed, teaching a class that the client attends, matchmaking or playing in the same recreational league, do entail dual relationships. The latter are examples of the types of topics that comprise the focus of our book.

Issues pertaining to boundaries and dual relationships were conspicuously absent among many of our forebears. Sigmund Freud, in a poignant and amusing exchange with Sandor Ferenczi, a prominent member of his inner circle, may be credited as being one of the first to recommend adherence to an obvious boundary. Ferenczi made no secret of the fact that he kissed his patients and let them kiss him, a detail that distressed and troubled his mentor. A letter to Ferenczi written by Freud on December 13, 1931 states:

"Now picture what will be the result of publishing your technique. There is no revolutionary who is not driven out of the field by a still more radical one. A number of independent thinkers in matters of technique will say to themselves: why stop at a kiss? Certainly one gets further when one adopts 'pawing' as well, which after all doesn't make a baby" (Jones, 1957, p. 175). In his letter, Freud went on to say that bolder clinicians would resort to "peeping and showing," which would lead to "petting parties, resulting in an enormous increase of interest in psychoanalysis among both analysts and patients." Regarding the "kissing technique," he cautioned that the younger analysts might find it difficult to stop at the point they had originally intended. Freud then stated, "And God the Father Ferenczi gazing at the lively scene he has created will perhaps say to himself: maybe after all I should have halted in my technique of motherly affection *before* the kiss."

Despite his strong words of caution, by today's standards, Freud himself would have faced possible penalties from ethics committees and licensing boards on several fronts. He gave some of his patients gifts, provided financial support to several others, entered into a matchmaking arrangement with two of his clients, gave legal advice, and offered a meal to the Rat Man. In keeping with current thinking, he would almost certainly have lost his license for having committed the boundary transgression and violation of analyzing his own daughter!

Carl Jung, according to the historians, had engaged in a sexual dual relationship. Sabina Spielrein had consulted Jung for therapy. She soon became not only his patient, but also his student, colleague, and according to her diary, lover. This resulted in confusion and suffering for both. When Frederick Perls, Paul Goodman, and Ralph Hefferline launched Gestalt Therapy in the 1950s, this movement, mainly under the aegis of Perls, became enormously popular in the 1960s during the sexual revolution and the flower child era. Blatant boundary crossings were openly espoused. For example, at Esalen in California, where Perls et al. established a training and therapy institute, therapists and clients often became playmates and even lovers. Again, by today's standards, it is not far-fetched to look upon many of their dealings as flagrant acts of malpractice.

Probably in response to this extreme laissez-faire climate of therapeutic interaction, concerned professionals became aware of the emotional damage that was being wrought and sought to establish a code of ethics and to lay down basic ground rules for practitioners. Terms such as "boundaries," "boundary violation," and "standard of care" entered the vernacular.

Today it is the mandate of the state licensing boards and professional ethics committees to oversee that no client is harassed, exploited, or harmed. There is almost universal agreement, for example, that therapists should not enter into a client-therapist sexual relationship of any kind. Clinicians who do not follow these rules can face severe penalties, including state investigation, public humiliation, loss of their licenses and livelihoods, and even criminal indictments. Many of these regulations are necessary and sensible, especially those that enforce strict consequences for sexual exploitation; but over the years, the rulebook has become needlessly stringent and rigid, and so inflated that at times it undermines effective therapy.

The impetus for this book arose out of our awareness that many punitive and picayune thinkers serve on regulatory boards and ethics committees, and they are apt to impose extreme penalties for minor infractions. Even worse, they have labeled various benevolent acts "unethical" and have chastised clinicians for engaging in them (e.g., driving a client to a railroad station during a taxicab strike, accompanying an anxious client to a dental visit, going to lunch with an anorexic client, or helping a client acquire a better sense of self by socializing with him or her).

Years ago, we believed that membership in a professional association such as the American Psychological Association (APA) would play a protective role in our professional lives. If a client ever made false allegations against us, we imagined that we could look to the APA for protection. Instead, as we learned from friends and colleagues, far from protecting us, the APA patrols and polices the conduct of its members and imposes penalties for alleged violations of its codes. The APA Ethics Committee plays a Big Brother role, often meting out severe punishments for minor transgressions or for engaging in dual relationships even whey they are clinically sound. It is obvious that tremendous bias and abuse of power can easily occur when a committee or board serves as the investigator, prosecutor, judge and jury. The APA Code of Ethics, like the codes of ethics of the American Counseling Association (ACA), the National Association of Social Workers (NASW), and the American Association for Marriage and Family Therapists (AAMFT), has also become the national and states' standard for almost all licensing boards and has far-reaching clinical, ethical, and legal ramifications.

Accountability is imperative. If such acts as harassment, exploitation, or sexual unions with clients are proved beyond a reasonable doubt, a therapeutic and educational program of rehabilitation may be decreed, and in some instances, expulsion from the APA, NASW, ACA, or other professional associations and the revocation of one's license would seem fitting and proper.

In this book we focus on *nonsexual dual relationships*, or what has come to be known as "multiple relationships." In our opinion, too many members of our profession compromise and undermine their true healing potential by forfeiting the benefits that selected clients can gain from a dual relationship. Most psychotherapists have a negative knee-jerk reaction to the idea of entering into any association with a client beyond the formal therapist-client relationship. Responses from many colleagues, both in private and in the correspondence columns of journals and periodicals, have been extremely critical of our published contentions that it is often extremely beneficial, with selected clients, to step outside the bounds of a sanctioned healer and work with people within the community, dine together, play tennis, or socialize in other capacities.

Interestingly, in the summer 2001 issue of the *Clinical Psychologist*, Alexander Chapman states, "The success of the rural practitioner may depend largely on his or her willingness to establish multiple relationships with potential clients through involvement in community committees, establishing informal community networks, etc." (p. 6). This statement is also true for many small communities, such as the military, deaf, church, gays, and certain ethnic minorities where dual relationships are not only unavoidable but in fact increase trust and often are essential for therapeutic effectiveness. It is also true of the 12-step community, which is millions strong throughout the U.S.A. and many other countries. It would include Alcoholics Anonymous, Narcotics

Anonymous, Gamblers Anonymous, CO-DA (Codependents Anonymous) and Adult Children of Alcoholics (ACOA) meetings. In those settings, a therapist or counselor may treat a fellow member.

We reiterate that none of the codes of ethics of any major professional association states that nonsexual dual relationships are unethical. They all acknowledge that some are unavoidable, but they have yet to endorse the fact that they can be beneficial. Several colleagues, who told us that they have found dual relationships with certain clients to be extremely helpful, how it had expedited treatment outcomes, were only willing to publish anonymous chapters. Although we decided not to include anonymous chapters, we nevertheless wish to share some poignant excerpts that a well-respected colleague sent us about her tribulations.

"When Arnold and Ofer asked me to write a chapter for their book on dual relationships, I actually shuddered with fear. Flashbacks. Traumas. I wanted nothing to do with this topic, didn't want my name associated with this book. I had nearly lost my license when the larcenous daughter of an elderly patient had her mother wrongfully declared incompetent so that she could take over the estate of one of the richest families in the country. When I intervened to try to help, her daughter filed a malicious complaint about me, charging me with what has become the most popular way to strip psychologists of their livelihoods, 'Boundary Violations.' This 'boundary' is defined so arbitrarily and absurdly, as in the case of a hungry psychologist giving up his lunch hour when a patient asked for an emergency visit, charged with 'eating a sandwich' during the visit. How could this be harmful?"

This anonymous writer goes on to narrate a tale of horror in which she was indicted by a state attorney general's office on two counts: (a) for "having lunch" with her 75-year-old patient (she had accepted a sandwich during a home visit), and (b) for "taking her shopping" (she had taken her to a local grocery store when her daughter had refused and it was her housekeeper's day off). The daughter's cousin, a psychotherapist who knew the ins and outs of licensing boards, had fueled this. "After 5 tortuous years, when my attorneys told me they could not help and I would never be able to work as a psychologist again, I myself wrote a letter to the governor of the state. Two weeks later the board dismissed the case and the assistant attorney general who prosecuted me was fired." We have heard many horror stories of this kind, and part of the raison d'être for this book is to challenge the aforementioned mentality, to broaden the scope of what is meant by establishing an effective therapeutic alliance, and to promote a truly humanistic perspective. This is the first book devoted entirely to nonsexual dual relationships.

The prohibition of dual relationships in therapy comes from four sources: (a) federal and state professional regulatory agencies instituted the prohibition in an attempt to protect consumers from harm by exploitative therapists; (b) traditional psychoanalysts embraced this prohibition for the purpose of ensuring the degree of detachment and neutrality that is necessary for the "analysis of the transference"; (c) our litigious culture induces fear in therapists of courts, boards, ethics committees, and attorneys. This fear manifests itself through the blind application of strict risk-management guidelines and compels most therapists to employ defensive practices that include extreme measures, such as the absolute avoidance of all dual relationships; and (d) the mainstream, traditional, urban psychotherapeutic model (vs. the rural community model), which, like the analytic model, emphasizes privacy, anonymity, separation, and strict boundaries in therapy.

Risk management is, according to a commonly held belief, one of the main reasons why dual relationships ought to be avoided. Risk management is the process whereby therapists avoid certain behaviors and interventions—not because they are clinically ill advised, harmful, or wrong, but because they may appear improper in front of judges, boards, or ethic committees. In addition to dual relationships, scheduling clients at the end of the day, self-disclosure, leaving the office together, or giving a client a comforting hug have all been placed high on the "don't do" list in the advice columns of attorneys and ethicists. The fear of lawsuits and of many hypervigilant regulatory and consumer protection agencies have created much dread and trepidation for therapists, especially around the issue of dual relationships.

"Risk management" may sound like practical or pragmatic advice but in fact, as Zur (2000) states, "It is a misnomer for a practice in which fear of attorneys and boards, rather than clinical considerations, determines the course of therapy" (p. 99). Therapists are trained, hired, and paid to provide the best care possible for clients. They are not paid to act defensively. Lazarus (1994) claims that "One of the worst professional or ethical violations is that of permitting current risk-management principles to take precedence over humane interventions" (p. 261). Clinical interventions must be determined by carefully constructed and, whenever possible, empirically based treatment plans, and not by fear of boards' and attorneys' advice. According to each client's problems, situation, personality, degree of functionality, history, and culture, such treatment plans may or may not include dual relationships. Clinically sound and clearly articulated treatment trajectories, combined with excellent clinical records and well-documented consultations, provide a more ethical and moral way of managing the risk of dual relationship interventions without losing professional integrity.

There is a fair amount of repetition in this book. We had considered wielding our editorial prerogative by trimming them out, but few people tend to read a book such as this from cover to cover. They are apt to focus on selected chapters that pique their attention. Thus, for example, the term "dual relationships" is defined and explicated in several chapters.

In various chapters throughout this book readers will find many of the issues in this introduction documented, amplified, and often poignantly confirmed.

REFERENCES

Chapman, A. L. (2001). Mental health service provision in rural communities: A challenging opportunity for growth in our profession. *Clinical Psychologist, 54,* 3–8.

Jones, E. (1957). *Sigmund Freud: Life and work.* London: Hogarth.

Lazarus, A. A. (1994). How certain boundaries and ethics diminish therapeutic effectiveness. *Ethics & Behavior, 4,* 255–261.

Zur, O. (2000). In celebration of dual relationships: How prohibition of nonsexual dual relationships increases the chance of exploitation and harm. *Independent Practitioner, 20* (3), 97–100.

Overview and Controversies of Dual Relationships and Psychotherapy

Part 1 provides an overview of the controversies of dual relationships, answers some of the most common objections, and demonstrates the situations in which dual relationships are inevitable or beneficial to clients. Chapter 1 commences with a provocative account by Zur and Lazarus that addresses the heart of the matter by examining and rebutting the most widespread arguments against dual relationships. Next, Lazarus (see chapter 2) argues that inflexible therapists who strictly avoid any boundary crossings or extensions are likely to undermine the very fabric of psychotherapy and thus subvert positive treatment outcomes. (Eight experts harshly critiqued this article, and Lazarus vigorously rebutted their contentions. The reader might well enjoy reading the entire interchange in *Ethics & Behavior*, 1994, *4*, 255–306.) In chapter 3, Tomm clarifies and amplifies aspects of the foregoing chapters by delving into the questionable ethics behind dual relationships per se. Chapter 4 presents a lucid account of the constructive power behind judicious boundary crossings and selected dual relationships. Zur clearly elucidates how exploitation and harm may ensue from the total eschewal of such interactions.

CHAPTER 1

Six Arguments Against Dual Relationships and Their Rebuttals

Ofer Zur, PhD and
Arnold A. Lazarus, PhD, ABPP

THE ORIGIN OF THE OPPOSITION
TO DUAL RELATIONSHIPS

Dual relationships between psychotherapists and clients have been frowned upon and denounced by the majority of therapists, ethicists, courts, licensing boards, ethics committees, and educators. The main reasons given for this proscription are that clients must be protected from exploitative and harmful therapists and that dual relationships, according to some, are not only harmful to clients but also compromise the integrity of the therapeutic process.

Issues of exploitation in general and sexual or business exploitation in particular are appropriately at the forefront of consumer advocates' agendas. The valid concern is that service professionals, such as psychotherapists, physicians, pastors, or attorneys, can easily exploit their clients by using their positions of authority or power for personal gain. Clients seeking help with mental health are often in crisis and likely to be highly vulnerable and suggestible. Many regard trust in and vulnerability to the therapist as an inherent part of the healing process (Barnett,

1996; Canter, Bennett, Jones, & Nagy, 1994; Caudill & Pope, 1995; Corey, Corey, & Callahan, 1984; Koocher & Keith-Spiegel, 1998; Zur, 2000b).

In view of clients' potential vulnerability and the numerous reports of harm inflicted on them by sexual dual relationships, the attempt to curtail exploitation and protect consumers from damage is reasonable and essential (Borys & Pope, 1989; Herlihy & Corey, 1992; Pope, 1988; Williams, 1997). Accordingly, most ethical guidelines for licensed mental health care providers include warnings against any exploitation and harm of patients by therapists, and a specific caution against sexual relationships with clients (e.g., American Association for Marriage and Family Therapists, 2001; American Psychological Association, 1992; National Association of Social Workers, 1999). (For a verbatim account of the Codes of Ethics on dual relationships, see chapter 5 in this volume.) Most states have developed civil and penal codes that, similar to professional ethical codes, aim to discourage therapists from entering into sexual relationships with clients. Practitioners who are reported for having violated these rules, especially those who inflict damage on their clients, are duly punished (Caudill & Pope, 1995).

ARGUMENTS AGAINST DUAL RELATIONSHIPS AND REBUTTALS

The traditional reasons for imposing negative sanctions on dual relationships stem from theoretical, ethical, and pragmatic reasoning. This chapter provides details of the principal arguments used by advocates for the prohibition of dual relationships:

1. The concern with boundaries
2. The slippery slope
3. Power and exploitation
4. Familiarity and issues pertaining to transference
5. Risk management
6. Leaving the office and incidental encounters

Each of the above six segments offers a description of the argument against dual relationships and a rebuttal. Following the critique of each predication, the reader is referred to relevant book chapters for further reading on the topic.

THE CONCERN WITH BOUNDARIES

The Argument Against Dual Relationships

At the heart of the opposition to dual relationships is an argument that places immense importance on clear boundaries in therapy. Accordingly, supporters of this line of reasoning view any deviation from these boundaries as a threat to the therapeutic process and regard such transgressions as potential if not inevitable precursors to harm, exploitation, and sexual relationships between therapists and clients (Borys, 1994; Brown, 1994; Katherine, 1993; Koocher & Keith-Spiegel, 1998; Pope, 1989; Pope & Vasquez, 1998; Sonne, 1989; Strasburger, Jorgenson, & Sutherland, 1992). Gutheil and Gabbard (1993) describe the critical areas relevant to boundary issues: time, place, space, money, gifts, services, clothing, language, self-disclosure, and physical contact.

The effect of dual relationships on the therapeutic frame is a major concern for almost all psychoanalysts and psychoanalytically oriented therapists. Many conceive this effect to be intrinsically negative and hence believe that they invariably interfere with and undermine clinical work (Epstein & Simon, 1990; Langs, 1976; Simon, 1992). Accordingly, they view all dual relationships as inherently harmful and advocate their complete avoidance. Psychoanalytic theory emphasizes the importance of boundaries and the neutral stance of the analyst. According to traditional analysts, effective management of transference and other therapeutic work requires clear and consistent boundaries that enable the therapist to preserve the analytic frame of therapy (Langs, 1988). Transgressions that detract from therapists' neutrality are said to contaminate the transference and hence are a detriment to analysis. Langs (1976) is an avid supporter of tight boundaries as a necessity for therapeutic progress. His work has been widely quoted by ethicists and those who view dual relationships as harmful. He testifies that "poor boundary management" impedes transference work and has other serious ramifications, such as the dilution of the therapist's influence. He also maintains that boundary variations, such as dual relationships, that deviate from the traditional practice of analysts are serious mistakes with a significant negative impact on the therapeutic process. Simon (1995) operates from a similar perspective and has numerous publications that epitomize the case against boundary crossings or dual relationships. Adhering to traditional analytic principles, his main guidelines state:

Maintain therapist neutrality. Foster psychological separateness of the patient. Obtain informed consent for treatment and procedures. Interact only verbally with clients. Ensure no previous, current, or future personal relationships with patients. Minimize physical contact. Preserve relative anonymity of the therapist. (Simon, 1994, p. 514)

The concern with boundaries is not limited to analytically oriented therapists. Most texts advocate rigid adherence to strict boundaries. Koocher and Keith-Spiegel (1998) claim in their widely used ethics text, " . . . we are convinced that lax professional boundaries are often a precursor of exploitation, confusion and loss of objectivity" (p. 171). Similarly, Borys and Pope (1989), Brown (1985), Kagle and Giebel-hausen (1994), Katherine (1993), Kitchener (1988), Pope and Vasquez (1998), Simon (1995), Sonne (1994), and many others view dual relationships as a detrimental boundary violation. They all view professional distance between therapist and client as essential, indeed as a sine qua non for effective clinical work.

Rebuttal

In discussing boundaries, it is imperative that boundary crossings are distinguished from boundary violations. Boundary violations refer to actions on the part of the therapist that are harmful, exploitative, and in direct conflict with the preservation of clients' dignity and the integrity of the therapeutic process. Examples of boundary violations are sexual or financial exploitation of clients. A boundary crossing is a benign and often beneficial departure from traditional therapeutic settings or constraints. Examples of boundary crossings are making home visits to a bedridden sick client; taking a plane ride with a client who has a fear of flying; attending a client's wedding, bar mitzvah, or other function; or conducting therapy while walking on a trail with a person who requests it and seems to benefit from it. Boundary crossings that also constitute dual relationships, such as socializing with clients or bartering, are the focus of this book.

Rigid boundaries often conflict with acting in a manner that is clinically helpful to clients. Rigidity, distance, and coldness are incompatible with healing. Lambert (1992) and many others affirm, through outcome research, the importance of rapport and warmth for effective therapy. Boundary crossings are likely to increase familiarity, understanding, and connection and hence increase the likelihood of success for the clinical work. Whitfield (1993) also describes how the most serviceable boundaries are those that are flexible, as opposed to those that are implemented in such a rigid manner as to cause harm through excessive and inappropriate distance.

We contend that exclusive reliance on analytic theory, which results in the eschewal of virtually all boundary crossings, has been detrimental to the overall impact of psychotherapy. Behavioral, cognitive-behavioral, humanistic, group, family, and existential therapeutic orientations are the most practiced orientations today. These treatment approaches tend to endorse what are considered clear boundary violations by most ethicists, psychoanalysts, and risk management advocates (Williams, 1997). In fact, feminist, humanistic, and existential orientations view the tearing down of artificial boundaries as essential for therapeutic effectiveness and healing (Greenspan, 1995).

As this book documents extensively (e.g., see chapter 4), the maintenance of rigid boundaries between therapists and patients in many close-knit communities is unrealistic and impossible. These communities include the *military* (Hines, Ader, Chang, & Rundell, 1998; Johnson, 1995; Staal & King, 2000); *rural* (Hargrove, 1986; Jennings, 1992; Schank & Skovholt, 1997); *religious* (Geyer, 1994; Montgomery & DeBell, 1997); *feminist* (Greenspan, 1995; Lerman & Porter, 1990; Stockman, 1990); *gay* (Brown, 1991; Smith, 1990); and *ethnic minorities* (Sears, 1990). Social norms in these communities include flexible and permeable boundaries and often favor mutuality between professionals, including therapists and their customers.

Interventions and the treatment plans, including the nature of boundaries, should be constructed according to the client's idiosyncratic situation, condition, problems, personality, culture, and history. It is preferable to base treatment plans on empirical research when available. The unduly restrictive analytic risk-management emphasis on clear, rigid, and inflexible boundaries interferes with sound clinical judgment, which ought to be flexible and personally tailored to clients' needs rather than to therapists' dogma or fear.

Throughout this book, the reader will discover many arguments of when boundary extensions and crossings increase therapeutic effectiveness. See, for example, chapters 23, 26, and 30, and parts 3, 5, 6, and 7.

THE "SLIPPERY SLOPE" ARGUMENT

The Argument Against Dual Relationships

The term "slippery slope" refers to the idea that failure to adhere to rigid standards, most commonly based on analytic and risk-management approaches, will undeniably foster relationships that are sexual or otherwise exploitative and harmful. This process is described by Gabbard (1994) as follows: " . . . the crossing of one boundary without obvious catastrophic results (making) it easier to cross the next boundary" (p. 284). Pope (1990), whose endorsement of the slippery slope idea has significantly contributed to its popularity, expresses a similar opinion: " . . . nonsexual dual relationships, while not unethical and harmful per se, foster sexual dual relationships" (p. 688). Strasburger et al. (1992) conclude, "Obviously, the best advice to therapists is not to start (down) the slippery slope, and to avoid boundary violations or dual relationships with patients" (pp. 547–548). Also in agreement is Simon (1991), who decrees that "The boundary violation precursors of therapist-patient sex can be as psychologically damaging as the actual sexual involvement itself" (p. 614). This poignant statement summarizes the opinion that the chance for exploitation and harm is reduced or nullified only by refraining from engaging in any dual relationship or boundary crossing. Many writers describe a long list of therapists' behaviors (e.g., self-disclosure, hugs, home visits, socializing, longer sessions, lunching, exchanging gifts, walks, playing in recreational leagues) that they believe to be precursors to sexual dual relationships (Borys & Pope, 1989; Craig, 1991; Keith-Spiegel & Koocher, 1985; Lakin, 1991; Pope, 1991; Pope & Vasquez, 1998; Rutter, 1989; St. Germaine, 1996). It was along these lines that Epstein and Simon (1990) developed the Exploitation Index, which has since become a frequently quoted reference in the field.

Sonne (1994) discusses how a therapist and client who are sports teammates can easily move their relationship to encompass activities, such as carpooling or drinking. She concludes that "With the blurring of the expected functions and responsibilities of the therapist and client comes the breakdown of the boundaries of the professional relationship itself" (p. 338). Similarly, Woody (1998) asserts, "In order to minimize the risk of sexual conduct, policies must prohibit a practitioner from having any contact with the client outside the treatment context and must preclude any type of dual relationships" (p. 188). The "slippery slope" argument is even more pronounced in the work of Evans (1997), who contends that from an ethical, legal, and clinical perspective, nonsexual and sexual dual relationships are absolutely equal and ought to be dealt with in the same manner.

Rebuttal

The slippery slope argument is grounded primarily in the assumption that any boundary crossing, however trivial it may be, inevitably leads to boundary violations. To assert that self-disclosure, a hug, a home visit, or accepting a gift are actions likely to lead to sex is like saying that doctors' visits cause death because most people see a doctor before they die (Zur, 2000a). Lazarus calls this thinking "an extreme form of syllogistic reasoning" (1994, p. 257). We learn in school that sequential statistical relationships (correlations) cannot simply be translated into causal connections. The fear that any boundary crossing will end up with sex is described by Dineen (1996) as part of the more inclusive problem of psychotherapists' sexualizing of all boundaries.

It is important to reiterate that whereas the analytic contingent underscores that crossing boundaries will nullify therapeutic effectiveness and hence cause harm, many other orientations have a different viewpoint. Behavioral, humanistic, group, family, existential, feminist, or gestalt therapies at times stress the importance of tearing down interpersonal boundaries and strongly dispute that this will lead to exploitation and harm (Greenspan, 1995; Williams, 1997; Zur, 2000a, 2000b, 2001a).

Contrary to popular expectations, dual relationships and familiarity with clients tend to reduce the probability of exploitation and do not increase it. The power differential in a more egalitarian relationship becomes attenuated so that the client is more likely to forestall any improprieties that may arise. (This is also amplified in the next section.) As concluded in studies of cults, exploitation flourishes in isolation (Singer & Lalich, 1995). Those who vigorously propound the "only in the office" policy and the isolation it imposes on the therapeutic encounter are more likely to foster exploitation and sexual misconduct (Zur, 2000a, 2001b). When implemented with care and integrity, dual relationships with clients and the familiarity that follows are more likely to curb exploitation and harm than encourage them.

For a more comprehensive response to the concern with dual relationships and the "Slippery Slope," see chapters 6, 7, and 17.

POWER AND EXPLOITATION

The Argument Against Dual Relationships

The primary rationale for the argument to abstain from all dual relationships is that therapists may misuse their power to influence and exploit clients for their own benefit and to the clients' detriment (Bersoff, 1999; Borys, 1992; Herlihy & Corey, 1992; Koocher & Keith-Spiegel,

1998; Pope, 1991; Pope & Vasquez, 1998). The argument is that the power differential enables and encourages therapists to exploit and harm their clients upon entering into dual relationships, that to venture beyond the threshold of the purely professional therapeutic hour inevitably fosters exploitation by the more authoritative clinician or counselor (Austin, 1998; Woody, 1998).

Kitchener (1988) describes the power differential between therapists and clients as one of the three most important factors in determining the risk of harm to clients engaged in dual relationships with their therapists. Similarly, Gottlieb (1993) lists power differentials as the first dimension in the decision-making model for avoiding exploitative dual relationships in therapy. Pope (Pope & Vasquez, 1998), like his many followers, maintains that because of the power differential, the client is vulnerable and incapable of free choice and hence exploitation is likely and therapeutic benefits are significantly compromised.

Rebuttal

The concern with therapists' power is important and valid, as the power differential is true for many, if not most therapist-client relationships. This is because therapists are generally hired for their expertise, which in most cases gives them at least some measure of an expert-based power advantage over their clients.

Power differential has almost become interchangeable with exploitation and harm in the ethics literature. However, when dealing with issues of power, one must remember that many relationships with a significant differential of power, such as parent-child, teacher-student, or coach-athlete, are not inherently exploitative (Zur, 2000a). Parental power facilitates children's growth, teachers' authority enables students to learn, and coaches' influence helps athletes to achieve their full athletic potential. Few, if any, marriage, business, friendship, or therapy relationships are truly equal. Therapists' power, like that of parents, teachers, coaches, politicians, policemen, attorneys, or physicians, can be used or abused. The Hippocratic Oath of "first do no harm" attends exactly to such dangers. The problem of abusive or exploitative power in therapy does not lie within dual relationships, but in therapists' propensity to abuse their power for selfish gain. Tomm (1993) adds, "It is not the power itself that corrupts, it is the disposition to corruption (or lack of personal responsibility) that is amplified by the power" (p. 11).

In this argument, patients are portrayed as malleable, weak, and defenseless in the hands of their powerful, dominant, and compelling therapists. The disparity in power is regarded as extreme, which is disempowering to the client. It is possible that many therapists who cling to the false ideals of the segregated therapy session and avoid dual relationships because it increases their professional status (Dineen, 1996; Zur, 2000b, 2001a) are thereby imbuing themselves with undue power that can all too easily be translated into exploitation. Many therapists work with clients who are much more powerful than them. Some clients are CEOs of large corporations, judges, powerhouse attorneys, master mediators, or successful entrepreneurs. Often, these clients do not regard their therapists as particularly powerful or persuasive, and their therapists experience them as the more powerful and successful half of the dyad. Such cases are a prime example of when therapists have to work hard at cultivating an aura of power so as to appear credible.

Many of America's businesses are family operated, wherein the members experience the complexities of dual relationships, power differentials, and the balancing of blood and money. Similarly, a therapist working professionally with clients whom they also know outside the office experience richness, various challenges, and creative difficulties, but this certainly does not inevitably lead to exploitation (Zur, 2000a).

As alluded to in the previous section, contrary to the general belief that dual relationships encourage exploitative behavior by therapists, it has been argued that the opportunity for exploitation is proportional to the amount of isolation in a given therapeutic relationship. The absence of relationships other than those developed in the traditional therapeutic session results in increased isolation. A therapist's power is increased in isolation because clients tend to idealize and idolize them. Most instances of exploitation occur in isolation, including spousal and child abuse (Walker, 1994). Sexual exploitation is less likely to occur if the therapist is also working with the client's spouse, friend, or parent or has another community connection with the client, either directly or through the client's family and friends. Therapists are less inclined to exploit those with whom they have a long-term or significant relationship outside of therapy (Tomm, 1993).

For a more comprehensive response to the concern with dual relationships, power, and exploitation, see chapters 8, 27, and 29.

FAMILIARITY AND ISSUES PERTAINING
TO TRANSFERENCE

The Argument Against Dual Relationships

The traditional urban analytic risk-management model of therapy inter-prets familiarity with clients outside the consulting room as inimical to therapy (Epstein & Simon, 1990; Faulkner & Faulkner, 1997; Langs, 1976; Pepper, 1991; Pope & Vasquez, 1998). According to this argument, familiarity contaminates the therapeutic exchange. Faulkner and Faulk-ner advocate that even in rural settings, therapists should avoid becom-ing familiar with current or prospective clients. They maintain that an ethical rural therapist must "avoid engaging in behaviors with a client that lead to the development of familiarity" (p. 232). Thus, they veto all dual relationships and boundary crossings.

The fundamental proposition behind this prohibition assumes that therapists of all persuasions require a level of anonymity so that their clients can hold them in high esteem. They fear that familiarity may breed contempt if clients gain the opportunity to see some of their therapists' shortcomings or frailties. Hence it is deemed essential to afford the client little (if any) opportunity to discover any shortcomings, weaknesses, or failings in their therapists.

Among psychoanalysts, the injunction to avoid familiarity or self-disclosure is even more stringent because it is held that veridical knowl-edge about the analyst as a person will compromise the projections necessary for the analysis of transference. The original analytic concern stems from the initial belief and theory about the management of the transference and "securing the frame" of analysis (Lewis, 1959). Analytically oriented writers, such as Borys (1994), Epstein (Epstein & Simon, 1990), Lakin (1991), Langs (1976), Pepper (1991), and Simon (1989) are in agreement that dual relationships and familiarity nullify clinical effectiveness because the purity of the transference is negated and the very fabric of the analysis is undermined.

Rebuttal

Contrary to the recommendations of therapist anonymity that stem from the urban-based model, there are some communities in which this is not feasible or desirable. The unique bond between therapists and clients in small communities is described by Hargrove (1986), Lazarus (1998, 2001), Schank and Skovholt (1997), and Zur (2000a, 2001a, 2001b) as abundant with commitment, care, and trust that, in turn, promote significant increases in therapeutic effectiveness.

Communities in which this manner of relating to clients is closer to the standard than the exception include *rural* (Hargrove, 1986; Jennings, 1992; Schank & Skovholt, 1997), *religious* (Geyer, 1994; Montgomery & DeBell, 1997), *feminist* (Greenspan, 1995; Lerman & Porter, 1990; Stockman, 1990), *gay* (Brown, 1991; Smith, 1990), and *ethnic minorities* (Sears, 1990). Social norms in these communities include the unavoidable overlap of relationships, professional and otherwise.

In small and close-knit communities, such as those cited above, clinical effectiveness is increased by familiarity and dual relationships. Familiarity is closely associated with beneficial therapeutic relationships. They are linked positively mainly because therapeutic relationships have been one of the best predictors of clinical effectiveness (e.g., Bergin & Garfield, 1994; Frank, 1973; Lambert, 1992; Miller, Duncan, & Hubble, 1997). Clients frequently emphasize the benefits that accrue when therapists interact with them in the community, outside the office. This fuller picture of clients' history, family, and interactions within the community gives context to clients' accounts of their lives. For many cases, to commence therapy without utilizing the supplementary knowledge available would slow or halt therapeutic progress and fail to serve the client, particularly in cases in which clients have a distorted view of themselves and their surroundings (Zur, 2000a).

Compatibility of lifestyle, values, and spiritual orientation between therapist and client are known to positively affect the outcome of therapy (Lerman & Porter, 1990). Clients who select their therapists based on prior knowledge and familiarity are more likely to feel connected to their way of life. The trust that is vital for therapeutic progress is already in place for many clients who choose their therapists because of prior knowledge (i.e., familiarity). In small communities, therapists are chosen in much the same way that a minister, physician, or baby-sitter is selected. The findings of a study by Gruenbaum (1986) oppose the previously described stance of Faulkner and Faulkner (1997). The items most frequently cited as harmful were rigidity, coldness, and distance on the part of the therapist.

The overriding emphasis that psychoanalysis places on therapist neutrality and distance to preserve the purity of transference work should not be seen as a model or frame of reference for the entire edifice of psychotherapy. Most therapists do not practice psychoanalysis or devote extensive time to the analysis of the "transference" (Lazarus, 1994; Zur, 2001b), yet the bulk of the therapeutic community is often expected to follow its standards (Williams, 1997). It is preposterous to hold therapists to the ideology of an orientation that they do not practice or believe in (Lazarus, 1994; Zur, 2000a).

For a more comprehensive response to the concern with dual relationships, familiarity, and transference see chapters 10, 11, and 20.

RISK MANAGEMENT

The Argument Against Dual Relationships

Risk management is the course by which therapists refrain from practicing certain behaviors or interventions because they may be misinterpreted and questioned by boards, ethics committees, and courts (Gutheil & Gabbard, 1993; Lazarus, 1994, 1998; Williams, 1997, 2000). Given the litigious climate in which we live, it has been argued that the fewer risks a therapist takes, the better. It is safer to adhere to a strict code of ethics, to cross no boundaries, and to avoid any transaction that might be viewed askance by licensing boards, ethics committees, or in a court of law. According to this argument, entering into a dual relationship with a client is a high-risk enterprise. It opens the door for inquiries into and suspicions about the therapist's conscious or unconscious motives. This vulnerability renders therapists susceptible to a host of accusations pertaining to proper treatment and the avoidance of exploitation. It is all too easy for some clients to read nefarious motives into the therapist's behavior in any extratherapeutic setting or situation.

Risk management advocates advise against any controversial interventions, regardless of their ethical or legal standing. Accordingly, bartering, hiking, or socializing with clients are high on the risk-management list of unadvisable actions. Gutheil and Gabbard (1993) claim that "From the viewpoint of current risk-management principles, a handshake is about the limit of social physical contact at this time" (p. 195). As the culture has become more litigious in the late 1990s, a whole industry of postgraduate seminars and texts have developed around the concept of risk management. In his book, *Danger for Therapists: How to Reduce Your Risk*, Austin (1998) equates dual relationships with exploitation and accordingly advises "Avoid any dual relationship with a client or former client" (p. 55). Woody has published several books on risk management, one of which is *Fifty Ways to Avoid Malpractice,* where he advocates the practice of "healthy defensiveness" (1998, p. 123).

Rebuttal

Though it sounds reasonable at face value, risk management results in practices that are based on fear of attorneys and boards rather than clinical considerations. Around the issue of dual relationships much fear has been planted in therapists of board investigations (Ebert, 1997; Peterson, 2001; Saunders, 2001; Williams, 2001). Clarkson (1994) states, "An unrealistic attempt to avoid all dual relationships in psychotherapy may be defensively phobic or repressive" (p. 32). Therapists are hired to provide services that include the best possible care for clients, not the implementation of defensive practices. As described by Lazarus (1994), "One of the worst professional or ethical violations is that of permitting current risk-management principles to take precedence over human interventions" (p. 260).

This fear of board investigations inspires therapists to take protective measures. Schank and Skovholt (1997) discuss the repercussions of this fear in rural areas, one of which is that therapists refrain from seeking consultation about unavoidable dual relationships, which lowers the quality of care for the client.

Relevant factors for the implementation of clinical interventions include the client's personality, situation, gender, history, culture, and degree of functionality. Treatment plans based on these considerations and available empirical research will far better serve the client than clinical decisions based on the advice of attorneys and the fear or terror of licensing boards. Accurate clinical records, well-documented consultations, and clearly articulated and clinically sound treatment plans are probably the best means of assuaging risk-management fears and ensuring that clients derive significant therapeutic benefits.

For a more comprehensive response to the concern with dual relationships and risk management, see chapters 3, 4, 14, and the guidelines in Appendix B.

ENCOUNTERS AND INTERACTIONS OUTSIDE THE OFFICE

The Argument Against Dual Relationships

Interacting with clients outside the office is often discouraged for *legal* (Bennett, Bricklin, & VandeCreek, 1994; Kitchener, 1988); *ethical*

(Gottlieb, 1993; Pope & Vasquez, 1991); and *clinical* (Borys & Pope, 1989; Epstein & Simon, 1990; Simon, 1991) reasons. Leaving the office is considered a boundary violation or boundary transgression (Gutheil & Gabbard, 1993; Kitchener, 1988; Koocher & Keith-Spiegel, 1998). "Seventy three percent of therapists were distressed about the fact that outside the safety of the office walls, they have little control over whether or not something is revealed about themselves or their lifestyle during these moments . . . " (Sharkin & Birky, 1992, p. 327). It is widely assumed that experience with clients outside the office leads to disruption of therapy, exploitation, harm, or sexual relationships. Common advice from consumer advocates includes a warning against leaving the office in order to discourage damaging behavior by exploitative therapists (Barnett, 1996).

The concern over incidental encounters with clients outside the office has received substantial attention by ethicists (Grayson, 1986; Sharkin & Birky, 1992; Spiegel, 1990). Analytically and psychodynamically oriented therapists are also extremely concerned about out-of-office encounters (Glover, 1940; Gody, 1996; Langs, 1988; May, 1988; Tarnower, 1966). The general message is for therapists to avoid all out-of-office encounters. Even rural therapists have been advised to avoid such encounters (Faulkner & Faulkner, 1997).

As previously discussed, the sensitivity of psychoanalysts to the issue of chance or incidental encounters is based on the concern that it contaminates the transference and hence interferes with clinical work. They also speculate that clients and therapists alike wish to avoid such encounters so that clients' views of their therapists as omnipotent are not disrupted. Avoidance of such out-of-office encounters seems to also be justified also in order to defend the therapists from them experiencing anxiety (Strean, 1981). Strean's concern is that extratherapeutic encounters are likely to provoke the type of transference and countertransference fantasies that evoke oedipal desires and sadistic urges, and significantly interfere with the analysis.

From an ethical point of view, the primary argument against incidental encounters is to avoid the invasion of a client's privacy or any breech in confidentiality. Sixty percent of respondents in Sharkin and Birky's survey reported "being concerned about the violation of confidentiality during incidental encounters" (1992, p. 327). Privacy and confidentiality have been known to contribute to trust in psychotherapy. In many instances, the private and insulated office setting provides an extremely important milieu in helping clients reveal meaningful clinical material that is essential for effective therapy. Privacy in therapy allows clients to be honest and have a sense of safety and security in the therapeutic exchange, and accordingly is associated with positive clinical outcomes (Lambert, 1991). Thus, the concern about dual relationships and other interactions outside the clinical setting most often raised by therapists and ethicists pertains to issues of confidentiality. According to this apprehension, being seen with a client in public, or even acknowledging a client by saying a simple "hello," may constitute a violation of the confidential therapeutic ethic.

Rebuttal

There appears to be a widespread belief that "privacy" and "confidentiality" are synonymous. Though they are connected, they are not identical. This was underscored by Lazarus in the January/February 2001 issue of the *National Psychologist* after being assailed by a critic who claimed that the very act of socializing with a client is a breach of confidentiality. Lazarus responded as follows: "When I am sitting at a lunch counter and socializing with a patient at his request, how does this violate his privacy or confidentiality? I get the feeling that [my critic] believes that I may be overcome by the urge to turn to the person alongside me and blurt out, 'This is Tim Smith, a patient I am treating for guilt over his extramarital affairs' " (p. 10).

In discussing situations in which therapists interact with their clients outside the office one must differentiate between three types of out-of-office experiences. As Zur (2001a) illustrates, the first type is where the out-of-office experience is part of a thought-out, carefully constructed, research-based treatment plan, such as eating lunch with an anorexic patient, taking an airplane ride with a client who has a fear of flying, or going to the local market with an agoraphobic client. The second is where the out-of-office experience is geared toward enhancing therapeutic effectiveness, such as attending a play to see a client who had overcome a fear of public speaking playing a role, or visiting a client's new art exhibit. The third type is comprised of encounters that constitute dual relationships, or what have been referred to as overlapping relationships (Schoener, 1997). These are relationships that naturally occur as part of normal living in rural, military, deaf, or other small communities. Examples of this include attending church, socializing, or playing in a recreational league with a client. All three types are boundary crossings, but not boundary violations.

Interacting with clients outside the office may not only be ethical but may actually be clinically desirable in certain situations and often consistent with Behavioral, Systems, Humanistic, Cognitive-Behavioral, Multimodal, and other nonanalytic orientations (Williams, 1997). Lazarus (1994) states, "I have partied and socialized with some clients, played tennis with others, taken long walks with some . . . " (p. 257). Jourard, a humanistically oriented therapist, states, "I do not hesitate to play a game of handball with a seeker or visit him in his home—if this unfolds in the dialogue" (cited in Williams, 1997, p. 242). Therapists' being known by their clients for their strengths and weaknesses can "humanize" the process and thus enhance the therapeutic relationship and the healing process.

Zur (2001a), in his article "Out-of-Office Experience" describes numerous instances in which he interacts daily with clients outside the consulting room in the small community where he resides. These interactions occur because these clients are also parents at the school that his children attend, clerks at the stores he frequents, or players at the recreational league in which he participates. Zur (2001b) also claims that out-of-office encounters do not, necessarily, interfere with so-called transference work. In his words, "it is all grist to the transference mill" (p. 203).

It is possible to manage incidental or chance encounters outside the office professionally and ethically. The first step is to discuss the possibility of meeting outside the office with clients early on in the treatment. Then the prudent therapist ought to ask the clients for their preferred way of handling it. While some clients prefer the therapist not to acknowledge them in public, others are quite open about the therapeutic relationship (Zur, 2001a). Clients with borderline, paranoid, or narcissistic personality disorders may have a strong reaction that must be anticipated and taken into account. It is also important to discuss any incidental encounter after it happens, at least for the first time, to make sure that clients' concerns are aired and clients are comfortable with the exchange. In complex situations or when chance encounters occur frequently, consultation with an expert colleague may be called for.

For a more comprehensive response to the concern with dual relationships and encountering clients outside the office, see chapters 4 and 7.

SUMMARY

This chapter outlines six of the main arguments against nonsexual dual relationships in psychotherapy and offers rebuttals to these points. For a more comprehensive exploration of the complexities involved in each argument, the reader is encouraged to peruse the specific book chapters cited at the end of each rebuttal.

REFERENCES

American Association for Marriage and Family Therapists. (2001). *AAMFT Code of ethics*. Retrieved July 8, 2001, from http://www.aamft.org/about/revisedcodeethics.htm

American Psychological Association. (1992). Ethical principles of psychologists and code of conduct. *American Psychologist, 47*, 1597–1611.

Austin, K. M. (1998). *Danger for therapists*. Redlands, CA: California Selected Books.

Barnett, J. E. (1996). Boundary issues and dual relationships: Where to draw the line? *The Independent Practitioner, 16* (3), 138–140.

Bennett, B. E., Bricklin, P. M., & VandeCreek, L. (1994). Response to Lazarus's "How certain boundaries and ethics diminish therapeutic effectiveness." *Ethics & Behavior, 4* (3), 263–266.

Bergin, A. E., & Garfield, S. L. (Eds.). (1994). *Handbook of psychotherapy and behavior change* (4th ed.). New York: Wiley.

Bersoff, D. N. (Ed.). (1999). *Ethical conflicts in psychology*. Washington, DC: American Psychological Association.

Borys, D. S. (1992). Nonsexual dual relationships. In L. Vandecreek, S. Knapp, & T. L. Jackson (Eds.), *Innovations in clinical practice: A source book* (Vol. 11, pp. 443–454). Sarasota, FL: Professional Resource Exchange.

Borys, D. S. (1994). Maintaining therapeutic boundaries: The motive is therapeutic effectiveness, not defensive practice. *Ethics and Behavior, 4* (3), 267–273.

Borys, D. S., & Pope, K. S. (1989). Dual relationships between therapist and client: A national study of psychologists, psychiatrists, and social workers. *Professional Psychology: Research and Practice, 20*, 283–293.

Brown, L. S. (1985). Power, responsibility, boundaries: Ethical concerns for the lesbian feminist therapist. *Lesbian Ethics, 1* (3), 30–45.

Brown, L. S. (1991). Ethical issues in feminist therapy. *Psychology of Women Quarterly, 15*, 323–336.

Brown, L. S. (1994). Boundaries in feminist therapy: A conceptual formulation. In N. K. Gartrell (Ed.), *Bringing ethics alive: Feminist ethics in psychotherapy practice* (pp. 29–38). New York: The Haworth Press.

Canter, M. B., Bennett, B. E., Jones, S. E., & Nagy, T. E. (1994). *Ethics for psychologists*. Washington, DC: American Psychological Association.

Caudill, O. B., & Pope, K. S. (1995). *Law and mental health professionals: California*. Washington, DC: American Psychological Association.

Clarkson, P. (1994). In recognition of dual relationships. *Transactional Analysis Journal, 24* (1), 32–38.

Corey, G., Corey, A. S., & Callahan, P. (1984). *Issues and ethics in the helping professions.* Pacific Grove, CA: Brooks/Cole.

Craig, J. D. (1991). Preventing dual relationships in pastoral counseling. *Counseling and Values, 36,* 49–55.

Dineen, T. (1996). *Manufacturing victims: What the psychology industry is doing to people.* Toronto: Robert Davies Publishing.

Ebert, B. W. (1997). Dual-relationship prohibitions: A concept whose time never should have come. *Applied & Preventative Psychology, 6,* 137–156.

Epstein, R. S., & Simon, R. I. (1990). The exploitation index: An early warning indicator of boundary violations in psychotherapy. *Bulletin of the Menninger Clinic, 54* (4), 450–465.

Evans, D. R. (1997). *The law, standards of practice, and ethics in the practice of psychology.* Toronto: Mond Montgomery.

Faulkner, K. K., & Faulkner, T. A. (1997). Managing multiple relationships in rural communities: Neutrality and boundary violations. *Clinical Psychology: Science and Practice, 4* (3), 225–234.

Frank, J. D. (1973). *Persuasion and healing: A comparative study of psychotherapy.* Baltimore: The Johns Hopkins University Press.

Gabbard, G. O. (1994). Teetering on the precipice: A commentary on Lazarus's "How certain boundaries and ethics diminish therapeutic effectiveness." *Ethics and Behavior, 4* (3), 283–286.

Geyer, M. C. (1994). Dual role relationships and Christian counseling. *Journal of Psychology and Theology, 22* (3), 187–195.

Glover, E. (1940). *An investigation of the technique of psychoanalysis.* Baltimore: Williams & Wilkins.

Gody, D. S. (1996). Chance encounters: Unintentional therapist disclosure. *Psychoanalytic Psychology, 13* (4), 495–511.

Gottlieb, M. C. (1993). Avoiding exploitative dual relationships: A decision-making model. *Psychotherapy, 30,* 41–48.

Grayson, P. A. (1986). Mental health confidentiality on the small campus. *Journal of American College Health, 34,* 187–191.

Greenspan, M. (1995). Out of bounds. *Common Boundary Magazine, July/August,* 51–56.

Gruenbaum, H. (1986). Harmful psychotherapy experience. *American Journal of Psychotherapy, XL* (2), 165–176.

Gutheil, T. G., & Gabbard, G. O. (1993). The concept of boundaries in clinical practice: Theoretical and risk-management dimensions. *American Journal of Psychiatry, 150,* 188–196.

Hargrove, D. S. (1986). Ethical issues in rural mental health practice. *Professional Psychology: Research and Practice, 17,* 20–23.

Herlihy, B., & Corey, G. (1992). *Dual relationships in counseling.* Alexandria, VA: American Association for Counseling and Development.

Hines, A. H., Ader, D. N., Chang, A. S., & Rundell, J. R. (1998). Dual agency, dual relationships, boundary crossings, and associated boundary violations: A survey of military and civilian psychiatrists. *Military Medicine, 163,* 826–833.

Jennings, F. L. (1992). Ethics of rural practice. *Psychotherapy in Private Practice (Special Issue: Psychological Practice in Small Towns and Rural Areas), 10* (3), 85–104.

Johnson, W. B. (1995). Perennial ethical quandaries in military psychology: Toward American Psychological Association and Department of Defense collaboration. *Professional Psychology: Research and Practice, 26,* 281–287.

Kagle, J. D., & Giebelhausen, P. N. (1994). Dual relationships and professional boundaries. *Social Work, 39* (2), 213–220.

Katherine, A. (1993). *Boundaries: Where you end and I begin.* New York: Fireside/Parkside.

Keith-Spiegel, P., & Koocher, G. P. (1985). *Ethics in psychology: Professional standards and cases.* New York: Random House.

Kitchener, K. S. (1988). Dual role relationships: What makes them so problematic? *Journal of Counseling and Development, 67,* 217–221.

Koocher, G. P., & Keith-Spiegel, P. (1998). *Ethics in psychology: Professional standards and cases.* New York: Oxford University Press.

Lakin, M. (1991). *Coping with ethical dilemmas in psychotherapy.* New York: Pergamon Press.

Lambert, M. J. (1991). Introduction to psychotherapy research. In L. E. Beutler & M. Cargo (Eds.), *Psychotherapy research: An international review of programmatic studies* (pp. 1–11). Washington, DC: American Psychological Association.

Lambert, M. J. (1992). Implications of outcome research for psychotherapy integration. In J. C. Norcross & M. R. Goldfried (Eds.), *Handbook of psychotherapy integration* (pp. 94–129). New York: Basic Books.

Langs, R. (1976). The therapeutic relationship and deviations in technique. In R. J. Langs (Ed.), *International journal of psychoanalytic psychotherapy* (Vol. 4, pp. 106–141). New York: Jason Aronson.

Langs, R. (1988). *A primer of psychotherapy.* New York: Gardner Press.

Lazarus, A. A. (1994). How certain boundaries and ethics diminish therapeutic effectiveness. *Ethics and Behavior, 4,* 255–261. *260*

Lazarus, A. A. (1998). How do you like these boundaries? *Clinical Psychologist, 51* (1), 22–25.

Lazarus, A. (2001). Not all 'dual relationships' are taboo; some tend to enhance treatment outcomes. *National Psychologist, 10,* 16.

Lerman, H., & Porter, N. (Eds.). (1990). *Feminist ethics in psychotherapy.* New York: Springer.

Lewis, P. (1959). A note on the private aspect of the psychoanalyst. *The Bulletin of the Philadelphia Psychoanalytic Association, 9,* 96–101.

May, R. (1988). *Psychoanalytic psychotherapy in a college context.* New York: Praeger.

Miller, S. D., Duncan, B. L., & Hubble, M. A. (1997). *Escape from Babel: Toward a unifying language for psychotherapy practice.* New York: Norton.

Montgomery, M. J., & DeBell, C. (1997). Dual relationships and pastoral counseling: Asset or liability? *Counseling and Values, 42* (1), 30–41.

National Association of Social Workers. (1999). *Code of ethics.* Retrieved July 27, 2001, from http://www.naswdc.org/Code/ethics.htm

Pepper, R. S. (1991). The senior therapist's grandiosity: Clinical and ethical consequences of merging multiple roles. *Journal of Contemporary Psychology, 21* (1), 63–70.

Peterson, M. B. (2001). Recognizing concerns about how some licensing boards are treating psychologists. *Professional Psychology: Research and Practice, 32* (4), 339–340.

Pope, K. S. (1988). Dual relationships: A source of ethical, legal, and clinical problems. *Independent Practitioner, 8* (1), 17–25.

Pope, K. S. (1989). Therapist-patient sex syndrome: A guide to assessing damage. In G. O. Gabbard (Ed.), *Sexual exploitation in professional relationships* (pp. 39–55). Washington, DC: American Psychiatric Press.

Pope, K. S. (1990). Therapist-patient sexual contact: Clinical, legal, and ethical implications. In E. A. Margenau (Ed.), *The encyclopedia handbook of private practice* (pp. 687–696). New York: Gardner Press.

Pope, K. S. (1991). Dual relationships in psychotherapy. *Ethics and Behavior, 1* (1), 21–34.

Pope, K. S., & Vasquez, M. J. T. (1991). *Ethics in psychotherapy.* New York: Random House.

Pope, K. S., & Vasquez, M. J. T. (1998). *Ethics in psychotherapy and counseling: A practical guide* (2nd ed.). San Francisco: Jossey-Bass.

Rutter, P. (1989). Sex in the forbidden zone: When men in power . . . betray women's trust. New York. *Psychiatric Annals, 21,* 614–619.

Saunders, T. R. (2001). After all, this is Baltimore—Distinguished Psychologist of the Year address. *The Independent Practitioner, 21,* 15–18.

Schank, J. A., & Skovholt, T. M. (1997). Dual-relationship dilemmas of rural and small-community psychologists. *Professional Psychology: Research and Practice, 28* (1), 44–49.

Schoener, G. R. (1997, September). *Boundaries in professional relationships.* Paper presented to the Norwegian Psychological Association, Oslo, Norway.

Sears, V. L. (1990). On being an "only" one. In H. Lerman & N. Porter (Eds.), *Feminist ethics in psychotherapy* (pp. 102–105). New York: Springer.

Sharkin, B. S., & Birky, I. (1992). Incidental encounters between therapists and their clients. *Professional Psychology: Research & Practice, 23* (4), 326–328.

Simon, R. I. (1989). Sexual exploitation of patients: How it begins before it happens. *Contemporary Psychiatry: Psychiatric Annals, 19* (2), 104–187.

Simon, R. I. (1991). Psychological injury caused by boundary violation precursors to therapist-patient sex. *Psychiatric Annals, 21,* 614–619.

Simon, R. I. (1992). Treatment boundary violations: Clinical, ethical, and legal considerations. *Bulletin of the American Academy of Psychiatry and the Law, 20,* 269–288.

Simon, R. I. (1994). Transference in therapist-patient sex: The illusion of patient improvement and consent, part 1. *Psychiatric Annals, 24,* 509–515.

Simon, R. I. (1995). The natural history of therapist sexual misconduct: Identification and prevention. *Psychiatric Annals, 25,* 90–94.

Singer, M. T., & Lalich, J. (1995). *Cults in our midst: The hidden menace in our everyday lives.* San Francisco: Jossey-Bass.

Smith, A. J. (1990). Working within the lesbian community: The dilemma of overlapping relationships. In H. Lerman & N. Porter (Eds.), *Feminist ethics in psychotherapy* (pp. 92–96). New York: Springer.

Sonne, J. L. (1989). An example of group therapy for victims of therapist-client sexual intimacy. In G. Gabbard (Ed.), *Sexual exploitation in professional relationships* (pp. 101–114). Washington, DC: American Psychiatric Press.

Sonne, J. L. (1994). Multiple relationships: Does the new ethics code answer the right questions? *Professional Psychology: Research and Practice, 25* (4), 336–343.

Spiegel, P. B. (1990). Confidentiality endangered under some circumstances without special management. *Psychotherapy, 27,* 636–643.

St. Germaine, J. (1996). Dual relationships and certified alcohol and drug counselors: A national study of ethical beliefs and behaviors. *Alcoholism Treatment Quarterly, 14* (2), 29–45.

Staal, M. A., & King, R. E. (2000). Managing a multiple relationship environment: The ethics of military psychology. *Professional Psychology: Research and Practice, 31* (6), 698–705.

Stockman, A. F. (1990). Dual relationships in rural mental health practice: An ethical dilemma. *Journal of Rural Community Psychology, 11* (2), 31–45.

Strasburger, L. H., Jorgenson, L., & Sutherland, P. (1992). The prevention of psychotherapist sexual misconduct: Avoiding the slippery slope. *American Journal of Psychotherapy, 46* (4), 544–555.

Strean, H. S. (1981). Extra-analytic contacts: Theoretical and clinical considerations. *Psychoanalytic Quarterly, 56,* 238–257.

Tarnower, W. (1966). Extra-analytic contacts between the psychoanalyst and the patient. *Psychoanalytic Quarterly, 35,* 399–413.

Tomm, K. (1993). The ethics of dual relationships. *The California Therapist, January/February,* 7–11.

Walker, L. E. A. (1994). *Abused women and survivor therapy: A practical guide for psychotherapists.* Washington, DC: American Psychological Association.

Whitfield, C. L. (1993). *Boundaries and relationships.* Deerfield Beach, FL: Health Communications.

Williams, M. H. (1997). Boundary violations: Do some contended standards of care fail to encompass commonplace procedures of humanistic, behavioral, and eclectic psychotherapies? *Psychotherapy, 34* (3), 238–249.

Williams, M. H. (2000). Victimized by "victims": A taxonomy of antecedents of false complaints against psychotherapists. *Professional Psychology Research & Practice, 31* (1), 75–81.

Williams, M. H. (2001). The question of psychologists' maltreatment by state licensing boards: Overcoming denial and seeking remedies. *Professional Psychology: Research and Practice, 32* (4), 341–344.

Woody, R. H. (1998). *Fifty ways to avoid malpractice.* Sarasota, FL: Professional Resource Exchange.

Zur, O. (2000a). In celebration of dual relationships: How prohibition of nonsexual dual relationships increases the chance of exploitation and harm. *Independent Practitioner, 2* (3), 97–100.

Zur, O. (2000b). Going too far in the right direction: Reflections on the mythic ban of dual relationships. *The California Psychologist, 23* (4), 14–16.

Zur, O. (2001a). Out-of-office experience: When crossing office boundaries and engaging in dual relationships are clinically beneficial and ethically sound. *Independent Practitioner, 21* (1), 96–100.

Zur, O. (2001b). On analysis, transference and dual relationships: A rejoinder to Dr. Pepper. *The Independent Practitioner, 21* (3), 201–204.

CHAPTER 2

How Certain Boundaries and Ethics Diminish Therapeutic Effectiveness

Arnold A. Lazarus, PhD, ABPP

Civilized interactions depend heavily on recognizing and respecting boundaries. To violate a boundary, whether of an entire nation or one individual, is to usurp someone's legitimate territory and invade his or her privacy by disregarding tacit or explicit limits. In quality relationships, people honor one another's rights and sensibilities and are careful not to intrude into the other's psychological space. It is therefore not surprising that the literature on psychotherapy continues to dwell on this important issue from many different perspectives.

Ethical considerations are closely related to matters of personal and interpersonal boundaries. The recently revised ethical principles of psychologists (*American Psychologist,* 1992, Vol. 47, no. 12) spells out numerous specific boundaries that all professional psychologists are required to respect. Many of the ethical principles and proscriptions emphasize the avoidance of harassment, exploitation, harm, and discrimination and underscore the significance of respect, integrity, confidentiality, and informed consent. Nevertheless, when taken too far,

Lazarus, A. A. (1994a). How certain boundaries and ethics diminish therapeutic effectiveness. *Ethics and Behavior, 4,* 255–261.

these well-intentioned guidelines can backfire. Furthermore, some psychotherapists have constructed artificial boundaries and tend to embrace prohibitions that often undermine their clinical effectiveness.

During my internship in the 1950s I was severely reprimanded by one of my supervisors for allegedly stepping out of role (one type of boundary) and thereby potentially undermining my clinical effectiveness. (In many quarters, clearly demarcated client-therapist roles have been very strongly emphasized in recent years.) It had come to my supervisor's attention that at the end of a session I had asked a client to do me the favor of dropping me off at a service station on his way home. My car was being repaired, and I had ascertained that the client would be heading home after the session and that I would not be taking him out of his way. My supervisor contended that therapy had to be a one-way street and that clients should not be called upon to provide anything other than the agreed-upon fees for service. Given my transgression, my supervisor claimed that I had jeopardized the client-therapist relationship. Interestingly, I recall that my rapport with the client in question was enhanced rather than damaged by our informal chat on the way to the service station.

The extent to which some clinicians espouse what I regard as *dehumanizing* boundaries is exemplified by the following incident. During a recent couples therapy session, the husband mentioned that he had undergone a biopsy for a suspected malignancy and would have the result later that week. Our next appointment was 2 weeks away, so I called their home after a few days to ask about the laboratory findings. The husband answered the telephone, reported that all was well, and expressed gratitude at my interest and concern. The wife, a licensed clinical psychologist, had a different reaction. She told a mutual colleague (the person who had referred the couple to me) that she was rather dismayed and put out at what I had done, referring to it as the violation of a professional boundary. A simple act of human decency and concern had been transformed into a clinical assault.

A different boundary issue was raised in the columns of a state journal. A therapist was treating an adolescent and wanted to arrange a meeting with the boy's mother. A busy professional, the mother's schedule was such that the most convenient time was during a lunch break, and she suggested they meet to discuss the matter at a local restaurant. The position taken by various correspondents was that this would not only transgress various boundaries but constitute a dual relationship. I wondered whether meeting in the park, or at the mother's place of work, in a hotel lobby, or in a car would be similarly discounted. Or could the venue indeed be a restaurant if no food but only coffee were ordered?[1]

During more than 3 decades of clinical practice, I have emphasized the need for flexibility and have stressed the clinical significance of individual differences. Dryden (1991), in an interview with me that he aptly subtitled "It Depends," clearly accentuated my contention that blanket rules for one and all will often bypass important individual nuances that have to be addressed. With some clients, anything other than a formal and clearly delimited doctor-patient relationship is inadvisable and is likely to prove counterproductive. With others, an open give-and-take, a sense of camaraderie, and a willingness to step outside the bounds of a sanctioned healer will enhance treatment outcomes. Thus I have partied and socialized with some clients, played tennis with others, taken long walks with some, graciously accepted small gifts, and given presents (usually books) to a fair number. At times, I have learned more at different sides of a tennis net or across a dining room table than might ever have come to light in my consulting room. (Regrettably, from the viewpoint of present-day risk management, in the face of allegations of sexual impropriety, it has been pointed out that such boundary crossings, no matter how innocent, will ipso facto be construed as evidence of sexual misconduct by judges, juries, ethics committees, and state licensing boards.)

Out of the many clients that I have treated, the number with whom I have stepped outside the formal confines of the consulting room is not in the hundreds, but give or take a few dozen. And when I have done so, my motives were not based on capriciousness but arose from reasoned judgments that the treatment objectives would be enhanced. Nevertheless, it is usually inadvisable to disregard strict boundary limits in the presence of severe psychopathology; involving passive–aggressive, histrionic, or manipulative behaviors; borderline personality features; or manifestations of suspiciousness and undue hostility.

Some years back, I was treating a "difficult" patient who was combative and contentious. He arrived early for his appointment one morning while I was still having breakfast. An intuitive whim led me to invite him to pull up a chair and have some toast and tea.[2] This was a turning

---

[1]It has been argued that meetings outside the office, followed by sessions during lunch, often lead to dinner dates, movies, and other social events, finally culminating in sexual intercourse (see Gabbard, 1989; Simon, 1989).

[2]Except for a period of 5 years when I worked out of a professional office, my private practice has been conducted out of my home. This, for many, is in and of itself a transgression of a significant boundary.

point. The act of "breaking bread" resulted in a cooperative liaison in place of his former hostility. Let me not be misunderstood. I am *not* advocating or arguing for a transparent, pliant, casual, or informal therapeutic relationship with everyone. Rather, I am asserting that those therapists who always go by the book and apply predetermined and fixed rules of conduct (specific dos and don'ts) across the board will offend or at the very least fail to help people who might otherwise have benefited from their ministrations.

For example, a psychiatric resident was treating a young woman who often asked him personal questions. "How old are you?" "Where did you go to school?" "Do you enjoy the ballet?" "Are you married?" In keeping with his supervisor's counsel, he studiously sidestepped all of these questions and asked about their intent. But the therapy was going nowhere, and he joined one of my supervision groups. "I think the patient is about to drop out of therapy," he said. This matter was discussed at length, whereupon I advised him to apologize to his patient, to explain that he meant no disrespect but was merely following his previous supervisor's advice. I recommended that he answer each of her questions, even showing her the photo of his young son that he carried in his wallet. At the next supervisory meeting, he reported having carried out his assignment and stated that their therapeutic alliance seemed to have been greatly enhanced; for the first time ever, real gains had accrued. The patient continued making progress.

There is something demeaning and hostile about having one's questions dismissed and answered by another question.

Client:	"Have you seen the latest Tom Cruise movie?"
Therapist:	"Why is this important?"
Client:	"Is your car the blue Chevy with the white interior?"
Therapist:	"Why do you want to know?"

It is even more demeaning when therapists simply dismiss straightforward queries:

Client:	"Did you play hockey in high school?"
Therapist:	"We are here to discuss you, not me."

Unless there are valid reasons for not being forthright, or unless the question goes beyond the bounds of propriety, why not answer it candidly and then inquire as to its significance? "Yes, I was quite an avid hockey player in high school. Why do you ask?"

An example of what strikes me as an excessive boundary issue was related by one of my students. He was seeing a client who had written a short poem that she wished to share with him. According to my student, his supervisor was concerned that he may have taken the poem and read it, rather than having asked the client to read it to him. The supervisor had allegedly stated, "It's best not to touch or handle clients' personal possessions." This type of rigid professionalism is most unfortunate and seems likely to breed alienation and distance and is apt to rupture the therapeutic relationship rather than foster it.

My thesis is that it doesn't hurt to temper rules and regulations with a touch of common sense. Thus a colleague referred a couple to me. After two sessions, it seemed that their individual agendas took priority over their dyadic transactions, and I suggested to my colleague that she might want to work with the wife while I treated the husband. A few weeks later, I asked my colleague if she felt, as I did, that the marriage was probably bankrupt. "I can't discuss this with you because I have not obtained [the wife's] permission to do so," she replied. Ethically, my colleague was certainly toeing the line, but to my way of thinking, she exercised poor clinical judgment. My question was not an idle, voyeuristic attempt to pry into her client's privacy. It was geared toward a potentially helpful collegial exchange of information. Besides, having seen the wife myself, I was not a casual outsider, but someone who was concerned about and involved with the dyadic system.

By contrast, I was approached by a colleague who was treating one of my former clients and wanted specific information about him. Strictly speaking, I should first have obtained a written release from the client. Instead of wasting time, I simply told my colleague about traps and barriers that the client had erected that had undermined the therapy. I was able to alert her to various pitfalls that the client was likely to dig and into which she (like I) would probably fall unless she exercised due caution. She subsequently informed me that my caveats were of enormous clinical value in forestalling a self-sabotaging client from destroying his life. My motives behind this collegial interchange were obviously entirely in the client's best interests.

I have crossed many boundaries to good effect. I have even treated relatives and friends in addition to colleagues and acquaintances, and some of my closest friends are former clients. Nevertheless, my plea for flexibility and my defense of unorthodoxy are not completely heretical. I remain totally opposed to any form of disparagement, exploitation, abuse, or harassment, and I am against any form of sexual contact with clients. But outside of these confines, I feel that most other limits and proscriptions are negotiable. But the litigious climate in which we live has made me more cautious in recent years. I would not take certain risks that I gave no thought to in the 1960s. For example, I accepted two clients into my home (at different times). One lived with my family for several weeks, the other for several days. Both were men from out of state who had relocated and were looking for a place to live. Similarly, I would have thought nothing of offering a client our spare bedroom on a snowy night or furnishing a couple of aspirins if someone asked for them. But like most of my colleagues, I have attended seminars on how to avoid malpractice suits that have made my blood run cold. It is difficult to come away from those lectures without viewing every client as a potential adversary or litigant. Fortunately, the effects tended to wear off after a few days, and I regained my spontaneity. But the ominous undertones remain firmly implanted and are reinforced by passages in books that explain how innocent psychologists can protect themselves against unwarranted lawsuits (Keith-Spiegel & Koocher, 1985). Consequently, being more guarded has rendered me a less humane practitioner today than I used to be in the 1960s and 1970s.

It is interesting that Freud gave some patients gifts, loaned them books, sent them postcards, offered a meal to the Rat Man, and even provided financial support in a few cases. Perhaps Freud's most striking boundary violation was the analysis of his own daughter, Anna. According to Gutheil and Gabbard (1993), "these behaviors are no longer acceptable practice regardless of their place in the history of our field" (p. 189).

While reading a book on psychodrama by Kellermann (1992), I was particularly impressed with his account of a client who had participated in psychodrama groups for many years. When asked what she had found most helpful, the client stated,

> The most important thing for me was that I established a close relationship with Zerka,[3] a kind of friendship which extended beyond the ordinary patient-therapist relation. She took me to restaurants and on trips and treated me like my own mother had never done. That friendship had such a great impact on me that I can feel its effects to this very day! (p. 133)

It is, of course, safer and easier to go by the book, to adhere to an inflexible set of rules, than to think for oneself. But practitioners who

---

[3]Psychodrama was founded by J. L. Moreno (1889–1974). His wife Zerka, son Jonathan, and many enthusiasts have carried on and extended the overall tradition.

hide behind rigid boundaries, whose sense of ethics is uncompromising, will, in my opinion, fail to really help many of the clients who are unfortunate enough to consult them. The truly great therapists I have met were not frightened conformists but courageous and enterprising helpers, willing to take calculated risks. If I am to summarize my position in one sentence, I would say that one of the worst professional or ethical violations is that of permitting current risk-management principles to take precedence over humane interventions. By all means drive defensively, but try to practice psychotherapy responsibly—with compassion, benevolence, sensitivity, and caring.

ACKNOWLEDGMENT

I am most grateful to Allen Fay, MD and Clifford N. Lazarus, PhD for their criticisms of the initial draft.

REFERENCES

Dryden, W. (1911). *A dialogue with Arnold Lazarus: "It depends."* Philadelphia: Open University Press.

Gabbard, G. O.(Ed.). (1989). *Sexual exploitation in professional relationships.* Washington, DC: American Psychiatric Press.

Gutheil, T. G., & Gabbard, G. O. (1993). The concept of boundaries in clinical practice: Theoretical and risk-management dimensions. *American Journal of Psychiatry, 150,* 188–196.

Keith-Spiegel, P., & Koocher, G. P. (1985). *Ethics in psychology: Professional standards and cases.* New York: Random House.

Kellermann, P. F. (1992). *Focus on psychodrama.* Philadelphia: Jessica Kingsley.

Simon, R. I. (1989). Sexual exploitation of patients: How it begins before it happens. *Psychiatric Annals, 19,* 104–122.

CHAPTER 3

The Ethics of Dual Relationships

Karl Tomm, MD

In my opinion, the American Association for Marriage and Family Therapy (AAMFT) Ethics Committee and the AAMFT Board are attending to the wrong issue in actively discouraging dual relationships in the field of family therapy. The focus in the *AAMFT Code of Ethics* should remain centered on the avoidance of exploitation and not be shifted onto the avoidance of dual relationships. I acknowledge the importance of finding ways to protect the dependency and trust of clients. However, a more specific means of doing so is required than simply avoiding dual relationships. An ethical injunction to avoid duality not only fails to address the exploitation that occurs within professional relationships, it introduces some of its own problems.

Exploitation and dual relationships are very different phenomena. To exploit is "to use selfishly for one's own ends" (Webster, 1989). In the context of a professional discipline it refers to taking advantage of one's professional relationship to use, or abuse, another person. Exploitation in relationships is always exploitation, regardless of whether it occurs in a dual relationship, a therapy relationship, a supervisory relationship, or a research relationship. A dual relationship is one

Reprinted by permission. Tomm, K. (1993). The ethics of dual relationships. *The California Psychologist, January/February*, 7–19. First published in *The Calgary Participator, A Family Therapy Newsletter*, Winter 1991, Volume 1, Number 3.

in which there are two (or more) distinct kinds of relationships with the same person. For instance, a therapist who has a relationship with someone as a client and who also has another relationship with that person, such as as an employer, an employee, a business associate, a customer, a colleague, a supervisee, a research subject, a neighbor, a friend, or a relative, is involved in a dual relationship. While dual relationships always introduce greater complexity, they are not inherently exploitative. Indeed, the additional human connectedness through a dual relationship is far more likely to be affirming, reassuring, and enhancing, than exploitative. To discourage all dual relationships in the field is to promote an artificial professional cleavage in the natural *patterns that connect* us as human beings. It is a stance that is far more impoverishing than it is protective.

The concern about dual relationships has been evident in the *AAMFT Code of Ethics* for some time. However, it has emerged even more strongly in the latest version of the *Code*, which was approved by the AAMFT Board in March 1991 and came into effect on August 1, 1991. This version explicitly urges the avoidance of dual relationships in three areas: (a) with clients, (b) with students, supervisees, and employees, and (c) with research participants. As such, the present *Code* imposes a pervasive restraint upon the nature and complexity of interpersonal relationships that are acceptable in the field. I regard this broad restrictive stance as counterproductive and believe the relevant issues need to be explored more rigorously and discussed more widely so that the statements in the *Code* can be reconsidered, and hopefully will be rewritten. In the reflections that follow, I will cite the pertinent sections of the current *Code*, raise concerns about the restrictions, draw attention to the potential benefits of dual relationships, and suggest that the issue be reexamined and the *Code* be revised.

RELEVANT SECTIONS OF THE 1991 AAMFT CODE OF ETHICS

Under the first principle, *Responsibility to Clients*, Subprinciple 1.2 states

> Marriage and family therapists are aware of their influential position with respect to clients, and they avoid exploiting the trust and dependency of each person. Therapists, therefore, make every effort to avoid dual relationships with clients that could impair professional judgment or increase the risk of exploitation. When a dual relationship cannot be avoided, therapists

take appropriate professional precautions to ensure judgment is not impaired and no exploitation occurs. Examples of such dual relationships include, but are not limited to, business or close personal relationships with clients. Sexual intimacy with clients is prohibited. Sexual intimacy with former clients for two years following the termination of therapy is prohibited.

On the surface this seems like a reasonable statement and I certainly agree that exploitation of clients and sexual intimacy with clients are unethical. However, I find the logical implication (introduced with "Therapists, therefore . . . ") that dual relationships are the source of exploitation extremely misleading. Even if one denies such a causal interpretation, one is still left with "guilt by association." The overall statement begins by encouraging an avoidance of exploitation; suggests this could be achieved by avoiding dual relationships; and concludes by prohibiting sexual intimacy with clients. By inserting the issue of dual relationships in the text between the general issue of exploitation and the specific issue of sexual exploitation, any relationship with a client outside the therapeutic relationship is given a very strong negative connotation. Indeed, there is no acknowledgment whatsoever of any potential benefit of dual relationships. The committee has turned a *blind eye* to the personal affirmation, improved reality testing, and mutual enrichment that often emerges through such relationships.

In my view, it is not duality that constitutes the ethical problem; it is a therapist's personal propensity and readiness to exploit clients (and occasionally a client's readiness to exploit therapists) that is central. Having a second relationship with the client only provides another avenue for exploitation to take place, if a therapist or client already happens to be so inclined. Duality per se does not create nor encourage exploitation. Yet, it appears that the AAMFT Ethics Committee would have us believe it does. In promulgating this view the committee is obfuscating the core ethical issue. It is shifting the focus from exploitation to duality and is promoting a treacherous illusion that exploitation can be prevented by simply avoiding dual relationships. Therapists could become complacent about their power and influence if they believed that they could not exploit clients by virtue of not having dual relationships with them. A therapist who is inclined to exploit clients does not need a dual relationship to do so. Various forms of exploitation and abuse, including sexual abuse, can take place within the therapeutic relationship and in the therapy room itself. Fortunately, the statement in the *Code* prohibiting sexual exploitation is clear and to the point and is not confused with duality.

But why would the Ethics Committee shift the focus from exploitation to duality? Do the members of the committee believe that dual relationships are, in fact, inherently problematic and therefore wrong? If so, this needs to be fully explained. Is it because there is a concern that the dependency and trust in the professional relationship will be transferred to and exploited in the dual relationship? This is a legitimate concern, but why give priority to exploitation in a dual relationship over exploitation in the professional relationship? Exploitation needs to be challenged wherever it occurs. Or is it simply because so many of the complaints that come to the attention of the committee entail dual relationships? The possibility that many complaints about therapists first arise through dual relationships does not mean that the dual relationship is the primary source of the problem. It usually is easier for clients to recognize exploitation in a nontherapeutic relationship than in a therapeutic relationship. This obtains because a therapeutic relationship tends to be unique in the client's experience, while the dual relationship can be compared with other similar (business or personal) relationships that the client has or has had. The availability of these comparisons is one reason why dual relationships actually may be protective.

They serve as a potential means for identifying subtle forms of exploitation so that appropriate restraints can be initiated. I suspect that if there is exploitation in a dual relationship there is also exploitation in the therapeutic relationship. The dual relationship route for client recognition of exploitation may have contributed to the Ethics Committees erroneous conclusion that a major source of exploitation is duality itself. Another possible reason for the committee's focus on duality may be administrative expediency. It is relatively easy for an ethics panel to determine whether or not a dual relationship has existed while it is sometimes quite difficult to determine whether or not exploitation has taken place. However, such expediency alone would not justify an ethical principle to avoid such relationships.

Under the fourth principle, *Responsibility to Students, Employees and Supervisees,* Subprinciple 4.1 states:

Marriage and family therapists are aware of their influential position with respect to students, employees and supervisees, and they avoid exploiting the trust and dependency of such persons. Therapists, therefore, make every effort to avoid dual relationships that could impair professional judgment or increase the risk of exploitation. When a dual relationship cannot be avoided, therapists take appropriate professional precautions to ensure judgment is not impaired and no exploitation occurs. Examples of such dual relationships include, but are not limited to, business or close personal relationships with students, employees, or supervisees. Provision of therapy to students, employees, or supervisees is prohibited. Sexual intimacy with students or supervisees is prohibited.

Besides perpetuating further obfuscation of duality as a source of exploitation, this statement again shifts the focus away from the more important issue, namely the increased interpersonal *power* available to the person in the dual positions of, for instance, supervisor and therapist. There is a significant power differential in all of the relationships referred to; between therapist and client, between teacher and student, between supervisor and supervisee and between employer and employee. The core ethical concern should be whether the power differential (in any one or combination of these relationships) is used to empower the personal and professional development of the other, or is used to exploit him or her. Obviously the more power one holds, the more devastating the possibilities for destructiveness. However, the converse is also true. The more power one holds, the greater the possibilities for constructive initiatives as well. It is not the power itself that corrupts, it is the disposition to corruption (or lack of personal responsibility) that is amplified by the power. If a training supervisor cum therapist is genuinely disposed to be helpful (an orientation which is presupposed for these social roles), the increased power will empower his or her helpfulness. Thus, the ethical focus in this principle should be on whether the increase in interpersonal power is exercised responsibly and on how one can build in more accountability when dual relationships do happen to emerge.

If the Ethics Committee was less preoccupied with duality and, instead, was more concerned about the imbalance of power in professional relations (which is intensified when a supervisor also becomes a therapist), it would have proposed a different means of taking "precautions." For instance, it would have proposed a means of increasing the power of the supervisee/client as a counterbalance. This could be done by proposing that the therapist/supervisor empower the client/supervisee to select a third party to review or monitor any disturbing complexities in the relationship. The commentary on the new *Code* which appeared in the April 1991 issue of *Family Therapist News* (p. 20) proposed virtually the opposite. It advised that the therapist obtain supervision of a dual relationship with a client (cf. Subprinciple 1.2) and the supervisor obtain supervision of supervision of a dual relationship with a supervisee (cf. Subprinciple 4.1). To give the therapist or supervisor the authority to select the additional resource (whom the client or supervisee may never know about) is to give even more covert power to the therapist or supervisor. It would be far more ethical for the committee to give responsibility to the therapist or supervisor to openly discuss with clients and supervisees the increased potential for both enrichment and exploitation through dual relationships and to invite clients and supervisees to bring in third parties of *their* choice at any time to clarify any concerns that might arise. The therapist or supervisor could be given the additional responsibility to assist in making such arrangements but would be expected to respect the client's and supervisee's priority in choosing which additional resources would be brought in.

I believe that any student, supervisee, or employee as well as any teacher, supervisor, or employer should retain a personal entitlement to turn down any invitation from the other for therapeutic involvement if they prefer to avoid the complexities entailed. But for AAMFT to categorically prohibit the provision of therapy to students, employees, or supervisees is unnecessarily restrictive in patterns of interprofessional relationships. Furthermore, such a prohibition implies that there is no continuity or overlap between supervision and therapy. It fosters the idea that the conduct of therapy can be separated from the person of the therapist. This reflects a reductionistic perspective. In keeping with the systemic review, I prefer a more holistic perspective which allows for the synergistic and integrative possibilities that arise when supervision is supported with therapy and vice versa. I have had several experiences of providing brief therapy for trainees where each process has enabled and enriched the other.

Under the fifth principle, *Responsibility to Research Participants*, Subprinciple 5.3 states:

> Investigators respect participants' freedom to decline participation in or to withdraw from a research study at any time. This obligation requires special thought and consideration when investigators or other members of the research team are in positions of authority or influence over participants. Marriage and family therapists, therefore, make every effort to avoid dual relationships with research participants that could impair professional judgment or increase the risk of exploitation.

Once again, dual relationships are brought forth as problematic and their constructive possibilities are ignored. There are some advantages to the presence of dual relationships in research. For instance, an investigator is far less likely to carry out questionable studies or to conduct potentially harmful experiments when he or she has another meaningful relationship with some of the research participants. This effect arises because there is a more direct and personal basis from which to become mindful about and to care about the possible negative effects of the study. Furthermore, the investigator may be able to interpret a participant's responses more coherently if collateral knowledge about the research participant is available through the other relationship. Dual relationships also provide a valuable conduit for feedback about unexpected effects of the study. Research participants often can offer a richer and more comprehensive description of their experience in the study (and its subsequent effects upon them) through the dual relationship because such reporting is not structured by the research. To discourage such feedback, during and/or after a study by discouraging dual relationships, is to diminish the possibility that investigators would become aware of some totally unanticipated effects of their investigations. In other words, by discouraging dual relationships in research, not only are participants less protected, the potential richness of the new knowledge generated also is liable to suffer.

In pointing out these potential positive influences of dual relationships in research, I am not saying that investigators should be actively encouraged to have dual relationships with their research participants. Appropriate decisions would depend upon the specific nature of the study and on the particular individuals involved. Seriously problematic biases could be introduced in some studies by both researchers. This is an issue for research design and methodology and the ethics of any particular study should be left to the local research ethics committee to adjudicate. With respect to the *AAMFT Code of Ethics*, the relevant focus should remain squarely on the avoidance of coercion and exploitation, and not be displaced onto duality.

THE NEED TO RECONSIDER DUAL RELATIONSHIPS

As currently written, the *AAMFT Code of Ethics* does not acknowledge any possibility that a dual relationship can be constructive. Dual relationships are seen only as potentially exploitative and, hence, should be avoided. Indeed, the repeated use of the phrase, "could impair professional judgment" gives me the impression that the Ethics Committee has come close to regarding duality as something analogous to a *toxic substance*, so that having a dual relationship is rather like being intoxicated by alcohol or being impaired with drugs. An alternative perspective could be that the members of the committee are so *intoxicated* with the idea that dual relationships are hazardous that they can no longer see anything positive in them.

In my experience, involvement in dual relationships actually can and often does contribute toward *improved*, rather than *impaired*, professional judgment. The improved judgment can be manifest in the specific case and/or it can be incorporated in one's overall patterns of decision making. Interestingly, this mode of professional development usually takes place after one has graduated and established a practice. This makes the value of dual relationships even more significant. Any process of improving one's professional judgment after one's *official* training is complete, is extremely important in any profession.

Just how do dual relationships contribute to improved professional judgment? Duality provides an important pathway for corrective feedback; a means to improve understanding and consensuality that enables greater wellness in human social systems in general. Dual relationships serve to *open space* for increased connectedness, more sharing, greater honesty, more personal integrity, more responsibility, more social integration, more complete healing, and more egalitarian human interaction. Furthermore, dual relationships tend to *reduce space* for exclusion practices, for covert manipulation, for deception, and for special privilege. When persons relate to each other in multiple contexts there is greater opportunity to recognize each other as ordinary human beings. There is less probability of either party persisting in distorted perceptions of the other, such as attributions of exaggerated insight and wisdom in therapists (by their clients), or attributions of pervasive personal limitations and deficits in clients (by their therapists). It is through a dual relationship that one's "reality testing" about another person has a whole new domain in which to operate. Through the integration of collateral experiences in the two relationships one benefits from the "depth perception of double description" (Bateson, 1972) and can form impressions that are better grounded. In other words, duality generally creates improved conditions for greater sanity and health all around.

Should these constructive possibilities be curtailed in our field simply because there is also the possibility of exploitation in dual relationships? I think not. Has the Ethics Committee "thrown out the duality baby along with the exploitation bath water?" I think so. Given the current *Code*, the positive aspects of dual relationships cannot even be explored without the risk of ethical censure.

But the present AAMFT position against duality is more serious than a simple injunction against relationship complexities that have the potential to be constructive. Not only is the "baby" being thrown out; a pathologizing social process is being introduced to take its place. It is a process that gives priority to professionalism over personal connectedness. This priority is pathologizing because it fosters human alienation and promotes an increase in interpersonal hierarchy. In the name of professionalism, we, as marriage and family therapists, are being encouraged to avoid becoming involved in the personal lives of our clients, students, trainees, employees, or research participants. In effect we are being told to maintain our "professional distance." The active maintenance of this interpersonal distance draws attention to and emphasizes the power differential between the persons involved. This distancing promotes a process of objectification and disposes us toward more of a vertical hierarchy in human relations. When social systems are restructured in this way, it is the professional whose status is raised. Consequently, the status of those being "served" is lowered in a reciprocal manner. This is one of the more sinister aspects of professionalism. Thus, while the policy of avoiding dual relationships ostensibly is in the service of protecting the vulnerability of clients, trainees, employees, and research participants, it actually privileges professionals instead. I question the ethics of such a policy.

The alienating effect of professionalism is intensified when we begin to respond to others as *occupants* of a position or role rather than as unique persons. In other words, when the person or the other is rendered irrelevant or unethical to relate to, we tend to relate to the role or position he or she occupies instead. The professional relationship becomes a process of interacting roles rather than interacting persons. Being treated as a mere *occupant* of a position (e.g., as "the patient" or as "the student") rather than as a unique individual is a profoundly dehumanizing experience. A professional disposition or attitude of avoiding the possibility of dual relationships inadvertently supports such alienating practices. This kind of professionalism enstructures a significant break in "the patterns that connect" us with one another as human beings. It separates and alienates us instead. Ironically, the professional who turns down invitations to be involved in a dual relationship can now cite the AAMFT *Code of Ethics* self-righteously as the basis for his or her action. Anyone who has used such grounds to turn down a friend's request for therapy can attest to the uncomfortable alienating effects of such a response.

EXPERIENCE IN DUAL RELATIONSHIPS

I personally have experienced dual relationships, both as a client/ trainee and as a professional. In the most significant experience that I have had as a client (i.e., 2 years of personal analysis during psychiatric residency training), I had concurrent advisory and preceptor relationships with my therapist. Each relationship seemed to augment the other. For instance, the advisory relationship enabled the initiation of therapy. My learning as a student of my therapist's theoretical work in clinical skills was enhanced and energized by my therapeutic relationship with him. While in the therapeutic relationship I felt more valued as a whole person because of the other relationships I had with him. Without these additional relationships I suspect that I would have struggled much more with feelings of being a "defective" human being simply by virtue of being in the "demeaning" client role. The dual relationships helped me preserve a better sense of personal worth. The long-term effects were also positive. An egalitarian collegueship and friendship subsequently emerged between us and has continued over the years to be a significant source of ongoing validation for me, both personally and professionally.

As a professional, I have had predominantly positive experiences in dual relationships as well. I have found that participation in such relationships constitutes a strong covert invitation for me to strive toward greater personal integrity, in both the personal and professional aspects. The dual involvement seems to activate a nonconscious process in me toward becoming more honest and authentic with the other. It is much more difficult to "hide behind the cloak of professionalism" when I allow a dual relationship to emerge. My mindfulness grows as I automatically become more aware of the potential significance of a wider scope of my behaviors in the experiences of the other. For instance, when I see a friend as a client, I become mindful of the potential consequences of my behavior as a therapist for the friendship. I also become more mindful of the relevance of my behavior as a friend for the therapeutic relationship. I find myself naturally seeking more congruence in these relationships and am stretched in the direction of more consistency, coherence, integrity, and authenticity. As a result, I seem to be evolving toward becoming both a more friendly therapist and a more therapeutic friend. This has been a welcome development, and, in my opinion, has enhanced the clarity and humanness of my professional judgment.

The majority of the feedback that I have received from clients, students, and supervisees about the dual relationships that I have had with them has been positive. Indeed, one trainee whom I saw briefly with his wife in therapy felt that it would have been unethical for me to turn down his request for therapy, given the importance of the training relationship I had with him at the time. In my view, the therapy enabled his training and the training enabled the therapy. This is not to say that my involvement in dual relationships always has been a simple, or an easy process. In a rather complicated situation of long-term therapy, one client felt she had lost me as a clinical resource when personal friendships emerged between our respective families. I supported her decision to find another therapist, but could understand her experience of loss in choosing to no longer see me as a therapist.

Thus, complications do occur but they are not necessarily exploitative. Whenever I invest the time and energy to sort out such complications, I usually find they enrich my personal and professional development to a significant degree. Thus, I concur with Ryder and Hepworth (1990) that we should not simply avoid the complexities involved in dual relationships but regard them as a means to facilitate our continued learning about and understanding of human relationships.

CONCLUDING COMMENTS

It is my opinion that the AAMFT is doing our field and our communities a major disservice by imposing such pervasive restraints on dual relationships through the *Code of Ethics*. Far more research and exploration into the nature, complexities, and consequences of a wide range of dual relationships is needed before such a broad restriction on duality is allowed to become entrenched in our professional attitudes. Not only is the issue of exploitation being confused, but human enrichment possibilities are being restrained, professional hierarchy is being privileged, and social alienation is being enhanced. In view of these effects, I propose that the existing statements on dual relationships in the *Code* be rescinded and the issue of exploitation be addressed more directly and explicitly. The Ethics Committee should redirect its focus to differentiating and clarifying the various forms of exploitation that commonly occur within primary and/or dual relationships and articulate additional principles like the statement prohibiting sexual intimacy. Clear statements about the specific kinds of exploitation (egoistic, emotional, voyeuristic, financial, authoritarian, ideological, etc.) that can occur would help professionals and clients alike to know what complications to look out for. The past experience of the Ethics Committee in responding to actual complaints from clients, trainees, and research participants would be one major resource in developing such statements.

I believe the complexities of dual relationships should be addressed somewhere in the *Code* as well; preferably in a separate section to curtail any continuing identity with exploitation. Opportunities for possible enrichment should be noted as well as risks for possible exploitation. One important example of the latter is the nonconscious transfer of the power differential (including dependency and trust) from one relationship to the other. This implicit process enhances the vulnerability to exploitation and should be disclosed explicitly and brought into the conscious awareness of professionals as well as those with whom they work. Whether a separate section on dual relationships is introduced into the *Code* or not, any future restatement of the issue needs to be far more differentiated and balanced than what currently exists.

I am clearly opposed to a general prohibition of dual relationships. However, I also am opposed to a general prescription of such relationships for the enrichment that is possible through them. Dual relationships often are very taxing in personal time and energy. Hence, each individual therapist and client, teacher and student, supervisor and supervisee, employer and employee, or research investigator and participant should be entitled to exercise free choice about whether or not he or she is ready and/or willing to enter into a particular dual relationship or not. Any such person also should be free to enter into a dual relationship with some persons, without being obliged to do so with others. In addition, if after having entered into a dual relationship, the persons involved wish to change their minds and would like to discontinue such involvements, they should be entitled to do so. What does seem reasonable to expect, however, is that any desires or decisions to avoid, initiate, and/or relinquish dual relationships be openly discussed, so that the parties involved can expand their awareness of the potential consequences, and, hence, become more responsible.

REFERENCES

AAMFT Code of Ethics. (1991). Washington, DC: American Association for Marriage and Therapy.

Bateson, G. (1972). *Steps to an ecology of mind.* New York: Ballantine.

Ryder, R., & Hepworth, J. (1990). AAMFT Ethical code: Dual relationships. *Journal of Marriage and Family Therapy, 16,* 127–132.

Webster's Unabridged Dictionary of the English Language. (1989). New York: Portland Press.

CHAPTER 4

In Celebration of Dual Relationships

How Prohibition of Nonsexual Dual Relationships Increases the Chance of Exploitation and Harm

Ofer Zur, PhD

ON BEING AN OCEANOGRAPHER IN THE WINE COUNTRY

Jack and I have played basketball for several years in our local recreational league. His wife, Janet, and I chaperone our children on field trips together and are on the same educational committee. When they called me seeking help to save their marriage, I delivered my sermon about dual relationships, objectivity, and ethical guidelines. In short, I told them I was not the man for the job. I had taught ethics, research, and clinical courses at the graduate and postgraduate level for over a decade, and my sermon was polished and substantiated with quotes,

Reproduced by permission of the Division of Psychologists in Independent Practice of the American Psychological Association. Zur, O. In celebration of dual relationships: How prohibition of nonsexual dual relationships increases the chance of exploitation and harm. *The Independent Practitioner, 20,* 97–100.

references, and court cases. To my surprise Jack and Janet were outraged rather than being understanding. "We have known you for a long time," they said, "we know your values and how you treat your wife, your children and your friends. We know of several marriages you have helped put on the right path. We choose you *because* we know you and *because* you know us well. Besides, we have already tried several other counselors to no avail, we are on the brink of divorce *and do not have the time* to tell our stories once again to another stranger."

Moving to a serene, small town in the Northern California wine country was significantly less serene than I had anticipated, as far as my private practice was concerned. Psychodynamically oriented and cognitively trained, I had great difficulty dealing with the lack of customary professional boundaries between my clients and myself. It was a shocking realization that people were choosing me as their therapist *because* they knew me and I knew them. Everything I had learned in graduate school, and from my supervisors, or had absorbed from the professional literature, led me to believe this was perilous.

Alarmed, I consulted with attorneys, supervisors, experts on ethics, and experienced therapists regarding my dilemma. How, I asked them, could I work with people who are part of my community? We discussed the ethical, legal, and clinical implications of such relationships on transference, countertransference, therapeutic alliance, boundaries, conflict of interest, objectivity, standard of care, power, freedom of choice, and so forth. We also analyzed in detail the potential clinical risks and benefits of entering into therapy with these people. The near consensus seemed to be that what I was doing was clinically, legally, and ethically inappropriate, and even dangerous. Although all my clients were fully informed about the complexities of dual relationships through my office policies, verbal explanations, and through receiving an actual copy of the APA Ethics Code, I was not engaged in sexual or business interactions with them, nor exploited or harmed them in any way, I was warned that I was walking into a minefield.

Despairingly, I started looking for a job in my former professions of oceanography and deep sea diving. To my dismay, I found no ads in the local paper stating: "A local winery is looking for an experienced deep sea diver."

PLAYING RUSSIAN ROULETTE WITH THE SOUL

Some clients' systematic search for a therapist-consultant is as sensible as it is rare. One client of mine, a physician, spent a couple of years observing me, reading my publications, meeting my wife and children, and following up closely on cases he referred to me. All this, admittedly, for the purpose of checking me out as a potential therapist for himself. When people contact me through the *Yellow Pages* or from the list provided by my psychological association, I am shocked at the cavalier lottery-type approach they are taking to the care of their psyches. In fact, they are playing Russian roulette with their souls.

THE ORIGINAL PROHIBITION

"Dual relationship" refers to any situation where multiple roles exist between a therapist and a client. Besides having sex with a client, other examples of dual relationships are engaging in therapy with a student, friend, or business associate.

The original prohibition against dual relationships in therapy emerged from two sources. Professional, federal, and state regulatory agencies developed the prohibition in an attempt to prevent therapists from exploiting and harming clients. Traditional psychoanalysis developed such prohibition for theoretical-analytic and clinical-transferential reasons.

Issues of exploitation in general, and sexual or business exploitation in particular, are appropriately at the forefront of consumer advocates' agendas. The valid concern is that helping professionals, especially psychotherapists, can easily exploit their clients by using their positions of power for personal gain. Hence, the effort to curtail exploitation and to protect consumers from harm is indeed essential.

GOING TOO FAR IN THE RIGHT DIRECTION: THE DEMONIZATION OF DUAL RELATIONSHIP

Professional organizations, consumer protection agencies, and legislators use the therapist-client sexual prohibition and the concern with exploitation as the basis for all their protective policies and guidelines. The original intent of the regulatory agencies to protect the welfare of clients by putting forth a straightforward ban on sexual relationships between therapists and clients (Ebert, 1997), mushroomed into a massively broad prohibition of all dual relationships. *As a result, the absolute avoidance of dual relationships has become a magical amulet guarding against any and all possible harm to patients involved in therapeutic treatment.* Consequently, the term "dual relationship" has been used interchangeably in the professional literature as a synonym for "exploitation," "harm," "abuse," "damage," and "sexual abuse."

As we are repeatedly reminded, the primary rationale for the avoid-all-dual-relationships argument is that therapists may misuse their power, and influence and exploit clients for their own benefit and to the clients' detriment. A power issue is certainly a valid concern. But is it reasonable to view the dual relationship as the sole source of exploitative interaction? Such unilateral responsibility can only be assigned where there is a belief in the domino theory or snowball effect of dual relationships; one thing inevitably leads to another. An initially innocent hug will inevitably progress to sexual intercourse and a gift will inevitably lead to a business relationship.

Kenneth Pope, a leading expert in ethical matters, makes a claim that has become a strict standard of therapeutic ethics and law: " . . . non-sexual dual relationships, while unethical and harmful per se, foster sexual dual relationships" (1990, p. 688). Simon (1991) agrees that "The boundary violation precursors of therapist-patient sex can be as psychologically damaging as the actual sexual involvement itself" (p. 614). These chilling words epitomize the notion that by avoiding any semblance of dual relationships we necessarily avoid all forms of exploitation and harm.

To assert that self-disclosure, a hug, a home visit, or accepting a gift is likely to lead to sex is like saying doctors' visits cause death because most people see a doctor before they die. One of the few master therapists who brings refreshing critical thinking to the field of ethics is Dr. Arnold Lazarus, the founder of Multimodal therapy who calls this thinking "an extreme form of syllogistic reasoning" (1994, p. 257). Sequential statistical relationships, as my undergraduate research professor emphasized, cannot simply be translated to causal ones.

WHEN FEAR OVERRIDES CLINICAL JUDGMENT

Therapists are tyrannized by their fear and by the dogmas promulgated by the rigid philosophies of 19th century analyis, as well as regulatory and consumer protection agencies. As a result, courses and publications on risk management have become big business. "Risk Management" may sound like practical advice, but often, it is a misnomer for a practice where fear and attorneys determine the course of therapy.

IF DUAL RELATIONSHIPS AREN'T UNETHICAL, WHY ISN'T THE PROHIBITION DEAD?

Due to the concern of rural and military therapists that dual relationships are unavoidable in such small and interwoven communities, most professional associations, among them the American Psychological Association (APA), have revised their ethical guidelines regarding dual relationships, discarding the traditional strict prohibition of dual relationships.

The revised *APA Ethical Guidelines of 1992*, in section 1.17 simply states:

> In many communities and situations, it may not be feasible or reasonable for psychologists to avoid social or other nonprofessional contacts with persons such as patients. . . . A psychologist refrains from entering into or promising another personal, scientific, professional, financial, or other relationship with such persons if it appears likely that such a relationship reasonably might impair the psychologist's objectivity or otherwise interfere with the psychologist's effectively performing his or her functions as a psychologist, or might harm or exploit the other party.

To most readers it will come as a surprise that the *1992 Revised Ethics Code does not consider dual relationships unethical*. Nevertheless, the changes in ethics codes have not put a dent in the professional and public opinions regarding the evils of dual relationships. Even today, this prohibition is erroneously assumed and implemented by most professional organizations, licensing boards, ethical committees and the courts.

Even the more relaxed 1992 version has been challenged for it's constitutionality, surprisingly, by Ebert (1997), a psychologist, attorney, and former chairman of the California Board of Psychology. He challenges the constitutionality of the prohibition due to the vagueness and the excessive breadth of the prohibition and how it may violate the constitutional right for privacy and association.

ON BEING THE FLASHER IN ALASKA

Flying with a client who has a fear of flying is a mandated exposure-intervention for the behavioral therapist, but is a boundary violation to the psychoanalyst and most ethicists. Seeing a wife and husband in joint and individual therapy simultaneously can be part of well-articulated systems-based therapy, but constitutes a serious boundary violation to the psychodynamic therapist. A walk on a trail might be part of a strategically planned intervention for the humanistically based therapist, but a transgression to the interpersonal practitioner.

Staying in the office regardless of the presented problem may seem right to analysts, ethicists or attorneys, but may not help those who suffer from agoraphobia, social phobia, or fear of flying. They respectively require leaving the office and going to open places, mixing with the crowd, or getting on an airplane. Practicing risk management by staying in the office cold, aloof, and detached is like the story about the flasher in Alaska where it is too cold to flash, so he just describes it. It neither works for the flasher nor for our clients.

IN PRAISE OF DUAL RELATIONSHIPS

Familiarity and Therapy.   Unlike the common myth that familiarity is an obstacle to therapy, I have found it to be extremely helpful. Relying on a neurotic or psychotic clients' distorted reports is futile and a set up for failure. Also, clients' familiarity with my spiritual beliefs and personal ethics helps them trust me more readily and realistically. Familiarity often shortens the length of therapy and increases its effectiveness.

Transference and Dual Relationships.   There is an unsubstantiated myth that familiarity and dual relationships interfere with the transference analysis. Transference occurs anywhere and anytime, not only when facing a "blank wall." Whether or not I know the people or they know me outside of therapy, transference and countertransference take place and, if the clinician is so inclined, the analysis can take place.

Isolation, Power, Duality, and Exploitation.   While privacy is often an important component in increasing psychotherapeutic effectiveness, it can also be a double-edged sword when it is used as an excuse for isolation. The privacy-secrecy argument has been also used to justify many therapists' attempts to hide, assert power inappropriately, or exploit. Sexual exploitation is less likely to occur if the therapist is also working with the spouse of a client, or has an outside connection to the family, perhaps through church. *In other words, sexual and other forms of exploitation are less likely to occur in therapy if dual relationships exist.* Similarly, isolating clients in therapy gives the therapist undue power and an easier opportunity to exploit clients.

Isolation and the "Resistance" Excuse.   In the isolation of the office without dual relationships, therapists can easily blame the clients for their own ineffectiveness by using the famous "resistance" charge. The prohibition of dual relationships enables incompetent therapists to avoid accountability for long periods of time while they charge, exploit, and harm clients by continuing therapy even when the clients do not get better. So, we not only fraudulently charge them for services rendered, but, far more detrimental, we give them the sense that they are permanently and hopelessly damaged.

Exploiting Therapists Will Exploit.   The problem of exploitation and harm lies not within the dual relationship, but in the therapist's propensity to exploit and harm. Therapists who tend to exploit will exploit clients with or without dual relationships. The Ethics Code must ban harm and exploitation, not dual relationships.

Dual Relationships in a Healthy Society.   In a healthy society, unlike our modern culture, people celebrate their reliance on each other. The more multiple the relationships, the richer and more profound the individual and cultural experience. The witch doctor, the wise elder, and the practical neighbor all contribute advice, guidance, and physical and spiritual support. In ministering to the needs of the members of the community, therefore, the healers, rabbis, priests, or therapists don't shun dual relationships, but rather rely on them for the insight and intimate knowledge that such relationships provide.

On Power Differential.   One must remember that neither dual relationships nor any relationship with a differential of power (i.e., parent-child, teacher-student) are inherently exploitative. While unpleasant to contemplate, it is altogether possible that many therapists cling to the false ideals of the segregated therapy session because it increases their professional status, imbuing them with undue power which can all too easily be translated into exploitation.

Dual Relationships Are Normal and Complex.   More than half of America's businesses are family run. In these businesses, people experience the complexities of dual relationships, balancing blood and money. Similarly, working professionally with people I know outside of the office adds richness and unavoidable difficulties to our lives.

CONCLUSION

The ban and demonization of dual relationships has come from an attempt to protect the public from exploiting therapists. Regretfully, it has emerged as a simplistic solution to a wide and complex problem. Even worse, the ban on dual relationships and the isolation it imposes on the therapeutic encounter tends to increase the chance of exploitation and decrease effectiveness of treatment. It enables incompetent therapists to wield their power without witnesses and accountability. In addition it buys into the general cultural trend towards isolation and disconnection. We have been frightened into accepting the ban, but now it is time to think critically, be courageous, and dare to be known by our clients. If we dare to cultivate multiple, nonsexual and nonexploitive relationships with our clients when appropriate, we can be better, more effective therapists.

REFERENCES

American Psychological Association. (1992). *Ethical principles for psychologists.* Washington, DC: American Psychological Association.

Ebert, W. B. (1977). Dual-relationship prohibition: A concept whose time never should have come. *Applied & Prevention Psychology, 6,* 137–156.

Lazarus, A. A. (1994). How certain boundaries and ethics diminish therapeutic effectiveness. *Ethics & Behavior, 4,* 255–261.

Pope, K. S. (1990). Therapist-patient sexual contact: Clinical, legal, and ethical implications. In E. A. Margenau (Ed.), *The encyclopedia handbook of private practice.* New York: Gardner Press.

Simon, R. I. (1991). Psychological injury caused by boundary violation precursors to therapist-patient sex. *Psychiatric Annals, 21,* 614–619.

The Ethics of Dual Relationships

Part 2 focuses on the general ethics of dual relationships, including concerns with the Codes of Ethics, standards of care, boundaries, and the primary responsibility of therapists to their clients. Chapter 5 presents Zur's cogent examination of the exact content of 14 professional organizations' codes of ethics in regard to dual relationships and describes the intent behind the codes that guide the sanctity of the client-therapist relationship in psychotherapy. He clarifies the mistaken construal that many practitioners have placed on the ethical realities of dual or multiple relations with selected clients. Chapter 6 is a penetrating rebuttal of the one-size-fits-all prescription of an intelligent standard of care. Williams lucidly explains why it can be harmful to ignore the extent of diversity among different psychotherapeutic approaches and how the rigid prohibition of boundary excursions can easily undermine humane and sensible interactions. In chapter 7, Zur provides a raison d'être for crossing office boundaries and engaging in extramural activities with some clients. He presents ethical grounds and describes clinical benefits that may ensue when venturing beyond the confines of the consulting room. Finally, in chapter 8, Rubin underscores the multiplicity of loyalties and relationships that extend across the realms of psychotherapy. He lucidly addresses how all therapists must maintain their clients' fidelity, and why, in so doing, multiple relationships are often necessary.

CHAPTER 5

The Truth About the Codes of Ethics

Dispelling the Rumors That Dual Relationships Are Unethical

Ofer Zur, PhD

The codes of ethics of psychotherapists' professional associations have evolved through the years to suit the increasing awareness and knowledge of the field. Like other codes during the midtwentieth century and ensuing decades, the Code of Ethics of the American Psychological Association (APA, 1953) concentrated on the general points of promoting client welfare and discouraging abuse of power by therapists. Years later, when the codes changed to provide more specific guidelines and restrictions, therapists were instructed to make every effort to avoid dual relationships (APA, 1977, 1981). In the late 1980s, the realization began to spread that dual relationships were unavoidable in some circumstances, such as living in rural areas, the military, and among constituents of definite individual communities, such as the deaf, gay, and other minorities. To reflect this fresh awareness about and acceptance of dual relationships, *all* major professional associations (e.g., ACA, 1996; APA, 1992; NASW, 1996) have revised their codes of ethics in recognition of the fact that dual relationships are neither always avoidable nor always unethical (Barnett & Yutrzenka, 1994; Ebert,

1997; Williams, 1997; Zur, 2000). This shift of recognition that dual relationships are unavoidable and can be ethical seems to have made little impression on the widespread opinion that dual relationships are inherently unethical and should be avoided (Hedges, 1993).

The common misapprehension about the ethics of nonsexual dual relationships results from lack of familiarity with, misunderstanding of, or a biased attitude toward the content of the codes themselves. These obstacles are inspired primarily by the analytic urban risk-management approach to therapy. Those still under the false impression that dual relationships are essentially unethical include the majority of therapists, judges, members of ethics committees, and attorneys. Notably, the most significant groups that demonstrate lack of clarity on this issue are scholars and ethicists, many of whom operate under the misinterpretation of dual relationships as innately unethical, exploitative, and harmful (Ebert, 1997; Hedges, 1993; Lazarus, 1994; Williams, 1997; Zur, 2001).

To circumvent the possibility of contributing to the confusion surrounding the codes of ethics, the next section is composed of *exact quotes* about dual relationships, lifted verbatim from the codes of ethics of the major professional associations. Because sexual dual relationships with current clients have always been unethical in the codes of ethics of all psychotherapists' professional associations, the passages that follow contain only those principles that directly relate to nonsexual dual relationships.

THE CURRENT CODES OF ETHICS, VERBATIM

1a. American Psychological Association (APA) *Ethical Principles of Psychologists and Code of Conduct* (1992), Section 1.17 states:

> In many communities and situations, *it may not be feasible or reasonable for psychologists to avoid social or other nonprofessional contacts* with persons such as patients, clients, students, supervisees, or research participants. . . . A psychologist refrains from entering into or promising another personal, scientific, professional, financial, or other relationship with such persons if it appears likely that such a relationship reasonably *might impair* the psychologist's objectivity or otherwise interfere with the psychologist's effectively performing his or her functions as a psychologist, or *might harm or exploit* the other party. (b) Likewise, whenever feasible, a psychologist refrains from taking on professional or scientific obligations when preexisting relationships *would create a risk of such harm*. (p. 1601 [emphasis added])

1b.   American Psychological Association (APA) *Ethics Code Draft Published for Comment* (2001), Section 3.05 titled, Multiple Relationships states:

> (a) A multiple relationship occurs when a psychologist is in a professional role with a person and (1) at the same time is in another role with the same person, (2) at the same time is in a relationship with a person closely associated with or related to the person with whom they have the professional relationship, or (3) promises to enter into another relationship in the future with the person or a person closely associated with or related to the person.
>
> A psychologist refrains from entering into a multiple relationship if the multiple relationship *could reasonably be expected to impair the psychologist's objectivity, competence, or effectiveness in performing his or her functions* as a psychologist or *otherwise risks exploitation or harm* to the person with whom the professional relationship exists.
>
> Multiple relationships that *would not reasonably be expected to cause impairment or risk exploitation or harm are not unethical.*
>
> (b) If a psychologist finds that, due to unforeseen factors, a potentially harmful multiple relationship has arisen, the psychologist attempts to resolve it with due regard for the welfare of the affected person and maximal compliance with the Ethics Code (p. 82 [emphasis added])

2.   American Psychiatric Association (APA) *Principles of Medical Ethics. With Annotations Especially Applicable to Psychiatry* (2001) does *not* mention dual or multiple relationships. It simply outlines the general principles that appear in all other codes, of the mandate to avoid exploitation and harm to patients.

3. ˙ American Association of Marriage and Family Therapists (AAMFT) *Code of Ethics* (2001), Section 1.3, states:

> Marriage and family therapists are aware of their influential positions with respect to clients, and they avoid exploiting the trust and dependency of such persons. Therapists, therefore, make every effort to avoid conditions and multiple relationships with clients that could impair professional judgment or increase the risk of exploitation. Such relationships include, but are not limited to, business or close personal relationships with a client or the client's immediate family. When the risk of impairment or exploitation exists due to conditions or multiple roles, therapists take appropriate precautions (Responsibility to Clients Section, para. 4.)

4.   The National Association of Social Workers (NASW) *Code of Ethics* (1999), Standard 1.06.c, states:

> Social workers should not engage in dual or multiple relationships with clients or former clients in which there is a risk of exploitation or potential harm

to the client. In instances when dual or multiple relationships are unavoidable, social workers should take steps to protect clients and are responsible for setting clear, appropriate, and culturally sensitive boundaries. (Dual or multiple relationships occur when social workers relate to clients in more than one relationship, whether professional, social, or business. Dual or multiple relationships can occur simultaneously or consecutively.) (Conflict of Interest Section, para. 3.)

5.   American Counseling Association (ACA) *Code of Ethics and Standards for Practice* (1996), Section A.1.d. of Family Involvement, states: "Counselors recognize that families are usually important in clients' lives and *strive to enlist family* understanding and involvement as a positive resource, when appropriate" (emphasis added). Section A.6.a, Dual Relationships, states:

> *Avoid when possible.* Counselors are aware of their influential positions with respect to clients, and they avoid exploiting the trust and dependency of clients. Counselors make every effort to avoid dual relationships with clients *that could impair professional judgment or increase the risk of harm* to clients. (Examples of such relationships include, but are not limited to, familial, social, financial, business, or close personal relationships with clients.) When a dual relationship *cannot be avoided,* counselors take appropriate professional precautions such as informed consent, consultation, supervision, and documentation *to ensure that judgment is not impaired and no exploitation occurs* (The Counseling Relationship Section, para. 6 [emphasis added])

6.   Feminist Therapy Institute (FTI) *Feminist Therapy Code of Ethics* (1987), Section III, Overlapping Relationships, states:

> (a) Feminist therapist *recognizes the complexity and conflicting priorities inherent in multiple or overlapping relationships.* The therapist accepts responsibility for monitoring such relationships to prevent potential abuse of or harm to the client. (b) *A feminist therapist is actively involved in her community.* As a result, she is especially sensitive about confidentiality. Recognizing that her client's concerns and general well-being are primary, she self-monitors both public and private statements and comments (p. 2 [emphasis added])

7.   Canadian Psychological Association (CPA) *Code of Ethics for Psychologists* (2000), Section III.33, states:

> Avoid dual or multiple relationships (e.g., with clients, research participants, employees, supervisees, students, or trainees) and other situations that *might present a conflict of interest or that might reduce their ability to be objective and unbiased* in their determinations of what might be in the best interests of others (Avoidance of Conflict of Interest Section, para. 3 [emphasis added])

Section III.34, states:

> Manage dual or multiple relationships that are unavoidable due to cultural norms or other circumstances in such a manner that bias, lack of objectivity, and risk of exploitation are minimized. This might include obtaining ongoing supervision or consultation for the duration of the dual or multiple relationship, or involving a third party in obtaining consent (e.g., approaching a client or employee about becoming a research participant). (Avoidance of Conflict of Interest section, para. 4.)

8. National Association of Alcoholism and Drug Abuse Counselors (NAADAC) *Ethical Standards* (1995), Principle 9.b states:

> The NAADAC member shall not engage in professional relationships or commitments that conflict with family members, friends, close associates, or others whose *welfare might be jeopardized* by such a dual relationship (Client Relationships section, para. 3 [emphasis added])

9. American Association of Pastoral Counselors (AAPC) *Code of Ethics* (1994), Section III.E, states:

> We avoid those dual relationships with clients (e.g., business or close personal relationships) *which could impair our professional judgement, compromise* the integrity of the treatment, and/or use the relationship for our own gain (Client Relationships section, para. 5 [emphasis added])

10. Canadian Counseling Association (CCA) *Code of Ethics* (1999), Section B, Counselling Relationships, subsection B8, Dual Relationships, states:

> Counsellors make every effort to avoid dual relationships with clients that could impair professional judgment or increase the risk of harm to clients. Examples of dual relationships include, but are not limited to, familial, social, financial, business, or close personal relationships. When a dual relationship can not be avoided, counsellors take appropriate professional precautions such as informed consent, consultation, supervision, and documentation to ensure that judgment is not impaired and no exploitation occurs.

11. California Association of Marriage and Family Therapists (CAMFT) *Ethical Standards for Marriage and Family Therapists* (1997), Section 1.2 states:

> Marriage and family therapists are aware of their influential position with respect to patients, and they avoid exploiting the trust and dependency of

such persons. Marriage and family therapists therefore avoid dual relationships with patients that are *reasonably likely to impair professional judgment or lead to exploitation.* A dual relationship occurs when a therapist and his/her patient engage in a separate and distinct relationship either simultaneously with the therapeutic relationship, or during a reasonable period of time following the termination of the therapeutic relationship. *Not all dual relationships are unethical, and some dual relationships cannot be avoided.* When a dual relationship cannot be avoided, therapists take appropriate professional precautions to insure that judgment is not impaired and that no exploitation occurs.

Section 1.2.2 adds:

Other acts *which would result in unethical dual relationships* include, but are not limited to, borrowing money from a patient, hiring a patient, engaging in a business venture with a patient, or engaging in a close personal relationship with a patient (Responsibility to Patients section, para. 2 [emphasis added])

12.   National Board for Certified Counselors (NBCC) *Code of Ethics* (1997) does *not* mention specific prohibition of dual or multiple relationships. It simply outlines the general principles that appear in all other codes, of the mandate to avoid exploitation and harm to patients.
13.   Northamerica Association of Masters in Psychology (NAMP) *Ethical Standards and Code of Conduct* (1997), Standard 3.2 states:

The Masters in *Psychology shall not engage* in "dual relations" of any kind *and should avoid* social contact with individuals such as clients, students, and supervisees (p. 6 [emphasis added])

14.   American Art Therapy Association (AATA) *Ethics Document* (1995), Standard 1.5 states:

Art therapists shall not engage in dual relationships with patients. Art therapists shall recognize their influential position with respect to patients, and they shall not exploit the trust and dependency of persons. A dual relationship occurs when a therapist and patient engage in separate and distinct relationship(s) or when an instructor or supervisor acts as a therapist to a student or a supervisee either simultaneously with the therapeutic relationship, or less than two (2) years following termination of the therapeutic relationship. Some examples of dual relationships are borrowing money from the patient, hiring the patient, engaging in a business venture with the patient, engaging in a close personal relationship with the patient, or engaging in sexual intimacy with a patient. (Responsibility to patients section, para. 6)

THE ETHICS CODES IN SOLIDARITY

Among the codes of all major psychotherapists' organizations, there is no blanket prohibition of nonsexual dual relationships. The American Psychiatric Association (2001) and the National Board for Certified Counselors (1998) exclude dual and multiple relationships from their codes altogether. These codes appropriately concentrate on preventing harm and exploitation of patients by therapists, as opposed to dictating a uniform course of action for therapists about dual relationships.

The position taken by the Northamerica Association of Masters in Psychology (NAMP, 1997) of absolute avoidance of dual relationships contradicts the stance of all major professional organizations. Either it is a reflection of outdated, unrealistic thinking or a significantly restrictive measure taken in an attempt to help masters-level psychologist-therapists gain equality with doctoral-level psychologists.

Similarly, the American Association of Art Therapists (AATA, 1995), in its quest to achieve legitimate standing among the rest of the professions, has also imposed ethical guidelines that are unreasonable, excessively limiting and impossible to follow in certain settings and situations.

There are unified principles among the codes of ethics of all major professional organizations concerning dual relationships in psychotherapy. Once the hindering factors of misinformation and prejudice are discarded, the platform of these codes is clear:

1. Sexual dual relationships with present clients are always unethical.
2. Nonsexual dual relationships are not always avoidable.
3. Nonsexual dual relationships are not always unethical.
4. Therapists must avoid only the dual relationships that might:

    • Impair their judgment and objectivity.
    • Interfere with performing therapy or supervision effectively.
    • Harm or exploit patients.

SUMMARY

By contrast to the widespread belief that nonsexual dual relationships are inherently unethical, the codes of ethics of all major professional organizations place no ban on nonsexual dual relationships and in fact acknowledge dual relationships as sometimes unavoidable. Instead of supporting the opinion that dual relationships are unethical under any circumstances, the codes dictate that only those relationships likely to impair judgement and objectivity interfere with the therapeutic work or harm or exploit patients ought to be avoided.

Understanding the ethics codes is imperative in order to make informed decisions about dual relationships. Blind trust in other practitioners' interpretations of these codes does not constitute a thorough process of gathering information. Therapists familiar with the ethics codes will realize that nonsexual dual relationships are neither always unethical nor always avoidable, and thus will be better prepared to make choices about dual relationships that attend to the needs of the client. When the propensity to practice based on fear of litigation or licensing boards is set aside and replaced by firsthand knowledge of the ethics codes themselves, dual relationships can be accurately regarded as yet another opportunity to help clients.

REFERENCES

American Art Therapy Association. (1995). *Ethics document.* Retrieved August 26, 2001, from http://www.arttherapy.org/ethics2.html

American Association for Marriage and Family Therapists. (2001). *AAMFT code of ethics.* Washington, DC: Author. Retrieved July 8, 2001, from http://www.aamft.org/about/revisedcodeethics.htm

American Association of Pastoral Counselors. (1994). *Code of ethics.* Fairfax, VA: Author. Retrieved July 8, 2001, from http://www.aapc.org/ethics.htm

American Counseling Association. (1996). *Code of ethics and standards of practice.* Alexandria, VA: Author. Retrieved July 8, 2001, from http://www.cacd.org/codeofethics.html.

American Psychiatric Association. (2001). *The principles of medical ethics. With annotations especially applicable to psychiatry.* Retrieved August 26, 2001, from http://www.psych.org/apa_members/medicalethics2001_42001.cfm

American Psychological Association. (1953). *Ethical standards of psychologists.* Washington, DC: Author.

American Psychological Association. (1977). *Ethical standards of psychologists.* Washington, DC: Author.

American Psychological Association. (1981). Ethical principles of psychologists. *American Psychologist, 36,* 633–638.

American Psychological Association. (1992). Ethical principles of psychologists and code of conduct. *American Psychologist, 47,* 1597–1611.

American Psychological Association. (2001). Ethics code draft published for comment. *Monitor on Psychology, February,* 76–89.

Barnett, J. E., & Yutrzenka, B. A. (1994). Nonsexual dual relationships in professional practice, with special applications to rural and military community. *The Independent Practitioner, 14* (5), 243–248.

California Association of Marriage and Family Therapists. (1997). *Ethical standards for marriage and family therapists.* San Diego, CA: Author. Retrieved July 8, 2001, from http://www.camft.org/StaticContent/1/sitemap.html.

Canadian Counseling Association. (1999). *Code of ethics.* Retrieved August 26, 2001, from http://www.ccacc.ca/coe.htm

Canadian Psychological Association. (2000). *Code of ethics for psychologists.* Retrieved July 8, 2001, from http://www.cpa.ca/ethics2000.html

Ebert, B. W. (1997). Dual-relationship prohibitions: A concept whose time never should have come. *Applied & Preventive Psychology, 6,* 137–156.

Feminist Therapy Institute. (1987). *Feminist therapy code of ethics.* Denver: Author.

Hedges, L. E. (1993). In praise of the dual relationship. *The California Therapist, May/June,* 46–50.

Lazarus, A. A. (1994). How certain boundaries and ethics diminish therapeutic effectiveness. *Ethics & Behavior, 4* (3), 255–261.

National Association of Alcoholism and Drug Abuse Counselors. (1995). *Ethical standards.* Retrieved July 8, 2001, from http://www.naadac.org/ethics.htm

National Association of Social Workers. (1996). *NASW code of ethics.* Washington, DC: Author.

National Association of Social Workers. (1999). *NASW code of ethics.* Retrieved July 18, 2001, from http://www.naswdc.org/Code/ethics.htm

National Board for Certified Counselors. (1998). *NBCC code of ethics.* (Approved 1997). Greensboro, NC: Author.

Northamerica Association of Masters in Psychology. (1997). *Ethical standards and code of conduct.* Norman, OK: Author.

Williams, M. H. (1997). Boundary violations: Do some contended standards of care fail to encompass commonplace procedures of humanistic, behavioral and eclectic psychotherapies? *Psychotherapy, 34,* 239–249.

Zur, O. (2000). In celebration of dual relationships: How prohibition of nonsexual dual relationships increases the chance of exploitation and harm. *The Independent Practitioner, 20,* 97–100.

Zur, O. (2001). Out-of-office experience: When crossing office boundaries and engaging in dual relationships are clinically beneficial and ethically sound. *The Independent Practitioner, 21* (2), 96–100.

CHAPTER 6

Boundary Violations

Do Some Contended Standards of Care Fail to Encompass Commonplace Procedures of Humanistic, Behavioral, and Eclectic Psychotherapies?

Martin H. Williams, PhD

One matter that may be discussed at malpractice proceedings—before a civil court, licensing board, or ethics committee—concerns the inappropriate crossing of boundaries by the psychotherapist. These "boundary violations" include, but are not limited to: hugging, dining with, self-disclosing personal information or feelings to, making house calls to, exchanging gifts with, engaging in

Reprinted by permission of the Division of Psychotherapy (29) of the American Psychological Association. Williams, M. H. (1997). Boundary violations: Do some contended standards of care fail to encompass commonplace procedures of humanistic, behavioral and eclectic psychotherapies? *Psychotherapy: Theory/Research/Practice/Training, 34,* 239–249.

nonsexual socializing with, or lending books to patients during treatment. The most egregious boundary violation is sexual intercourse during treatment—something that virtually all practitioners condemn. However, as discussed below, some contributors to the ethics literature assert that the occurrence of less severe boundary violations, like self-disclosure or gift-giving, lends validity to plaintiffs' contentions that sexual activity—denied by the therapist—must have actually occurred, and some contend that a series of minor boundary violations shows a pattern of negligence and justifies licensing sanctions or financial settlements even in the absence of sexual activity.

This chapter is intended to show that two distinct and contradictory positions exist regarding boundaries in psychotherapy. On the one hand, authors argue that ethics concerns dictate a need for careful maintenance of boundaries as well as a need to sanction practitioners who violate. On the other hand, the traditions and practices of some forms of psychotherapy dictate that certain boundaries be routinely crossed. These two positions do not coexist well. For example, the possibility exists that a humanistic or behavioral psychotherapist, who practices in accord with published techniques and traditions deriving from those theoretical orientations, may appear to violate community standards should his or her work be adjudicated by a licensing board consultant or plaintiff's expert who holds a conservative view of boundaries. To the extent that this occurs, behavioral, humanistic, or eclectic practitioners may be at risk for licensing sanctions or financial penalties should their practices be scrutinized by a sanctioning agency—regardless of the validity of the original allegations.

The discussion below is organized into three main parts. First, the viewpoint that holds that boundaries should be carefully maintained will be discussed. Second, humanistic and behavioral viewpoints on boundaries will be respectively presented. Next, surveys which depict therapists' boundary related behaviors will be used to identify the extent to which some therapists cross boundaries. Finally, the issue of risk management—changing one's practice to avoid the appearance of wrongdoing—will be discussed, and conclusions will be drawn.[1]

---

[1] This discussion largely focuses on humanistic and behavioral approaches to boundaries, as their literature includes the strongest advocacy for boundary crossing. However, many of the same issues apply to modern psychoanalytic approaches which, in contrast to classical psychoanalysis, may also include boundary crossing. As Stricker (1990) has pointed out with respect to the boundary of self-disclosure, "Contemporary developments in psychoanalytic theory allow for the possibility of therapist self-disclosure, leaving unanswered questions concerning the choice, timing and amount of material to disclose" (p. 279).

THE LOGIC OF BOUNDARY CONCERNS

Several authors have contributed arguments that emphasize the importance of maintaining boundaries in psychotherapy (Atkins & Stein,
1993; Bennett, Bricklin, & VandeCreek, 1994; Brodsky, 1989; Brown,
1994; Epstein & Simon, 1990; Epstein, Simon, & Kay, 1992; Folman,
1991; Gabbard, 1994; Gechtman, 1989; Goisman & Gutheil, 1992;
Gottleib, 1993, 1994; Gutheil, 1989, 1994; Gutheil & Gabbard, 1993;
Johnston & Farber, 1996; Katherine, 1993; Notman & Nadelson, 1994;
Pope, 1989, 1994; Simon, 1991, 1992, 1994, 1995; Smith & Fitzpatrick,
1995; Sonne, 1989, 1994; Strasburger, Jorgenson, & Sutherland, 1992).
The quotations which follow exemplify aspects of this viewpoint. Pope
(1994), for example, states the following:

> Establishing safe, reliable, and useful boundaries is one of *the most fundamental
> responsibilities of the therapist.* The boundaries must create a context in which
> therapist and patient do the work of therapy. (p. 70) [emphasis added]

Katherine (1993) expresses a similar view:

> A boundary violation is committed when someone knowingly or unknowingly
> crosses the emotional, physical, spiritual, or sexual limits of another.

> Whether a violation is intended or not, whether it is committed out of igno-
> rance or malice, it is still a violation. It still harms. (p. 86)

> More subtle violations occur when the caregiver initiates interaction that is
> only appropriate among peers. Your doctor is not your peer. Your therapist
> is not your peer. (p. 88)

> Professional distance between therapist and client gives the client her greatest
> safety. . . . Social contact between therapist and client muddies the bound-
> aries. I used to go to client weddings, but now I don't. . . . My presence in
> other contexts confuses the fact that I have a special, unique, protected role
> in her life with specific limitations. (p. 91)

Johnston and Farber (1996) in summarizing Langs' conservative psychoanalytic view of boundaries state:

> Consequences of poor boundary management include the communication
> of the therapist's intrapsychic conflicts to the patient, the contamination
> of the transference and consequent interpretations, the dissolution of the
> therapeutic "hold," and the possibility of inappropriate gratification resulting
> from countertransference problems. (p. 392)

Finally, Simon (1991) asserts the following regarding consequences of boundary violations:

> The boundary violation precursors of therapist-patient sex *can be as psychologically damaging as the actual sexual involvement itself.* Unfortunately, professional ethics codes are usually silent concerning the specific boundary violations that often precede therapist sexual misconduct. (p. 614) [emphasis added]

Most of the contributions listed above have included acknowledgment of the difficulty of establishing specific prohibitions on boundary crossing, considering that each case and each practice style is unique. As Smith and Fitzpatrick (1995) have written:

> The effects of crossing commonly recognized boundaries range from significant therapeutic progress to serious, indelible harm. The issues are further complicated by the wide range of individual variation that exists in a field where what is normal practice for one clinician may be considered a boundary violation by another. (p. 505)

A similarly catholic approach appears to be espoused by Simon (1992) when he writes:

> . . . considerable disagreement exists among psychiatrists concerning what constitutes treatment boundary violations. The therapy techniques of one therapist may be anathema to another therapist who considers such practices as clear boundary violations (p. 269). . . . boundary excursions inevitably occur in almost every therapy. (p. 286)

Finally, Brown (1994) exemplifies how attempted solutions to the problem of therapeutic boundaries can inadvertently become codified as rules. She states:

> What I have found, to my dismay, is that when I have shared strategies that evolved into solutions that work for me, carefully framing as my solutions and opinions rather than "the rule," I find myself quoted two journal articles later as saying that "such and so behavior is not okay." (p. 30)

However, one can also find in the literature statements that would seem to imply that widespread agreement exists concerning a prohibition of certain boundary crossing behaviors, as well as the need to sanction them. For example, Strasburger et al. (1992) write:

> The slippery slope of boundary violations may be ventured upon first in the form of small, relatively inconsequential actions by the therapist such as

scheduling a "favored" patient for the last appointment of the day, extending sessions with the patient beyond the scheduled time, having excessive telephone conversations with the patient, and becoming lax with fees. Violations can involve excessive self-disclosure by the therapist to the patient. . . . Gifts may be exchanged. The therapist may begin to direct the patient's work and personal life choices. . . . Meetings may be arranged outside the office for lunch or dinner. . . . Notice that in this scenario, the therapist has not touched the patient, nor has the therapist said or done anything that is overtly sexual. *The treatment, however, has already become compromised, and the therapist may be found liable civilly. The therapist is also vulnerable to action by a licensing board, should the patient wish to make a complaint.* (p. 547 [emphasis added])

In a similar vein, Simon (1995) has suggested that agreement exists among diverse schools of psychotherapy regarding boundaries. He states, "The boundary guidelines . . . , with appropriate clinical modifications, are a unifying element in the over 450 different forms of psychotherapy currently in existence" (p. 90). Simon provides the following list of "treatment boundary guidelines" which appears in several of his publications:

Maintain therapist neutrality. Foster psychological separateness of patient. Obtain informed consent for treatment and procedures. Interact verbally with clients. Ensure no previous, current, or future personal relationships with patients. Minimize physical contact. Preserve relative anonymity of the therapist. Establish a stable fee policy. Provide a consistent, private, and professional setting. Define length and time of sessions. (1994, p. 514)

Boundary Violations Versus Transference Abuse

Frequently mentioned in civil and licensing board actions to make reference to a standard of care, the term "boundary violation" has become prevalent during the past 10 years. Although psychotherapeutic boundaries have been conceptually useful to some practitioners for many years (e.g., Langs, 1976; Stone, 1976), the concept of boundary violations has recently supplanted that of "transference abuse" (e.g., Gabbard & Pope, 1988; Pope & Bouhoutsos, 1986) in the malpractice arena as one that describes unethical, overly close relations between therapist and patient. In Pope and Bouhoutsos' (1986) seminal work on therapist-patient sex, as in Bates and Brodsky's (1989) extensive case study, no mention is made in the index of the word "boundaries." In contrast, Pope's (1994) book on therapist-patient sex contains no fewer than 14 index citations under this term, perhaps giving some indication of the increasing popularity of this concept.

Transference abuse has been a problematic concept in malpractice litigation because of its overt theoretical linkage to psychoanalysis, causing the concept to be meaningless or offensive to numerous practitioners. As Gutheil (1989) has pointed out:

> It seems that professionals who belong to a school of thought that rejects the idea of transference, behaviorists, or psychiatrists who provide only drug treatment, are being held to a standard of care they do not acknowledge. (p. 31)

The greater courtroom utility of boundary violations, by contrast to that of transference abuse, may rest on the universality of the former concept. It is free from the criticism that it derives only from psychoanalysis with relevance only to practitioners espousing allegiance to that school.

A Therapeutic Rationale for Careful Boundary Maintenance

An argument relative to the import of maintaining boundaries in psychotherapy might be outlined as follows:

1. Psychotherapy is a powerful tool that can evoke powerful emotions.
2. Reported victims of therapist-patient sexual involvement often tend to be women and the perpetrators men.
3. Psychotherapy patients tend to regress to infantile and vulnerable states.
4. This regression places the patient in a situation which is reminiscent of a family, in which the child is vulnerable to the parent.
5. Consequently, the male therapist, as metaphorical father, must ensure that the vulnerability of the female patient, his metaphorical daughter, is not exploited. (This is equally true regardless of gender of patient or therapist, although most litigation involves this metaphorical "father–daughter" dyad (e.g., Pope, 1990a, 1990b).
6. Steps must be taken to give the patient clear messages that any vulnerability will not be exploited.
7. These steps include establishing *boundaries* between the therapist and patient, and between the professional and the social.

These boundaries include clearly demarcating starting and stopping times of sessions, having no social contacts with patients, not touching patients, not disclosing personal information to the patient, always billing patients, and doing all related activities to continually remind the patient and make abundantly clear that this is a professional, rather than social or sexually intimate, relationship.

8. Patients, because of their regressed and vulnerable state, may attempt to initiate behaviors that are more social or sexual than therapeutic. The therapist always bears the burden of preventing this from occurring. Because the patient's judgment may be impaired, the therapist bears the exclusive responsibility for setting limits.

9. Some patients, because of a prior history of childhood or adult sexual abuse, may become confused regarding the difference between that which is therapeutic and that which is social or sexual. Consequently, even apparently harmless forays into social or personal activity, which are not part of treatment, must be avoided to avoid confusing the patient as to the nature of the relationship.

10. In light of all of the above, even seemingly trivial "boundary violations," such as giving a patient a ride should her car be broken, can indicate a disregard for the import of boundaries and can be a sign of negligence. Such negligence can approach metaphorical incest considering the father-daughter metaphor which is attributed to these therapeutic dyads.

From this point of view, one of the most significant curative aspects of psychotherapy may be that the patient undergoes his or her initial lifetime experience of an interpersonal relationship in which boundaries are adequately maintained. By virtue of this, the patient comes to learn that the therapist is a separate person, not dependent on the patient for love or any other emotional needs, and that it is possible for the patient to have other, mature, adult, independent, and nonexploitative relationships. In addition, the patient learns that there can be healthy relationships such as psychotherapy in which the stated goals which gave rise to the relationship are in fact carried out without manipulation, hidden agendas, or abuse. While this approach shares many elements with the ground rules of classical psychoanalysis (Greenson, 1967; Gutheil & Gabbard, 1993), it is also informed by modern concepts such as family dysfunction and the incest survivor movement (e.g., Russell, 1986), feminist therapy[2] (e.g., Brown, 1994), and has become a cornerstone of the addiction-recovery movement (e.g., Katherine, 1993).

Although anecdotal reports provide support for arguments which hold that even nonsexual boundary violations lead to patient harm, for example, Simon (1991), the reliable occurrence of such harm has not been established. The difficulties in systematically associating resultant harm with previous boundary violations of a sexual nature have been discussed elsewhere (Pope & Bouhoutsos, 1986; Williams, 1992, 1995).

HUMANISTIC PSYCHOTHERAPY: A SOLUTION TO A DIFFERENT PROBLEM

Humanistic psychotherapists, and those eclectic therapists influenced by humanistic concepts and methods, practice from viewpoints which lead them routinely and intentionally to engage in what some might argue are grossly negligent boundary violations. Humanistic psychotherapy includes, but is not limited to, approaches such as Gestalt (e.g., Fagen & Shepherd, 1970; Perls, 1969; Smith, 1976), encounter group (e.g., Korchin, 1976; Rogers, 1970), Transactional Analysis (e.g., Berne, 1961, 1964), Existential (e.g., Yalom, 1980), and client-centered psychotherapy (e.g., Rogers, 1951, 1961). Bugental's work (1986, 1987) exemplifies a more recent, eclectic approach to humanistic psychotherapy.

It is of great significance that the humanistic movement, as described by Korchin (1976) and others, has been devoted *not to maintaining but to tearing down the boundaries between therapist and patient.* Korchin describes the essence of Humanistic Psychology as follows:

> Above all else, therapy involves an authentic encounter between two real individuals, free of sham and role-playing, rather than technical acts of an interpretive, advising, or conditioning sort. (1976, p. 352)

The following quotation from Bugental (1987) provides some insight into the humanistic ethos with respect to boundaries:

---

[2]Feminist therapists seem, at times, to advocate both careful boundary maintenance and a humanistic sort of closeness. Regarding the latter, Brown and Walker (1990) have stated "Some recent authors . . . have suggested that being overly distant may be as damaging and thus ethically problematic in therapy as is an overt violation of a boundary under the guide of 'closeness' " (p. 143).

Long-term therapy of some depth inevitably involves times of warm commu-
nion and times of great stress—for both participants. Living through these
together has a true bonding effect which is not always recognized by those
who teach or practice more objective modes. Nevertheless, therapist and
patient often have what can only be called a love relationship, which is by
no means simply a product of transference and countertransference. Patient
and therapist are two human beings, partners in a difficult, hazardous, and
rewarding enterprise; it is unreal to expect otherwise. (p. 258)

Humanistic practitioners might argue that for the therapist to be
self-disclosive makes the patient feel more equal to, rather than inferior
to, the therapist. It allows the patient to see that all people have failures
and other unresolved matters in their lives, and that there is no essential
difference, in fact, between those people who are psychotherapists and
those people who are patients. In discussing self-disclosure with patients,
Bugental (1987) advocates, "First and foremost: strict honesty is required" (p. 143).

In the context of group psychotherapy, Vinogradov and Yalom (1990)
offer the following recommendations:

Group psychotherapists may—just like other members in the group—openly
share their thoughts and feelings in a judicious and responsible manner,
respond to others authentically, and acknowledge or refute motives and
feelings attributed to them. In other words, therapists, too, can reveal their
feelings, the reasons for some of their behaviors, acknowledge the blind spots,
and demonstrate respect for the feedback group members offer them. (p. 198)

In a similar vein, humanists might argue that many other activities
that were excluded from classical psychoanalytic technique can take
place without harming the therapeutic process, and, in fact, will help
it. Some humanists, like Perls (e.g., 1969), largely defined their methods
in contrast to what they considered to be stagnant psychoanalytic doctrine and unnecessary psychoanalytic prohibitions. Consequently, patients are urged to call humanistic therapists by their first names,
therapists might socialize with patients—especially in the context of a
personal growth center or retreat, gift-giving is not unheard of, sessions
might take place outside of the office, and hugging, in sharp contrast
to analytic reserve, becomes the order of the day. Although these activities are not specifically prescribed by any particular humanistic theory,
they flourish in the open, innovative, and often spontaneous climate of
humanistic psychotherapy. This excerpt from Jourard (1971) provides
specific examples of the wide range of behaviors that might be part of
a humanistic practice style:

In the context of dialogue I don't hesitate to share any of my experience with existential binds roughly comparable to those in which the seeker finds himself (this is now called "modeling"); nor do I hesitate to disclose my experience of him, myself, and our relationship as it unfolds from moment to moment. . . . I might give Freudian or other types of interpretations. I might teach him such Yoga know-how or tricks for expanding body-awareness as I have mastered or engage in arm wrestling or hold hands or hug him, if that is the response that emerges in the dialogue.

I do not hesitate to play a game of handball with a seeker or visit him in his home—if this unfolds in the dialogue. (p. 159)

Humanistic approaches like Jourard's were part of the training of many psychotherapists during the 1970s. To what extent individuals trained in this approach continue to practice largely in this same manner is unknown, although it appears, at least to the author, that many of today's licensing board and malpractice defendants were trained during the 1960s and 1970s, when tearing down boundaries was encouraged. Survey research by Pope, Tabachnick, and Keith-Spiegel (1987) found that 14% of practitioners recently identified themselves as "humanistic," and Borys and Pope (1989) found a relationship between theoretical orientation and boundary-related behaviors. Further, one finds no indication in the humanistically oriented journals of a radical shift away from previous styles. In contrast, recent examples, like the following from the *Journal of Humanistic Psychology,* indicate that similar, boundary-blurring themes continue to prevail within the realm of humanistic psychotherapy:

At her moment of deep despair, this young woman found in her core the courage and strength to call the therapist to open herself to her as one human being to another. The therapist returned her embrace without words.

This moment of dialogue did not interfere in any way in the therapist's observation and evaluation. On the contrary—it added most valuable data that a moment later the therapist could bring into her psychological-observational stance. (Kron & Friedman, 1994, p. 71)

Recent humanistic writings have become less strident regarding the need to challenge therapeutic boundaries in contrast to humanistic publications of 2 or 3 decades ago. One wonders whether humanistic practice has become more conservative with respect to boundaries, or whether humanistic practitioners—fearing lawsuits or ethics enforcement—simply have become less forthcoming about their boundary-crossings. A relatively recent study by J. Simon (1990), although based on a small sample, indicates that the most self-disclosive therapists considered their mentors to be Albert Ellis, Carl Rogers, Fritz Perls, and Werner Erhard. This supports the notion that the basic humanistic ethos regarding boundaries may still be intact.

Recently, some psychoanalytic psychotherapists have adopted a liberal position regarding the boundary of self-disclosure. Some analysts now seek a "shared experience" between analyst and analysand. This requires authentic self-disclosure by the analyst, making aspects of this psychoanalytic approach indistinguishable from humanism, as illustrated by the following quotation from Fisher (1990):

> Further, I contend that for a genuine encounter to occur between patient and therapist, and for authentic growth in intimacy to emerge (which is at the heart of the need for therapy to begin with) a truly shared experience must take place. Again, the belief herein suggested is that the encounter between patient and therapist (like that between parent and child) should take place between (psychological) equals: between the co-participants of dyadic psychotherapy. Lastly, that the sharing of experiencing, which leads to intimacy, is achieved through the process of (mutual) self-disclosure. (p. 14)

One may surmise that the revised APA Ethics Code (1992), statutory changes, and changes in professional liability coverage (e.g., Pope, 1994) have had an impact on overt sexual boundary violations committed by humanistic therapists. Past examples of the humanistic approach to sexual boundaries, reckless at minimum and unethical by today's standards, have been provided by Finney (1975), regarding client-centered therapy, and Shepard (1975), regarding Gestalt therapy.

BEHAVIOR THERAPY: ANOTHER REBELLION AGAINST THE CULTURE OF PSYCHOANALYTIC TECHNIQUE

Behavior therapy is another approach to psychotherapy that arose, in part, as a rebellion against psychoanalysis (Korchin, 1976). Practitioners of behavior therapy, and eclectic therapists who have been influenced by this approach, might routinely commit what many today would call boundary violations. Many behavior therapists have never been part of the culture of psychoanalysis, and many have gone through their graduate school or residency training free from exposure to even the most basic ground rules of psychoanalysis, including those pertaining to boundaries. Indeed, should a behavior therapist-in-training encounter a list of psychoanalytic practice guidelines, the result might be little more than derisive laughter. Arnold Lazarus, the noted behavior therapist, has referred to psychoanalysis as a "speculative theory" and has called transference a "myth" (A. A. Lazarus, personal communication, September 27, 1990).

In practice, behavior therapists have cogent reasons to counter even the most basic of classical psychoanalytic dicta. For example, the analytic blank screen allows the patient to project fantasies as part of the transference. For this reason, classical psychoanalysts would not be self-disclosive; the less the patient actually knew about the analyst, the more the patient could project. Behavior therapists, in contrast, use the concept of modeling, which holds that the patient might learn from the therapist by copying behaviors or even attitudes and that this could be curative. To practice modeling, the behavior therapist might need to be self-disclosive. For example, a behavior therapist might tell the patient how that therapist overcame his or her own fear of flying (e.g., Ellis, 1977). In addition, while the psychoanalyst might prefer to leave the patient guessing about the degree and nature of his or her training—another source of material to analyze—the behavior therapist might carefully spell out the nature of his or her training and experience, to better be seen as a high status model, capable of influencing behavior. Indeed, a behavior therapist might, upon request, disclose his or her high success rate at treating similar cases to that for which the patient seeks help, while a classical psychoanalytically oriented practitioner would interpret such a request only in terms of the patient's psychodynamics.

From the viewpoint of behavior therapy, there has been little concern about socializing with patients outside of therapy sessions. Some behavior therapists have argued that they merely apply a set of technical procedures and, consequently, require no special rules for the therapist-patient relationship beyond those rules that would apply to one's relationship with one's architect (e.g., Marquis, 1972). As Marquis states, "The resulting relationship is one in which I have felt quite comfortable having good friends as clients and good clients as friends" (pp. 48–49).

Nothing in the theory of behavior therapy would or should preclude socializing with patients, taking meals with them, giving them gifts, or treating them at their homes, schools, or offices. Hugging patients might increase the therapist's potency as a reinforcer for the patient and thus might be support theoretically, and on the subject of touching patients. Marquis advises:

> The depth of relaxation is tested carefully by observing the client visually and by *manipulating the extremities.*

Psychologists and social workers are often reluctant to touch a client, but even most clients with phobias about being touched accept the procedure easily. (p. 55 [emphasis added])

A behavior therapist's viewpoint on self-disclosure is provided in the recent handbook by Burns (1990), a strong proponent of the currently popular cognitive behavior therapy. Burns advises, "Let the patient know how you feel about what he or she is saying. This will make you appear more genuine and real" (p. 514). He provides the following case example to illustrate his use of self-disclosure:

I told Ronda that I felt inadequate. I said I felt as if every sentence that came out of my mouth was wooden and useless to her. I said that although I usually felt I had something to offer, it didn't seem that way today. I told her I felt excluded and shut out, and that I felt angry with her. I said I wanted to give her something positive and I believed that the therapy could be successful, but I felt thwarted in my efforts. (p. 521)

In a similar vein, Dryden (1990) argues that therapist self-disclosure is an integral part of Rational Emotive Therapy (RET). Dryden states:

Given that the effective RET therapist would accept herself for her errors and flaws and for past and present emotional disturbances, she will, as often as is therapeutically advisable, show her client how she upset herself about experiences similar to those with which her client is concerned and how she used RET to overcome such emotional disturbances. (p. 66)

Lazarus (1994a, 1994b) recently took issue with those who would strictly enforce boundary maintenance. He provided numerous examples from his practice in which either treatment issues or common politeness dictated a need to dine with, self-disclose to, socialize with, or befriend patients and argued that such activities had either no ill effects on treatment or were helpful. Invited discussants reacted sharply, presenting Dr. Lazarus as naive and foolhardy and generally lucky to have managed his boundary crossings without adverse consequences (e.g., Gabbard, 1994; Gutheil, 1994), or they suggested that while he might possess the skill to negotiate these boundary crossings successfully, others who would follow his example might not (Bennett et al., 1994). None of the discussants seemed to accept his overriding point that *"one of the worst professional or ethical violations is that of permitting current risk-management principles to take precedence over humane interventions"* (p. 260 [emphasis added]).

Goisman and Gutheil (1992) provide a poignant example of what might occur when commonplace behavior therapy procedures are held up to psychoanalytic scrutiny regarding boundary maintenance:

> We are aware of a case currently in litigation where a number of the charges against an experienced behavior therapist flowed from the testimony of a psychoanalytically trained expert witness, who faulted the behavior therapist for assigning homework tasks to patients, hiring present and former patients for jobs in psychoeducational programs and other benign interventions, and performing a sexological examination and sensate focus instructions in a case of sexual dysfunction. From a psychoanalytic viewpoint all of these would likely constitute boundary violations of a potentially harmful sort, but from a behavioral viewpoint this is not the case. The legal system in this lawsuit had some difficulty, as is commonly the case, in grasping the distinctions between therapies and the variations of boundary norms appropriate to each type of treatment. (p. 538)

As with humanistic approaches, some of the most direct challenges to therapeutic boundaries by behavior therapists were published some years ago, leaving the reader to wonder about the extent to which practitioners who were trained during a more liberal era may have moved toward more careful boundary maintenance in their contemporary practices.

DIVERSITY OF PRACTICE

Research has demonstrated that practice is diverse with respect to boundaries. Table 6.1 shows the self-reported rates of some of the now controversial activities that Pope et al. (1987) found in the practices of a national sample of psychologists. Psychologists were asked to rate the frequency with which various boundary-blurring activities occurred in their practices, for example, lending money to patients, socializing with them, asking favors of them, and touching them in various ways. As Table 6.1 indicates, many of the controversial boundary-related activities were surprisingly prevalent in the practices of psychologists. An interesting aspect of this sample is that humanistic approaches only comprised 14% of the psychologists surveyed, behavioral only 2.6%, while practitioners identifying themselves as psychodynamic comprised 32.9%. Considering the theoretical positions taken by the various schools with respect to these boundary-blurring activities, one would suspect that homogeneous samples of either humanistic or behavioral practitioners

TABLE 6.1   Self-Reported Rates of Boundary-Related Behaviors

Description	Reported Rate of Occurrence
Telling a client you are angry with him or her	42.5% responded from "sometimes" to "very often"
Using self-disclosure as a therapy technique	69.4% responded from "sometimes" to "very often"
Having a client address you by your first name	96.2% responded from "rarely" to "very often"
Hugging a client	41.7% responded from "sometimes" to "very often"
Kissing a client	23.5% responded "rarely"
Accepting a client's gift worth at least $50	19.1% responded "rarely"
Accepting a gift worth less than $5 from a client	58.1% responded from "sometimes" to "very often"
Asking favors (e.g., a ride home) from clients	35.7% responded "rarely"
Lending money to a client	23.9% responded "rarely"
Inviting clients to a party or social event	15.4% responded "rarely" or "sometimes"

From "Ethics of Practice: The Beliefs and Behaviors of Psychologists as Therapists," by K. S. Pope, B. G. Tabachnick, and P. Keith-Spiegel, 1987, *American Psychologist, 42*, pp. 995–997. Adapted with permission.

might yield even higher reported rates. As it is, these authors found that the use of self-disclosure, at least on rare occasions, is an *"almost universal" aspect of psychotherapy* (p. 998 [emphasis added]). This is significant in view of Simon's (1994) injunction, noted above, that one must "preserve relative anonymity of the therapist," and it becomes especially significant considering the assertion by Simon (1991) and others that *the degree of self-disclosure in psychotherapy is a better predictor of sexual involvement with patients than is the degree of nonsexual touching.*

A similar study by Borys and Pope (1989) also supported the notion that practice is diverse with respect to boundaries. In this study, an interdisciplinary national sample of psychiatrists, psychologists, and social workers was surveyed. Table 6.2 shows the rates of occurrence of boundary-blurring behaviors in this sample. As was the case with the Pope et al. study (1987), these rates were much higher than one would expect were Simon's guidelines, listed above, to be widely observed. Both tables show that gift giving, dining together, nonsexual touching,

TABLE 6.2 Self-Reported Rates of Boundary-Related Behaviors

Description	Reported Rate of Occurrence
Disclosed details of current personal stresses to a client	38.9% did this with a few or more clients
Went out to eat with a client after a session	11.6% did this with a few or more clients
Accepted a client's invitation to a special occasion	35.1% did this with a few or more clients

From "Dual Relationships Between Therapist and Client: A National Study of Psychologists, Psychiatrists, and Social Workers," by D. S. Borys and K. S. Pope, 1989, *Professional Psychology: Research and Practice, 20,* p. 288. Adapted with permission.

asking favors, and self-disclosure are not uncommon in psychotherapeutic practice. Borys and Pope's findings also provided support for the present contention that maintenance of boundaries is related to therapeutic orientation, with a statistically significant relationship being found between "frequency of reported social involvements with clients . . . and theoretical orientation" (p. 288). Statistically significant differences in behavior were also found when psychodynamic practitioners were contrasted with humanistic ones.

A recent study by Johnston and Farber (1996) surveyed psychologists' attitudes and behaviors regarding "everyday" boundaries in psychotherapy, such as starting and ending sessions on time, requiring timely payment of fees, and demanding adherence to specified appointment times. Although this set of studied boundaries was subtle, and less likely to constitute behaviors that were of questionable ethics, therapists' behavior was once again diverse. Findings indicated that

> patients make relatively few demands and psychotherapists accommodate them most of the time. This finding stands in opposition to the generally accepted image of the psychotherapist standing firm in the face of persistent attempts by the patient to challenge existing boundaries and suggests a spirit of cooperation and good faith underemphasized in theoretical writings. (p. 397)

The particular set of boundaries investigated by Johnston and Farber did not show a relationship between boundary maintenance and any therapist variables, such as theoretical orientation. However, it should be noted that "humanistic" was not used as one of the choices for assigning theoretical orientation.

A Generation Gap

The possibility exists that attitudes are changing, and that psychotherapists who have been trained within the past few years may tend to more closely adhere to the boundary guidelines promulgated by Simon (1994) and others. Indeed, the survey by Borys and Pope (1989) found a significant relationship between therapists' years of experience and their ratings concerning the ethics of maintaining dual professional roles with patients, with less experienced therapists more likely to consider dual roles unethical. Perhaps professionals' attitudes regarding the ethics of certain boundary-related behaviors have changed dramatically over the past 2 decades. One consequence of this would be a schism between older and younger practitioners, with the older practitioners appearing to the younger ones to be less ethical. This possible interaction between experience and ethics is a matter that requires additional research. One implication of such a "generation gap" would be that a younger expert witness, in adjudicating behaviors that are not specifically enumerated by an ethics code, might honestly testify that an elder practitioner seems to have practiced negligently, when, in fact, the elder practitioner may have practiced well within the standard of care of the cohort with which he or she trained.

AVOIDING THE APPEARANCE OF WRONGDOING

An additional, very significant contribution to conceptualizations of boundaries has been proposed by Gutheil and Gabbard (1993). These authors reviewed a wide range of "boundary crossings," which may or may not constitute boundary violations, and they argued that even certain boundary crossings which are *justified and consistent with good care should be eschewed on the basis of their possible adverse appearance in court*. This process of avoiding behaviors, not because they are wrong, but only because they *appear* wrong, is known as "risk management." Gutheil and Gabbard state that plaintiff's attorneys will make these crossings appear to the jury to be incontrovertible evidence of wrongdoing. Thus, regarding the question of scheduling patients late in the day, they state:

> In the fog of uncertainty surrounding sexual misconduct (usually a conflict of credibilities without a witness), this factor has gleamed with so illusory a brightness that some attorneys seem to presume that because the patient had the last appointment of the day, sexual misconduct occurred! (p. 191)

On the subject of self-disclosure of matters which include information concerning the therapist's family, they advise that such behavior

> may be used by the legal system to advance or support a claim of sexual misconduct. The reasoning is that the patient knows so much about the therapist's personal life that they must have been intimate. (p. 194)

Finally, in discussing a case in which a psychiatrist, who was ultimately exonerated, was found guilty of sexual misconduct, they state that:

> recent court decisions suggest a trend toward findings of liability for boundary violations even in the absence of sexual contact. On this basis, the risk-management value of avoiding even the appearance of boundary violations should be self-evident. (p. 189)

Gutheil and Gabbard (1993) may be correct that avoiding behaviors in psychotherapy which, although harmless and appropriate, might appear negligent is a good risk-management strategy. However, one may question, in terms of both principle and practicality, whether practitioners ought to change their deeply held beliefs and established methods to avoid "looking bad." As a practical concern, modifying one's methods in the interest of risk management becomes a more difficult decision to the extent that one's practice relies on boundary-crossing techniques, as it becomes easier to the extent that one's practice does not. Indeed, some of the distinguishing characteristics of one's practice might be its boundary-crossing procedures. Prospective clients seeking treatment, or colleagues making referrals, might seek out a given practitioner only because that practitioner truly is a dyed-in-the-wool behaviorist or humanist, known to use methods specific to those approaches. Why, for example, would a patient seek treatment at a "humanistic growth center" if the psychotherapy offered were largely indistinguishable from that found in other offices? Clearly, there would be professional or business risks for some practitioners were they to adopt the risk-management strategies proposed by Gutheil and Gabbard.

As a final point, it should be noted that Gutheil and Gabbard (1993) have also advocated restraint in court regarding accusations of boundary violation, urging that attention be paid to the context in which the boundary crossing occurred prior to drawing conclusions regarding harmfulness or standard of care. However, as a practical matter, whether a boundary *crossing* is perceived as a boundary *violation* is very much in the eye of the beholder. The author's own consulting experience indicates that plaintiff and defense experts are capable of arriving at opposite, but equally firm, conclusions when confronted with the same clinical data. This, in the author's opinion, is *not* the result of the use of "hired guns" as expert witnesses who will testify on one side or the other for a fee. Instead, these experts appear to be sincere individuals who, like the authors quoted above, simply hold a range of divergent views of what constitutes appropriate psychotherapy.

The plaintiff has a purpose in establishing that nonsexual boundary violations occurred. In some legal cases the occurrence of sexual negligence is not contested, yet the occurrence of other boundary crossings is nevertheless disputed in court. The question arises as to why a plaintiff would bother to establish that self-disclosure, for example, had taken place in the context of psychotherapy that was known to have been grossly negligent because it had included sexual intercourse. The answer concerns the nature of malpractice insurance: Most, if not all, of today's malpractice insurance policies exclude coverage for damages resulting from therapist-patient sexual involvement. Thus, a finding for the plaintiff in a civil case that awards damages due to sexual transgressions would not result in payment by the insurance carrier. Many defendants lack the resources to pay such awards which can exceed a million dollars. To prevent such fruitless courtroom victories, plaintiffs often file complaints intended to establish, consistent with Simon's (1991) writings cited earlier, that the nonsexual boundary violations which occurred were harmful in and of themselves, constituted negligent psychotherapy in and of themselves, and would have, with a reasonable degree of certainty, resulted in equivalent damages to those observed even had sexual contact not taken place. This strategy places the insurance carrier in a position such that the damage award will be paid, even when sex was involved, because the sexual involvement had been shown not to be the only, or even chief, source of harm to the patient. In fact, one strategy would have the plaintiff intentionally omitting instances of documented sexual contact as part of the complaint, thereby enhancing the argument for insurance coverage as negligent psychotherapy.

CONCLUSION

With the above in mind, it may be argued that strict boundary maintenance, although supported by some authors, should not constitute a minimum standard of care. While there is a near unanimity among practitioners that therapist-patient sexual involvement is unethical during treatment (Pope et al., 1987), the other boundary-related behaviors which have been discussed are neither specifically prohibited by ethical guidelines, nor are they universally recognized as deviations from the standard of care.

The complex endeavor of psychotherapy, which includes dozens of theoretical perspectives, several different licensed professions with disparate training requirements, and innumerable continually evolving techniques, cannot facilely be delimited by an overly simple and restrictive set of rules (e.g., those proposed by Simon, 1994), deviation from which would seem to place one beneath the standard of care. This is no better exemplified than by the text of the Distinguished Professional Contribution Award presented by the American Psychological Association to Kenneth Pope in 1994 ("Awards," 1995). Although Pope's substantial contributions to the literature have emphasized the importance of maintaining clear boundaries in psychotherapy (e.g., 1989, 1994), his award biography describes several instances, in his treatment of a female patient, of what Gutheil and Gabbard (1993) might term boundary crossings (although not boundary violations). The exemplary treatment carried out by Pope had included daily meetings without fee and his arranging for a personal friend of his to lend the patient money and to provide her with an airline ticket and a place to stay. In the context of the particular case, these boundary excursions appeared to be both humane and sensible. However, some practitioners might, in the interest of risk management, avoid making similar modifications. Clearly, any efforts that would discourage the sort of flexibility of practice exemplified by Pope's case serve no end but to increase the likelihood that undue damage awards will be paid, that dedicated clinicians will be improperly sanctioned, and that the practice of psychotherapy will stagnate as practitioners become more concerned with risk management than with innovation.

REFERENCES

Atkins, E. L., & Stein, R. (1993). When the boundary is crossed: A protocol for attorneys and mental health professionals. *American Journal of Forensic Psychology, 11,* 3–21.

Awards for Distinguished Professional Contributions. (1995). *American Psychologist, 50,* 236–247.

Bates, C. M., & Brodsky, A. M. (1989). *Sex in the therapy hour: A case of professional incest.* New York: Guilford.

Bennett, B. E., Bricklin, P. M., & VandeCreek, L. (1994). Response to Lazarus's "How certain boundaries and ethics diminish therapeutic effectiveness." *Ethics and Behavior, 4,* 263–266.

Berne, E. (1961). *Transactional analysis in psychotherapy.* New York: Grove.

Berne, E. (1964). *Games people play.* New York: Grove.

Borys, D. S., & Pope, K. S. (1989). Dual relationships between therapist and client: A national study of psychologists, psychiatrists, and social workers. *Professional Psychology: Research and Practice, 20,* 283–293.

Brodsky, A. M. (1989). Sex between patient and therapist: Psychology's data and response. In G. Gabbard (Ed.), *Sexual exploitation in professional relationships* (pp. 15–26). Washington, DC: American Psychiatric Press.

Brown, L. S. (1994). Boundaries in feminist therapy: A conceptual formulation. *Women and Therapy, 15,* 29–38.

Brown, L. S., & Walker, L. (1990). Feminist therapist perspectives. In G. Stricker & M. Fisher (Eds.), *Self-disclosure in the therapeutic relationship* (pp. 135–154). New York: Plenum.

Bugental, J. F. (1986). Existential-humanistic psychotherapy. In I. L. Kutash & A. Wolf (Eds.), *Psychotherapist's casebook* (pp. 222–236). San Francisco: Jossey-Bass.

Bugental, J. F. (1987). *The art of the psychotherapist.* New York: W. W. Norton.

Burns, D. D. (1990). *The feeling good handbook.* New York: Plume.

Dryden, W. (1990). Self-disclosure in rational emotive therapy. In G. Stricker & M. Fisher (Eds.), *Self-disclosure in the therapeutic relationship* (pp. 61–74). New York: Plenum.

Ellis, A. (1977). *How to master your fear of flying.* New York: Institute for Rational-Emotive Therapy.

Epstein, R. S., & Simon, R. I. (1990). The exploitation index: An early warning indicator of boundary violations in psychotherapy. *Bulletin of the Menninger Clinic, 54,* 450–465.

Epstein, R. S., Simon, R. I., & Kay, G. G. (1992). Assessing boundary violations in psychotherapy: Survey results with the exploitation index. *Bulletin of the Menninger Clinic, 56,* 150–166.

Fagen, J., & Shepherd, I. L. (1970). *Gestalt therapy now.* New York: Harper & Row.

Finney, J. (1975). Therapist and patient after hours. *American Journal of Psychotherapy, 29,* 593–602.

Fisher, M. (1990). The shared experience and self-disclosure. In G. Stricker & M. Fisher (Eds.), *Self-disclosure in the therapeutic relationship* (pp. 3–15). New York: Plenum.

Folman, R. Z. (1991). Therapist-patient sex: Attraction and boundary problems. *Psychotherapy, 28,* 168–173.

Gabbard, G. (1994). Teetering on the precipice: A commentary on Lazarus's "How certain boundaries and ethics diminish therapeutic effectiveness." *Ethics and Behavior, 4,* 283–286.

Gabbard, G., & Pope, K. (1988). Sexual intimacies after termination: Clinical, ethical, and legal aspects. *Independent Practitioner, 8,* 21–26.

Gechtman, L. (1989). Sexual contact between social workers and their clients. In G. Gabbard (Ed.), *Sexual exploitation in professional relationships* (pp. 27–38). Washington, DC: American Psychiatric Press.

Goisman, R. M., & Gutheil, T. G. (1992). Risk management in the practice of behavior therapy: Boundaries and behavior. *American Journal of Psychotherapy, 46,* 533–543.

Gottleib, M. C. (1993). Avoiding exploitative dual relationships: A decision-making model. *Psychotherapy, 30,* 41–48.

Gottleib, M. C. (1994). Ethical decision making, boundaries, and treatment effectiveness: A reprise. *Ethics and Behavior, 4,* 287–293.

Greenson, R. (1967). *The technique and practice of psychoanalysis.* New York: International Universities Press.

Gutheil, T. G. (1989, November/December). Patient-therapist sexual relations. *The California Therapist, 6,* 29–39.

Gutheil, T. G. (1994). Discussion of Lazarus's "How certain boundaries and ethics diminish therapeutic effectiveness." *Ethics and Behavior, 4,* 295–298.

Gutheil, T. G., & Gabbard, G. O. (1993). The concept of boundaries in clinical practice: Theoretical and risk-management dimensions. *American Journal of Psychiatry, 200* (2), 188–196.

Johnston, S. H., & Farber, B. A. (1996). The maintenance of boundaries in psychotherapeutic practice. *Psychotherapy, 33,* 391–402.

Jourard, S. M. (1971). *The transparent self.* New York: D. Van Nostrand.

Katherine, A. (1993). *Boundaries: Where you end and I begin.* New York: Fireside/Parkside.

Korchin, S. (1976). *Modern clinical psychology.* New York: Basic.

Kron, T., & Friedman, M. (1994). Problems of confirmation in psychotherapy. *Journal of Humanistic Psychology, 34,* 66–83.

Langs, R. J. (1976). The therapeutic relationship and deviations in technique. In R. J. Langs (Ed.), *International journal of psychoanalytic psychotherapist* (pp. 106–141). New York: Jason Aronson.

Lazarus, A. A. (1994a). How certain boundaries and ethics diminish therapeutic effectiveness. *Ethics and Behavior, 4,* 255–261.

Lazarus, A. A. (1994b). The illusion of the therapist's power and the patient's fragility: My rejoinder. *Ethics and Behavior, 4,* 299–306.

Marquis, J. M. (1972). An expedient model for behavior therapy. In A. A. Lazarus (Ed.), *Clinical behavior therapy,* pp. 41–72.

Notman, M. T., & Nadelson, C. C. (1994). Psychotherapy with patients who have had sexual relations with a previous therapist. *Journal of Psychotherapy Practice and Research, 3,* 185–193.

Peals, F. S. (1969). *Gestalt therapy verbatim.* Lafayette, CA: Real People Press.

Pope, K. S. (1989). Therapist-patient sex syndrome: A guide for attorneys and subsequent therapists to assessing damage. In G. Gabbard (Ed.), *Sexual exploitation in professional relationships* (pp. 39–56). Washington, DC: American Psychiatric Press.

Pope, K. S. (1990a). Therapist-patient sex as sex abuse: Six scientific, professional, and practical dilemmas in addressing victimization and rehabilitation. *Professional Psychology: Research and Practice, 21,* 227–239.

Pope, K. S. (1990b). Therapist-patient sexual involvement: A review of the research. *Clinical Psychology Review, 10,* 477–490.

Pope, K. S. (1994). *Sexual involvement with therapists.* Washington, DC: American Psychological Association.

Pope, K. S., & Bouhoutsos, J. C. (1986). *Sexual intimacy between therapists and patients.* New York: Praeger.

Pope, K. S., Tabachnick, B. G., & Keith-Spiegel, P. (1987). Ethics of practice: The beliefs and behaviors of psychologists as therapists. *American Psychologist, 42,* 993–1006.

Rogers, C. R. (1951). *Client-centered therapy.* Boston: Houghton-Mifflin.

Rogers, C. R. (1961). *On becoming a person.* Boston: Houghton-Mifflin.

Rogers, C. R. (1970). *Carl Rogers on encounter groups.* New York: Harper & Row.

Russell, D. E. (1986). *The secret trauma: Incest in the lives of girls and women.* New York: Basic.

Shepard, M. (1975). *Fritz.* New York: Bantam.

Simon, J. C. (1990). Criteria for therapist self-disclosure. In G. Stricker & M. Fisher (Eds.), *Self-disclosure in the therapeutic relationship* (pp. 207–225). New York: Plenum.

Simon, R. I. (1991). Psychological injury caused by boundary violation precursors to therapist-patient sex. *Psychiatric Annals, 21,* 614–619.

Simon, R. I. (1992). Treatment boundary violations: Clinical, ethical, and legal considerations. *Bulletin of the American Academy of Psychiatry and Law, 20,* 269–287.

Simon, R. I. (1994). Transference in therapist-patient sex: The illusion of patient improvement and consent, part 1. *Psychiatric Annals, 24,* 509–515.

Simon, R. I. (1995). The natural history of therapist sexual misconduct: Identification and prevention. *Psychiatric Annals, 25,* 90–94.

Smith, D., & Fitzpatrick, M. (1995). Patient-therapist boundary issues: An integrative review of theory and research. *Professional Psychology: Research and Practice, 26,* 499–506.

Smith, E. W. (1976). *The growing edge of Gestalt therapy.* New York: Brunner/Mazel.

Sonne, J. L. (1989). An example of group therapy for victims of therapist-client. In G. Gabbard (Ed.), *Sexual exploitation in professional relationships* (pp. 101–114). Washington, DC: American Psychiatric Press.

Sonne, J. L. (1994). Multiple relationships: Does the new ethics code answer the right questions? *Professional Psychology: Research and Practice, 25,* 336–343.

Stone, M. H. (1976). Boundary violations between therapist and patient. *Psychiatric Annals, 6,* 670–677.

Strasburger, L. H., Jorgenson, L., & Sutherland, P. (1992). The prevention of psychotherapy sexual misconduct: Avoiding the slippery slope. *American Journal of Psychotherapy, 46,* 544–555.

Stricker, G. (1990). Self-disclosure in psychotherapy. In G. Stricker & M. Fisher (Eds.), *Self-disclosure in the therapeutic relationship* (pp. 277–290). New York: Plenum.

Vinogradov, S., & Yalom, I. (1990). Self-disclosure in group psychotherapy. In G. Stricker & M. Fisher (Eds.), *Self-disclosure in the therapeutic relationship* (pp. 191–204). New York: Plenum.

Williams, M. H. (1992). Exploitation and inference: Mapping the damage from therapist-patient sexual involvement. *American Psychologist, 47* (3), 412–421.

Williams, M. H. (1995). How useful are clinical reports concerning the consequences of therapist-patient sexual involvement? *American Journal of Psychotherapy, 49*(2), 237–243.

Yalom, I. D. (1980). *Existential psychotherapy.* New York: Basic.

CHAPTER 7

Out-of-Office Experience

When Crossing Office Boundaries and Engaging in Dual Relationships Are Clinically Beneficial and Ethically Sound

Ofer Zur, PhD

Conducting therapy outside the office, leaving the office with a client, and having nontherapeutic contact with clients out of the office have been frowned upon for legal (Bennett, Bricklin, & VandeCreek, 1994), ethical (Gottlieb, 1993; Pope & Vasquez, 1991), and clinical (Borys & Pope, 1989; Simon, 1991) reasons. They have been called boundary violations, boundary crossings, and boundary transgressions (Gutheil & Gabbard, 1993; Keith-Spiegel & Koocher, 1985).

Out-of-office experiences, whether part of a treatment plan or not, have also been placed high on the "slippery slope" list of items (Gut-

---

Reproduced by permission of the Division of Psychologists in Independent Practice of the American Psychological Association. Zur, O. (2001). Out-of-office experience. *The Independent Practitioner, 21* (2), 96–100.

heil & Gabbard, 1993; Simon, 1991; Strasburger, Jorgenson, & Suther-land, 1992). The term "slippery slope" alludes to a snowball dynamic and has been described as follows: " . . . the crossing of one boundary without obvious catastrophic results (making) it easier to cross the next boundary" (Gabbard, 1994, p. 284). Kenneth Pope, a leading expert in ethical matters, makes a claim that not only supports the "slippery slope" idea but has become a strict standard of therapeutic ethics and law: " . . . nonsexual dual relationships, while not unethical and harmful per se, foster sexual dual relationships" (1990, p. 688). Following this line of thinking, the conclusion is, "Obviously, the best advice to thera-pists is not to start (down) the slippery slope, and to avoid boundary violations or dual relationships with patients" (Strasburger et al., 1992, pp. 547–548).

Interacting with clients out of the office has traditionally been placed under the broad umbrella of dual relationships. A dual relationship in psychotherapy occurs when the therapist, in addition to his or her therapeutic role, is in another relationship with his or her patient. Since the early 1990s, the ethical codes of the American Psychological Association (APA) (1992) and all other major professional associations no longer impose a strict and uniform ban on dual relationships. In-stead, the changed codes acknowledge that dual relationships may not always be avoidable or unethical. While the absolute ban has been lifted, the belief in the prohibition is still prevalent (Faulkner & Faulkner, 1997; Gutheil & Gabbard, 1993; Strasburger et al., 1992). The revised code of ethics calls on therapists to avoid dual relationships only, " . . . if it appears likely that such a relationship reasonably might impair the psychologist's objectivity or otherwise interfere with the psychologist's effectively performing his or her function as a psychologist, or might harm or exploit the other party" (APA, 1992, p. 1601).

In response to an increase in client complaints and litigation, insur-ance companies, ethics committees, licensing boards, and attorneys have been advising therapists to "practice defensively" and to employ "risk management techniques" (Bennett et al., 1994; Keith-Spiegel & Koocher, 1985; Pope & Vasquez, 1991; Strasburger et al., 1992). Simon (1991) induces even more dread with his often-quoted, chilling, and ludicrous statement that "The boundary violation precursors of thera-pist-patient sex can be as psychologically damaging as the actual sexual involvement itself" (p. 614). As a result, therapists are acting out of fear of lawsuits and boards sanctions rather than according to what is effec-tive and helpful. Consequently, clinical judgment and treatment are often compromised (Ebert, 1997; Lazarus, 1994a, 1994b, 1998; Tomm, 1993; Williams, 1997; Zur, 2000a, 2000b).

Consumer advocates advise against leaving the office and against dual relationships in an attempt to protect the public from exploiting therapists (Barnett, 1996; Bennett et al., 1994). This argument is primarily based on psychoanalytic theory, which asserts that all clinical contacts must be strictly confined to the office. According to this theory, leaving the office interferes with the transference analysis, the hallmark of analytic work. While only a limited segment of therapists practice psychoanalysis, the rest of the therapeutic community is unfairly held to this standard (Williams, 1997). Holding therapists to such standards, which they neither believe in nor practice, is one of the biggest impediments in the field of psychotherapy (Lazarus, 1994a, 1994b; Zur, 2000a).

This chapter attempts to shed a new light on the rarely discussed issue of deliberate and strategic crossing of the office boundaries. It argues that leaving the office may not only be ethical and effective but may actually be clinically mandated in certain situations. This chapter describes how leaving the office can be consistent with behavioral, systems, humanistic, cognitive-behavioral, multimodal, and other non-analytic orientations. The chapter discusses three types of out-of-office experiences. The first type is where the out-of-office experience is part of a thought-out, carefully constructed, research-based, treatment plan. The second is where the out-of-office experience is geared to enhance therapeutic effectiveness. The third type is comprised of encounters that naturally occur as part of normal living in one's community. While the first two types do not constitute dual relationships, the third one does.

OUT-OF-OFFICE EXPERIENCES AS PART OF A TREATMENT PLAN

By the time he sought my services, John was on the brink of bankruptcy; his business was suffering gravely due to his debilitating fear of flying. I outlined behavioral, biological, and psychodynamic treatment options for him. His sense of urgency induced him to start with systematic desensitization. Following the standard behavioral protocol, I introduced him to gradual, progressive exposures to anxiety-eliciting images culminating with an in vivo experience of flying. To carry out this last step, he booked us on a round-trip flight from San Francisco to Los Angeles with an hour layover in LA. He was able to fly thereafter and salvaged his business.

Jean was anorexic and bulimic. She had undergone both cognitive and psychodynamic therapy without success. Wanting to try a different approach, we developed a family-systems and behavior-based treatment plan that included individual lunches and family dinners in which I participated. We discussed privacy concerns and ways to deal with the possibility of friends or colleagues approaching us during our restaurant meetings. Jean attributed the success of our therapy to the multiple approaches and the flexibility of the in- and out-of-office experiences.

I saw Mary and her husband over the course of a year for marital therapy. During therapy, Mary revealed a long history of abusive relationships with men, which included sexual molestation at a young age and, more recently, sex with a therapist. As we had achieved our original treatment goal of strengthening the marital unit, Mary requested to shift to individual therapy, aimed at dealing with the abuse issues. She set some clear conditions for her individual work with me. My suggestions for her to continue therapy with a female therapist were rejected. For obvious reasons, she would not meet with me, initially, alone in my office; therefore, we agreed to meet at a coffeehouse where she would feel safe due to its public nature. As with Jean, we discussed the potential ramifications of meeting in a public place. As with Jean, significant progress was achieved within a few months and we were able to shift therapy to the office.

Max was a young mechanic with unusual schizotypal features characterized by connecting with machines rather than human beings. He came to see me at the insistence of his mother who was concerned with his increased isolation and suicidality. He clearly did not like my office. Five minutes into the first session, on his way to the door, he offered to show me his newly restored car. I had to choose between stopping treatment before it had even started and accepting his offer. For the next couple of years, he would enter my waiting room punctually and from there we would depart to various destinations. As he welded and tinkered, I learned about his relationships with his parents, and between carburetors and distributor caps I found insights into his distrust of people and love of machines. As our "under the hood" therapy progressed, he gradually came to trust me, and a few others. He even developed his first (arm's-length) relationship with a woman. Since that first day, he has never entered my office.

Jerry has suffered from schizophrenia since childhood. Over the many years that we have been working together, at his request, we have spent many of our sessions walking and talking and marveling at the natural beauty of a nearby trail. In my office, he is often withdrawn, anxious, and distracted, while on the trail he is much more open and relaxed.

Twenty years after Jill's daughter died in a car crash, I accompanied her, at her request, on her very first visit to her daughter's grave. The psychiatrist whom Jill had seen immediately after the crash gave her Valium, to which she became addicted. Her second therapist dismissed her request to be accompanied to the grave as "resistance" and "acting out of the transference." Clearly neither was helpful in her hour of need and both proved to be harmful as they interfered with her grieving process.

Spending several years with John in psychoanalysis, exclusively *in* the office, immersed in transference interpretation or in an existential exploration of the meaning of his fear of flying would not have helped John avoid bankruptcy. Since Jean's eating disorder had not been helped by a couple of legitimate approaches; it was time to try something else. Refusing Mary's coffeehouse arrangement might have been good risk management practice, but would also have constituted abandonment—an ethical violation. Max would not meet anywhere but "under the hood." There was no choice in the matter if I wanted to help him. Jerry's requests for "walking and talking" sessions proved to be the most effective approach. Jill needed support and guidance in her grief, not drugs to numb her pain or analytic scolding. Other situations that would require leaving the office and making a home visit are working with those who are homebound, such as the elderly or those who are sick and bedridden.

The intent of the prior examples is not to advocate for therapists leaving the office indiscriminately or habitually. The intent is to present instances in which leaving the office was part of a clearly articulated treatment plan that constituted the most effective intervention for the specific situation. Such interventions are consistent with behavioral, humanistic, and cognitive-behavioral orientations (Lazarus, 1994a; Williams, 1997). They neither constitute dual relationships nor violate the APA's, or any other professional association's, ethics code. I could have followed numerous writers' advice to practice defensively by staying in the office no matter what. However, by following that advice I would have been providing substandard care and, in fact, I would have been committing ethical violations of the mandate to " . . . improve the condition of both the individual and society" (APA, 1992, p. 1597) and the mandate of "avoiding harm" (APA, 1992, p. 1601).

WHEN OUT-OF-OFFICE EXPERIENCE ENHANCES THERAPEUTIC EFFECTIVENESS

After 3 months of premarital, system-based therapy, a couple invited me to their wedding. I accepted the invitation and was surprised and honored when they publicly acknowledged my role in cementing their nuptial commitment.

An adolescent girl sought therapy to help her with her fear of public speaking, which prevented her from participating in her school play. Her performance on opening night, to which she invited me, was magnificent.

A sculptor came to see me for a severe artist's block. After 3 years of in-office, intensive, psychodynamically oriented therapy, he invited me to his first one-man show at a local gallery. It was an impressive exhibit.

After a couple of months of dealing with issues of work, creativity, and drug addiction, a landscape architect suggested that we spend a session viewing the actual gardens he had designed. The tour increased my understanding of him and my capacity to help him.

Several couples and individuals, over the years, have invited me to their housewarming parties, weddings, anniversaries, and funerals of loved ones. When appropriate, I have accepted these invitations.

It is important to note that I do not always accede to clients' requests to leave the office. In fact, there are just as many reasons not to leave the office including intentional manipulation and avoidance by the client. I declined to do so, for instance, in the cases of a borderline woman, a man in the midst of a paranoid breakdown, a relapsing drug user, and a woman who was overwhelmingly attracted to me.

All the interventions where I left the office were preceded by thorough consideration, were consistent with behavioral, humanistic, and existential treatment plans (Williams, 1997), and were geared to enhancing client welfare. All resulted in an increase of therapeutic alliance, knowledge of the clients, and, most important, enhanced effectiveness of treatment. Similarly, Robin Williams playing the therapist in the movie, *Good Will Hunting*, decided to effectively break the ice by taking the highly resistive and distrustful young client, played by Matt Damon, to the riverbank for a walk. None of these interventions constituted dual relationships or ethical violations. The "slippery slope" did not turn out to be slippery at all as neither exploitation nor harm nor sexual relationships resulted. Like the first type of out-of-office experience, none of these interventions comply with analytic or rigid risk management standards. After all, clients do not pay for defensive therapy, but for effective therapy.

OUT-OF-OFFICE EXPERIENCES AS PART OF HEALTHY DUAL RELATIONSHIPS IN THE COMMUNITY

Susan and I have children the same age. We have chaperoned field trips and sat on committees together at school. At the outset of therapy, we discussed the complexities and potential difficulties of our multiple relationships. She made it clear that she chose me *because* she knew and trusted me and appreciated my parenting methods and the importance I attach to marriage, family, and community. She thought that my knowledge of her would speed up therapy. The daily "Good morning" greetings at school neither interfered with therapy, which progressed well, nor with psychodynamic and transference work.

Sue is a retail clerk at one of the local stores that my wife and I frequent. Unbeknownst to me, she chose to tell my wife, as she checked us out of the store, how I "saved her marriage and helped her children." (My wife is used to it.)

David and Esther were a Jewish couple who had just moved to town. They sought my services due to marital and spiritual concerns. I invited them to my annual Chanukah party where they established several long-lasting connections and reported that the party was an important milestone on their spiritual and communal path.

The American Psychological Association's Ethics Code states clearly that "In many communities and situations, it may not be feasible for psychologists to avoid social or other nonprofessional contacts with persons such as patients, clients, . . . " (APA, 1992, 1601). Several authors have acknowledged that therapists who practice in rural, military, and small communities, or in subcultures of gays, the deaf, or other minorities, often have ongoing, unavoidable, yet not unethical, social, and other exchanges with their clients outside the office (Barnett, 1996; Keith-Spiegel & Koocher, 1985).

Unlike the first two types of out-of-office experiences, these community connections with clients constitute dual relationships. They are part of communal life where people are connected and interdependent in a healthy way and are neither isolated nor insulated from each other. Not only were these relationships nonsexual, nonexploitive, and nonharming, they enhanced therapeutic alliance, trust, and effectiveness. Still, therapists should be thoughtful when taking on clients within their community. Some situations and people are not suited to this kind of work. Such were the cases of a hostile man whose son did not get along with my child, a jealous colleague, and a close friend of an ex-lover. A couple of times I had to terminate treatment because the complexity of dual relationships unexpectedly interfered with the clinical work. These terminations provided valuable learning experiences to clients about the importance of reevaluating plans and rethinking boundaries.

While the analytic approach will eschew socializing with clients, the humanistic, cognitive, or behavioral approaches may not (Williams, 1997). Marquis (cited in Williams, 1997) writes: "The resulting relationship is one in which I have felt quite comfortable, having good friends as clients and good clients as friends" (pp. 48–49). Lazarus (1994a) states, "I have partied and socialized with some clients, played tennis with others, taken long walks with some . . . " (p. 257). Jourard states "I do not hesitate to play a game of handball with a seeker or visit him in his home—if this unfolds in the dialogue" (cited in Williams, 1997, p. 242).

RETHINKING "SLIPPERY SLOPE" AND BOUNDARIES IN THERAPY

Contrary to popular dogmatic expectation, I did not slide uncontrollably down the "slippery slope" and did not end up sleeping with John, Jean, Max, Susan, Sue, Jerry, or Jill. In fact, the out-of-office experiences reduced the probability of exploitation because they were carried out in public. The tyrannical creed propounding the "only in the office" policy and the isolation it imposes on the therapeutic encounter are main contributors to exploitation and sexual misconduct (Zur, 2000a).

Leaving the office is not the norm in my practice. It occurs only when there is clinical evidence that it would enhance effectiveness of treatment or it is unavoidable in the community. Like most professions, therapy involves contacts and reputation. Almost all of my clients chose therapy with me because they either know me personally or heard about me from a trusted friend. It may surprise the reader that one of the several therapeutic modalities I use with my clients is psychodynamic therapy and that none of the out-of-office experiences described in this article have interfered with transference and psychodynamic work when they were applied. Meeting outside the office, like knowing me personally, makes the transference more reality-based and just provides more "grist" for the (transference) mill.

Lazarus (1994a) has stated succinctly that "One of the worst professional or ethical violations is that of permitting current risk-management principles to take precedence over humane interventions" (p. 260). Indeed, in some situations, not leaving the office, due to defensive practice considerations, can constitute substandard care and an ethical violation.

One of the goals of this chapter is to free therapists to intervene according to clients' specific situations and presenting problems and not according to fear of attorneys, licensing boards, or analytic dogma. There are situations in which interacting with clients outside the office is the best intervention and there are situations where it is clearly counterindicative. As Lazarus (1994b) summarizes it simply: "It depends."

REFERENCES

American Psychological Association (APA). (1992). Ethical principles of psychologists and code of conduct. *American Psychologist, 47,* 1597–1611.

Barnett, J. E. (1996). Boundary issue and dual relationships: Where to draw the line? *The Independent Practitioner, 16* (3), 138–140.

Bennett, B. E., Bricklin, P. M., & VandeCreek, L. (1994). Response to Lazarus's "How certain boundaries and ethics diminish therapeutic effectiveness." *Ethics & Behavior, 4* (3), 261–266.

Borys, D. S., & Pope, K. S. (1989). Dual relationships between therapist and client: A national study of psychologists, psychiatrists, and social workers. *Professional Psychology: Research and Practice, 20,* 283–293.

Ebert, B. W. (1997). Dual-relationship prohibitions: A concept whose time never should have come. *Applied & Preventive Psychology, 6,* 137–156.

Faulkner, K. K., & Faulkner, T. A. (1977). Managing multiple relationships in rural communities: Neutrality and boundary violations. *Clinical Psychology: Science and Practice, 4,* 225–234.

Gabbard, G. O. (1994). Teetering on the precipice: A commentary on Lazarus's "How certain boundaries and ethics diminish therapeutic effectiveness." *Ethics & Behavior, 4* (3), 283–286.

Gottlieb, M. C. (1993). Avoiding exploitative multiple relationships: A decision-making model. *Psychotherapy, 30,* 41–48.

Gutheil, T. G., & Gabbard, G. O. (1993). The concept of boundaries in clinical practice: Theoretical and risk management dimension. *American Journal of Psychiatry, 150,* 188–196.

Jourard, S. M. (1971). *The transparent self.* New York: D. Van Nostrand.

Keith-Spiegel, P., & Koocher, G. P. (1985). *Ethics in psychology*. New York: Random House.

Lazarus, A. A. (1994a). How certain boundaries and ethics diminish therapeutic effectiveness. *Ethics & Behavior, 4,* 255–261.

Lazarus, A. A. (1994b). The illusion of the therapist's power and the patient's fragility: My rejoinder. *Ethics & Behavior, 4,* 299–306.

Lazarus, A. (1998). How do you like these boundaries? *The Clinical Psychologist, 51,* 22–25.

Marquis, J. M. (1972). An expedient model for behavioral therapy. In A. A. Lazarus (Ed.), *Clinical behavior therapy*, pp. 41–72.

Pope, K. S. (1990). Therapist-patient sexual contact: Clinical, legal, and ethical implications. In E. A. Margenau (Ed.), *The encyclopedia handbook of private practice* (pp. 687–696). New York: Gardner Press, Inc.

Pope, K. S., & Vasquez, M. J. T. (1991). *Ethics in psychotherapy and counseling*. San Francisco: Jossey-Bass.

Simon, R. I. (1991). Psychological injury caused by boundary violation precursors to therapist-patient sex. *Psychiatric Annals, 21,* 614–619.

Strasburger, L. H., Jorgenson, L., & Sutherland, P. (1992). The prevention of psychotherapist sexual misconduct: Avoiding the slippery slope. *American Journal of Psychotherapy, 84* (4), 544–555.

Tomm, K. (1993). The ethics of dual relationships. *The California Therapists,* Jan./Feb., 7–19.

Williams, M. H. (1997). Boundary violations: Do some contended standards of care fail to encompass commonplace procedures of humanistic, behavioral and eclectic psychotherapies? *Psychotherapy, 34,* 239–249.

Zur, O. (2000a). In celebration of dual relationships: How prohibition of nonsexual dual relationships increases the chance of exploitation and harm. *The Independent Practitioner, 20,* 97–100.

Zur, O. (2000b). Going too far in the right direction: Reflection on the mythic ban of dual relationships. *California Therapist, 23* (4), 14, 16.

CHAPTER 8

The Multiple Roles and Relationships of Ethical Psychotherapy

Revisiting the Ideal, the Real, and the Unethical

Simon Shimshon Rubin, PhD

This chapter suggests that current thinking about dual and multiple relationships may benefit from another look. The term "multiple role relationships" is proposed to allow for a reexamination of what is and what should be the proper management of professional relationships that generally are multidimensional. As will be shown, multiple roles and multiple allegiances characterize the interpersonal realities of practice for the mental health professional. As such, their management, not their prohibition, is the issue. The chapter is divided into three sections. It opens with current views of multiple relationships; considers representative sources and bases for prohibitions against dual or multiple relationships; and closes by arguing for a view that stresses the context of human relationships as one of involvement rather than functional interaction alone.

ROLES AND RELATIONSHIPS OF ETHICAL PSYCHOTHERAPY

The focus of this chapter is on redefining and possibly redirecting our thinking about dual and multiple relationships from a strict dichotomous outlook to a more graded response. By utilizing an alternative terminology of "multiple role relationships," the chapter sets forth a model that guides the conceptualization and management of the complicated role relationships of the professional. Multiple role relationships are seen as the reality and foundation of practice (Rubin, 2000). They are understood to include the professional roles that clinicians adopt vis-à-vis their clients, but are not limited to these. Multiple role relationships set out to encompass the gamut of involvements that the professional has with regard to clients. The term also includes the role relationships that the professional has with himself or herself, as well as his or her family as they may relate to treatment, the relationships with coworkers, third-party payers, the client's family, and so forth.

In his 1803 text on medical ethics, Percival addressed motives of personal gain and the need to balance them rather than to prohibit them (Percival, 1803). As such, this pioneering ethicist does much to allow for natural human experience to be included in the ethical discussion. Perhaps the ultimate dual relationship is to treat a client and be involved in a sexual liaison. This is clearly prohibited (American Psychological Association [APA], 1992; Pope, Sonne, & Holroyd, 1993). Yet, the individual health care provider is involved in a multiplicity of relationships with clients; he or she has a financial stake in the client being in treatment, an emotional stake in succeeding in work with the other, a wish to make a favorable impression on coworkers and bosses. In all those cases, the client's needs are not the only ones.

Unfortunately, in much of what has been written about dual or multiple relationships, anything other than the strict professional relationship with a client generally receives negative attention. This unduly constricts the interaction. Such a narrow approach may lead to greater misunderstanding and ultimately cause greater harm to professionals and clients alike (Sonne, 1994). Because this approach discourages professional consideration and monitoring of the complexity of the professional relationships of health care providers, the reality and complexity of these transactions are discarded in favor of simplistic guidelines (Lazarus, 1994; Williams, 1998).

CURRENT VIEWS OF MULTIPLE RELATIONSHIPS

The most recent revision of the APA Code of Ethics (1992) has taken a somewhat ambiguous position on multiple relationships. Reading and rereading the code and attendant literature, the impression one forms suggests that multiple relationships are generally unethical and should be avoided, but that it is acceptable to manage them if clients are protected (Catalano, 1997). The muddled message may leave room for creative management of the psychologist's professional practice, but it fails to assist psychologists to manage the ethical demands of the profession.

> In many communities and situations, it may not be feasible or reasonable for psychologists to avoid social or other nonprofessional contacts with persons such as patients, clients, students, supervisees, or research participants. Psychologists must always be sensitive to the potential harmful effects of nonprofessional contacts on those persons with whom they deal. A psychologist refrains from entering into or promising another personal, scientific, professional, financial, or other relationship if it appears likely that such a relationship might impair the psychologist's objectivity or otherwise interfere with the psychologist's ability to perform his or her functions. It remains important to avoid harming or exploiting the other party. (American Psychological Association, 1992, p. 1601, Principle 1.17 of the Ethics Code)

Should this principle be taken to mean that it is best never (or almost never) to have "nonprofessional" contacts? This judgment is often simply unreasonable or impossible given the circumstances of practice in real life. In rural communities, for example, clients and therapists frequently interact in various settings, but it is one thing to say "they have no choice" and quite another to say that "such a practice is eminently ethical."

It is fair to say that current standards of practice treat some varieties of multiple role relationships as so fraught with risk and complications as to demand complete abstinence from particular combinations of specific relationships (Koocher & Keith-Spiegel, 1998; Rubin & Dror, 1996). All seem to concur that the concomitant relationships of spouse or lover and psychotherapist are strongly contraindicated. Yet in nonsexual contexts, it should be equally apparent that the management of multiple-role relationships is actually the state of the art and the norm of what psychologists do most of the time. As I shall demonstrate shortly, while this point is particularly significant for psychotherapy and necessitates special understanding to be managed appropriately, the basic premise raised herein is generally applicable to most of the role relationships that psychologists undertake. It may be that the use of the term "multiple roles" may well be a more accurate description of the work of psychologists than multiple relationships.

It is not hard to see that the multiple responsibilities of professors whose duties as instructors ethically require them to teach competently and professionally may run counter to the administration's need to dramatically expand class size in order to keep a university program or department solvent. Another example is that of the health care provider whose duties as therapist in any family system is to multiple persons and multiple relationships. These competing responsibilities are not necessarily satisfied simultaneously and may involve considerable conflict when the member's goals are in opposition. The fact that all of the relationships and roles in such a therapy may be considered necessary for the clients' benefit should not obscure their multiple nature and potential for conflict.

The therapist has to balance client requests and needs, professional conceptualization and knowledge of the appropriate range of treatments, as well as constraints of external third-party payers who may be both a current referral source and also a future source of income. The multiple role of the professional here involves obligations to client welfare, professional standards, scientific bases, self-interest, and organizational-systemic demands that are all impacting on professionals as they attempt to remain true to the ethical aspirations of the profession (Beutler, Bongar, & Shurkin, 1998). These conflicts and conflicting demands will not go away no matter how severely dual "relationships" are criticized, for they are the reality rather than the theory of practice (Pelligrino & Thomasma, 1993).

The paradigmatic multiple "relationship" that has attracted the most attention is the complication of sexual relationships and a second primary relationship such as educator, therapist, supervisor, or administrator. While it is naïve to minimize the uniquely complicating features of sexual intimacy upon fiduciary relationships that require the client's interests to be protected, one cannot deny that the interplay of two people in an ongoing relationship links them together along multiple dimensions of involvement. As social beings primed to be involved with each other, it is the awareness of the involvement and its management that protect therapists and clients from error. The elements of the psychologist's professional stature, power, or ability to psychologically threaten the other are often complications in both the therapeutic as well as academic role relationships (Blevins-Knabe, 1992; Slimp, O'Connor, & Burian, 1994). Attention to boundary issues, for example not to enter into additional business dealings with clients (beyond the therapy business), may not be appropriate in educational settings. The external behavioral prohibitions against crossing certain boundaries, however, cannot and should not close off sensitivity to the involvement that is at the heart of human interaction. The attention that Pope (1994) and others have accorded to managing the experience of sexuality in the therapeutic relationship has spotlighted the need to confront and contain the pressures and confusions that sexuality engenders in therapy. I would argue that the multiple roles and relationships that are endemic to the psychotherapy relationship should be treated in analogous fashion. We should realize that therapy needs to be analyzed as role relationships that fundamentally involve multiple duties and responsibilities to multiple sources that can be confusing and anxiety provoking, as well as becoming harbingers of trouble if they are not explicated and recognized. In previous writings, I have addressed these issues both with regard to supervision in psychotherapy (Rubin, 1997) as well as in the context of direct provision of psychotherapy treatment (Rubin, 2000).

SOURCES OF THE PROHIBITIONS AGAINST DUAL AND MULTIPLE RELATIONSHIPS AND ROLES

The negative image of "dual relationships" stems from several sources. A paradigmatic model of the dual relationship for psychologists stems from the medico-professional origins of patient care. The view that breach of confidentiality as well as client-therapist sexual contact are unethical and detrimental have roots in the Hippocratic oath (Beauchamp & Walters, 1994). The roots of the prohibition stem from concern with power inequity and with the requisite conditions for patients to agree to submit to physician care (that their secrets be safe and that their sexuality be respected). There is no prohibition against friendship, however, or against entering into business dealings with patients. What is to be maintained is that the standard of care of client not be impaired. The understanding of what exactly is wrong with dual relationships and multiple roles has moved in a number of directions, and often many are invoked simultaneously (Baer & Murdock, 1995). Most are rooted in the sexual area. I will consider only three and attempt to show that either extreme positions, condoning all or condemning all such multiple relationships, are untenable.

Undoubtedly, the main source for the condemnation of multiple relationships focuses on sex with clients. One route has compared sexual contact with clients to a kind of quasi-incestuous behavior or normative violation. This linkage is one that touches upon deeply embedded notions of wrongful human behavior (Gabbard, 1994). Another route has focused on therapist-client sexual contact from a utilitarian risk benefit point of view. This has powerfully and convincingly demonstrated the consistently increased risk of harm inherent in such a dual therapeutic relationship (Pope et al., 1993). Still others have emphasized the dual relationship question with sexual (and other relationships) as a situation of unequal power lending itself to coercive outcomes (Koocher & Keith-Spiegel, 1998).

It is neither ethical nor logical to make a case for the total disregard of the risks and dangers of multiple relationships and roles. Yet one would not have to look far to find paradigms of dual relationships and multiple roles that enhance professional and personal relationships. If the family model that is set forth interdicting client therapist sexual contact has roots in boundary violations of incest, risk, and power inequity, perhaps we would do well to return to the family to look again at the multiple roles and relationships that are managed therein. After all, it is the management of these multiple roles and relationships that form the developmental pathways of psychologists long before they choose to work in the profession.

The schematic model of the functional nuclear family in its traditional role would see it as a unit that contains individuals linked together with both complimentary and conflicting goals. The nuclear family is a unit where full expression of sexuality is managed and expressed as for example in the couples unit. And yet, the couple's dyadic sexuality as well as other variations of sexual attraction are contained and not acted upon other members of the family. Correspondingly, the family unit beginning with the couples unit unites two people of different life experiences and genders, who must balance self-interest with the interest of the other and of the larger divisions (couple unit, family, extended family). Risks to the members are real, and power imbalance may be endemic; yet most of us continue to remain favorably disposed to the institution linking people together while working to improve it. The point I wish to make is not that the family unit is prototypical of all aspects of the contractual relationship of psychotherapy. However, I do wish to stress that the family is central to the formation of a template that recognizes that relationships are managed in complex, complicated, and yet, ethical ways.

The second source I wish to consider is the risk benefit model. When the free and open exchange of faculty and students in their nonsexual relationships are avoided as they go beyond strict meetings of an academic nature, the results are not uniformly positive. In conversations with a number of doctoral level psychology students enrolled in courses on professional ethics, they shared their perception that professors in the United States had minimal social and desirable out-of-class interactions with them because they feared that as faculty they might run afoul of the APA (1992) code of ethics (Graduate Students in Psychology, personal communication, 1994). If this perception is correct, and in some cases it probably is, then assessing the risk of multiple-role relationships with students would suggest that the risk is bimodal. Too intense a relationship outside of the educational mandate can lead to boundary blurring and an undesirable infringement on the autonomy of students, as well as confusion to both parties because of the often unequal status of the relationship. Too distant a relationship can lead to feelings of anomie, missed opportunities for the informal transfer of learning, and failure to facilitate a perspective across the divide of status, expertise, and experience.

Whether there is a parallel situation for the psychotherapy situation, and perhaps the small-town situation is an example of this, then too great an avoidance of multiple-role relationships may well work to build a sense of anomie and estrangement, rather than protection.

A third source for the perception of multiple relationships (again beginning with the sexualized relationship) emerges from attention to the unequal power of therapist and client in the therapeutic relationship (Gottlieb, 1993). Although sometimes couched in the language of individual rights and freedom to choose, for sexual contact between clinician and client the APA code and many state laws choose to emphasize the need to protect the client (Pope & Vasquez, 1998). The choice of client protection is couched in the language of ethical discourse as emphasizing the beneficent rather than the autonomous aspects of client welfare (Bersoff & Koeppel, 1993; Beauchamp & Childress, 1994). The perception is that in a situation of power differential, and particularly when one is in an institutional system, the client is at a serious disadvantage. In such situations, the "freedom to choose" may well be the "inability to refuse." The awareness of unequal power, status, and so forth in the psychotherapeutic relationship is an important part of the proper respect for the client (Rubin, 2000). The experienced therapist will not lightly disregard her knowledge base in considering alternatives with the patient, for this knowledge base has value. The need to recognize the potential disadvantage of the client who may not be able to either recognize or resist the "power" elements of the relationship is a part of the professional responsibility. The psychotherapy practitioner would do well to contemplate how those disparities of status, knowledge, and desirability limit the client. This weighing of professional responsibility to know better (with its parentalist connotation), as opposed to respecting clients' autonomy, is not easily achieved. In conversations with students sensitive to issues of power differentials, the difference between dominating the patient by virtue of the professional role and assisting the patient through the expertise of the professional role did not resolve easily.

In Emanuel and Emanuel's (1992) depiction of four types of physician-patient relationship modes, the role that may be most sensitive to power disparity and avoidance of parentalism casts the clinician's responsibility as one of presenting information with a studious avoidance of personal preference. Patients sometimes experience this stance as one that leaves them very much alone. An alternative viewpoint suggests a more equal relationship in which the physician takes patient preferences and background into account while interacting and exploring options with the patient. This model is attractive, but may not fully take into account the influence of physician influence and other experts in the health care system. Juggling the hats of service provider, bookkeeper, scientist, and consultant to the client retains the blending and combination of multiple roles addressed above. I believe that we shoulder our ethical responsibilities better by realizing and acknowledging that such multiple-role relationships are basically normative and extend far beyond the sexual relationships that have absorbed so much attention (Pearson & Piazza, 1997).

Looking to what it is that makes for the problems in the multiple-role relationship, we have identified issues of crossing boundaries along an incest paradigm, a utilitarian cost-benefit analysis model, and one concerned with power differentials. The summary of this section to this point, however, suggests that either extreme—too lax or too strict a view of multiple-role relationships—undermines and compromises the complexity of the therapeutic enterprise. Smith and Fitzpatrick's (1995) article examining boundary crossings and differentiating them from boundary violations is another step in this direction. It is not wrong to condemn the harmful and deleterious effects of client-therapist sexual activity, because that is grounded in empirical fact as well as in professional morality. It is, however, misleading and counterintuitive to sweepingly delegitimize the entire range of nonsexual multiple roles and relationships. Although the current code of ethics has taken some steps in the direction of specifying what types of multiple-role relationships may be acceptable, the fundamental multiplicity of human relationships and roles require further attention so as to realize the beneficial goals of a more relaxed view of certain boundary extensions. When the analysis of ethics and ethical behavior is considered from perspectives permitting alternative views of desirable behaviors serving constructive goals, then dialogue underlying professional training and practice is enriched (Cohen & Cohen, 1999). On issues of multiple roles and relationships, considering professional relationships that move beyond the most narrow contractual professional-client relationship opens many creative avenues. We cannot deny, however, that it may also necessitate a more careful consideration of the risks posed by a more broad-based analysis of acceptable behaviors on the other. In my critique of the professional behavior of the fictional Trotter in Yalom's (1997) *Lying on the Couch*, I address these issues in greater detail (Rubin, 2001).

In the next section, we shall consider professional interactions from the perspective of the relationship model. The balance of sensitivity to self and to others, considered within the matrix of peoples' concerns for one another, is seen as fundamental to the therapy enterprise. As a result, human caring and involvement is the underlying stratum that must be understood before moving to limit and sharpen boundaries in professional relationships. This perspective shares elements with feminist and relations of care discussions in the literature (Gilligan, 1982; Sherwin, 1992).

THE CONTEXT OF RELATIONSHIPS

In his opening to the psychiatric interview, Sullivan (1970) defines the clinical interview as a meeting between an "expert" and a patient that occurs for the client to obtain benefit. Whatever one's understanding of Sullivan's conception of the professional role of the psychiatrist, there is no denying that he consistently emphasized the human qualities of the professional insofar as they related to the basic vulnerabilities of all people. He repeatedly focused on how sensitivity to the other ("patient") was a source of threat to the self of the professional, and thus was a potential source for the mismanagement of the relationship. Sullivan's repeated points about the multiple sensitivities in the meeting of expert and patient are delivered in the framework of a viewpoint that sees multiple sensitivities and multiple sources for error arising from the meeting of two people. His exhortations to doctors and other professionals to not use the patient for self-aggrandizement and to place the needs of the patient as paramount are useful guidelines. Yet even a cursory reading of the participant-observer relationship will point the reader to an understanding that one is always interacting in a human context, and the notion of a disinterested scientific instrument is far from the reality of the situation (Havens, 1986). One is always operating in an interpersonal field in relationship to the other while responding from within the self. The balance of self-interest with client interest and professional goals are not impossible, but the avoidance of multiple relationship vis-à-vis the self, client, and a variety of societal and professional objectives is unattainable (Strupp & Hadley, 1977; Thompson, 1990).

To illustrate with an example: Dr. Y is referred a private client by her supervisor Dr. X due to her expertise with anxiety disorders. Although Dr. Y is aware that her skills are not commensurate with what this client needs, she is reluctant to reject a referral from her supervisor. Duty to self and duty to client need not remain opposed here (she might obtain additional supervision on this case, for example). The fact remains, however, that there is often a multiple matrix of competing loyalties that must be satisfied. It is the multiple roles that exist within this "single" relationship that have potential for trouble if they are delegitimized and ignored.

It is not only the interpersonal theorists such as Sullivan, of course, that speak to the multiplicity of dimensions of relationship in working with clients. Psychodynamic theorists have for years made the management of the patient relationship to the therapist, and the therapist relationship to the patient, the foci of study (e.g., Gill, 1987; Racker, 1974; Sandler, 1973). It is fair to say that the therapist is no longer seen as one who should avoid or analyze away countertransference reactions (Tansey & Burke, 1989). This branch of psychotherapy has moved to include and incorporate the insights available from the therapist's relationship to the client with particular attention to the multiplicity of stimuli that people have for one another.

> As analysis developed, transference, at first considered a major obstacle in treatment, came to be seen as the fulcrum on which the psychoanalytic situation rests. Similarly, countertransference, first seen as a neurotic disturbance in the psychoanalyst, preventing him from getting a clear and objective view of the patient, is now increasingly recognized as a most important source of information about the patient as well as a major element of the interaction between patient and analyst. (Segal, 1993, p. 13)

Paradoxically, it is the countertransferential reactions of therapists today that are seen as most dangerous when they are ignored rather than accepted and managed. Or in simple terms, believing or acting as if only professional and neutral responses are experienced by the therapist is untrue and increases the risk of therapeutic error.

The ethical analyses associated with feminine, feminist, and communitarian writings has asserted the value and importance of attention to issues of relationship and care (Sherwin, 1992). Gilligan's work emphasizing girls' and women's greater propensity to consider details of the relationship between people and the responsibility between them has been understood as an illustration of the way in which issues of relationship may take their place alongside (or supersede) analyses emphasizing abstract principles and reasoning (Benhabib, 1987). Although Sherwin's critique of ethics is assigned to women, one could argue that its scope is appropriate to caregivers irrespective of gender. It certainly serves as a powerful contrast to the abstract notion of "relationships" set forth in the ethical principles of the APA (1992) that focus on the topic.

> Ethical models based on the image of ahistorical, self sufficient, atom-like individuals are simply not credible to most women. Because women are usually charged with the responsibility of caring . . . and emotionally nurturing men both at work and at home, most women experience the world as a complex web of interdependent relationships, where responsible caring for others is implicit in their moral lives. The abstract reasoning of morality that centers on the rights of independent agents is inadequate for the moral reality in which they live. (Sherwin, 1992, p. 47)

Bowlby (1979) has commented on the centrality of relationship to the healing process. Perhaps a contemporary viewpoint blending love of work and love of client emerges from Loewald. I conclude the section on involvement and caring within therapy with the following:

> Scientific detachment in its genuine form, far from excluding love, is based on it. In our work, it can be truly said that in our best moments of dispassionate and objective analyzing, we love our object, the patient, more than at any other time and are compassionate with his whole being. In our field scientific spirit and care for the object [person] flow from the same source. . . . To discover truth about the patient is always discovering it with him and for him as well as for ourselves and about ourselves. And it is discovering truth between each other, as the truth of human beings is revealed in their interrelatedness. (Loewald, 1980, pp. 297–298)

CONCLUSION

In contrast to "multiple relationships" with the questionable connotations of the term, most of us would agree that a readiness for as well as the occurrence of personal involvement between two people, irrespective of professional status, are prototypical human and social responses. For psychotherapists, this means that we understand, expect, and encourage such involvement as a part of the human encounter. Included here is both the recognition and respect for boundaries. The fiduciary aspects of the relationship or the therapist's responsibility to the client, supervisee, or student remain. The recognition that the impact of psychological involvement upon one or both parties can contribute to difficulties in the relationship and cause harm to the vulnerable is a major contribution of the attention to multiple relationships (Anderson & Kitchener, 1998; Koocher & Keith-Spiegel, 1998; Pope & Vasquez, 1998; Rubin & Amir, 2000). Nonetheless, discussion of these features overshadows the numerous levels of meaning and involvements in the therapy relationship. In addition to reiterating the incompatibility of certain role responsibilities in therapy, we should concentrate on the management of human involvement and interdependence in the therapeutic spheres (Berman, 1997; Celenza, 1995; Renik, 1997, 1999; Rubin, 2001).

The ubiquitous and multiple involvement, meanings, and loyalties inherent in the professional relationships of psychologists and psychotherapists have more often been intuitively recognized than discussed in the literature (Thompson, 1990). Recognizing these involvements as ubiquitous and as possessing desirable elements of involvement and care, we might do better to accept the multiplicity of roles, involvements, and motivations as normative. Consideration should be given to the features and conditions likely to upset the management of the multiple involvements that may be operant in psychotherapy (Rubin, 2000). The harmful aspects of multiple involvements and relationships do not stem from their mere existence. More than anything else, the dangers to multiple features of our involvement with one another are also rooted in the failure to perceive and properly balance the complex motivations, feelings, and behaviors that characterize human interactions—professional or otherwise.

Professionals as people are involved with their superiors, peers, and clients in many ways. These involvements have the potential to help us at times and to hinder us at other times, but they are always present. It is the professional psychologist's responsibility to understand these involvements, to manage them properly, and to ensure that fidelity to the client is maintained. While fidelity to the self cannot be the only principle operant in professional work, fidelity to the client alone will also skew the basis of the professional undertaking. We are persons who contended with multiple loyalties and role relationships long before we became professionals. It would seem logical to base our work on a sensitive understanding of the relationship between the personal and the professional sides of our existence that do justice to human interdependence and vulnerability-involvement by finding the proper balance between the two.

REFERENCES

American Psychological Association. (1992). Ethical principles of psychologists and code of conduct. *American Psychologist, 47,* 1597–1611.

Anderson, S. K., & Kitchener, K. S. (1998). Nonsexual posttherapy relationships: A conceptual framework to assess ethical risks. *Professional Psychology, 29* (1), 91–99.

Baer, B. E., & Murdock, N. L. (1995). Nonerotic dual relationships between therapists and clients: The effects of sex, theoretical orientation, and interpersonal boundaries. *Ethics and Behavior, 5* (2), 131–145.

Beauchamp, T. L., & Childress, J. F. (1994). *Principles of biomedical ethics* (4th ed.). New York: Oxford University Press.

Beauchamp, T. L., & Walters, L. (1994). *Contemporary issues in bioethics* (4th ed.). Belmont, CA: Wadsworth.

Benhabib, S. (1987). The generalized and the concrete other: The Kohlberg-Gilligan controversy and moral theory. In E. F. Kittay & D. T. Meyers (Eds.), *Women and moral theory* (pp. 154–157). Totowa, NJ: Rowman & Littlefield.

Berman, E. (1997). Relational psychoanalysis: A historical background. *American Journal of Psychotherapy, 51* (2), 185–203.

Bersoff, D. N., & Koeppel, P. M. (1993). The relation between ethical codes and moral principles. *Ethics and Behavior, 3* (3–4), 345–357.

Beutler, L. E., Bongar, B., & Shurkin, J. N. (1998). *Am I crazy or is it my shrink?* New York: Oxford University Press.

Blevins-Knabe, B. (1992). The ethics of dual relationships in higher education. *Ethics and Behavior, 2,* 151–163.

Bowlby, J. (1979). *The making and breaking of affectional bonds.* London: Tavistock.

Catalano, S. (1997). The challenge of clinical practice in small or rural communities: Studies in managing dual relationships in and outside of therapy. *Journal of Contemporary Psychotherapy, 27* (1), 23–35.

Celenza, A. (1995). Love and hate in the countertransference. *Psychotherapy: Theory, Research and Practice, 32,* 301–307.

Cohen, E. D., & Cohen, G. S. (1999). *The virtuous therapist: Ethical practice of counseling and psychotherapy*. Belmont, CA: Wadsworth.

Emanuel, E. J., & Emanuel, L. L. (1992). Four models of the physician-patient relationship. *Journal of the American Medical Association, 267*, 2221–2226.

Gabbard, G. O. (1994). Psychotherapists who transgress sexual boundaries with patients. *Bulletin of the Menninger Clinic, 58* (1), 124–135.

Gill, M. M. (1987). *Analysis of transference*. New York: International Universities Press.

Gilligan, C. (1982). *In a different voice: Psychological theory and women's moral development*. Cambridge, MA: Harvard University Press.

Gottlieb, M. C. (1993). Avoiding exploitative dual relationships: A decision-making model. *Psychotherapy: Theory, Research and Practice, 30* (1), 41–48.

Havens, L. L. (1986). *Making contact: Uses of language in psychotherapy*. Cambridge, MA: Harvard University Press.

Koocher, G. P., & Keith-Spiegel, P. (1998). *Ethics in psychology: Professional standards and cases* (2nd ed.). New York: Oxford University Press.

Lazarus, A. A. (1994). How certain boundaries and ethics diminish therapeutic effectiveness. *Ethics and Behavior, 4*, 253–261.

Loewald, H. W. (1980). *Papers on psychoanalysis*. New Haven, CT: Yale University Press.

Pearson, B., & Piazza, N. (1997). Classification of dual relationships in the helping professions. *Counselor Education and Supervision, 37*, 89–99.

Pelligrino, E. M., & Thomasma, D. C. (1993). *The virtues in medical practice*. New York: Oxford University Press.

Percival, T. (1803). *Medical ethics; Or a code of institutes and precepts, adapted to the professional conduct of physicians and surgeons*. Manchester, NY: S. Russell.

Pope, K. S. (1994). *Sexual involvement with therapists: Patient assessment, subsequent therapy, forensics*. Washington, DC: American Psychological Association.

Pope, K. S., Sonne, J., & Holroyd, J. (1993). *Sexual feelings in psychotherapy: Explorations for therapists and therapists in training*. Washington, DC: American Psychological Association.

Pope, K. S., & Vasquez, M. J. T. (1998). *Ethics in psychotherapy and counseling: A practical guide* (2nd ed.). San Francisco: Jossey-Bass.

Racker, H. (1974). *Transference and counter-transference*. London: Hogarth Press and the Institute for Psychoanalysis.

Renik, O. (1997). The perils of neutrality. *Psychoanalytic Quarterly, 65*, 495–517.

Renik, O. (1999). Playing one's cards face up in analysis: An approach to the problem of self-disclosure. *The Psychoanalytic Quarterly, 68*, 521–539.

Rubin, S. (1997). Balancing duty to client and therapist in psychotherapy supervision: Clinical, ethical and training issues. *The Clinical Supervisor, 16* (1), 1–23.

Rubin, S. (2000). Differentiating multiple relationships from multiple dimensions of involvement: Therapeutic space at the interface of client, therapist and society. *Psychotherapy: Theory, Research and Practice, 37* (4), 315–324.

Rubin, S. (2001). Ethical dilemmas, good intentions and the road to hell: A clinical-ethical perspective on Yalom's depiction of Trotter's therapy. *Psychiatry, 64* (2), 146–157.

Rubin, S., & Amir, D. (2000). When expertise and ethics diverge: Lay and professional evaluation of psychotherapists in Israel. *Ethics and Behavior, 10* (4), 375–391.

Rubin, S., & Dror, O. (1996). Professional ethics of psychologists and physicians: Morality, confidentiality and sexuality in Israel. *Ethics and Behavior, 6* (3), 213–238.

Sandler, J. (1973). *The patient and the analyst.* New York: International Universities Press.

Segal, H. (1993). Countertransference. In A. Alexandris & G. Vaslamatzis (Eds.), *Countertransference: Theory, technique, teaching* (pp. 13–20). London: Karnac.

Sherwin, S. (1992). *No longer patient: Feminist ethics and health care.* Philadelphia: Temple University Press.

Slimp, P. A. O'Connor, & Burian, B. K. (1994). Multiple role relationships during internship: Consequences and recommendations. *Professional Psychology: Research and Practice, 25* (1), 39–45.

Smith, D., & Fitzpatrick, M. (1995). Patient-therapist boundary issues: An integrative review of theory and research. *Professional Psychology: Research and Practice, 26* (5), 499–506.

Sonne, H. L. (1994). Multiple relationships: Does the new ethics code answer the right questions? *Professional Psychology: Research and Practice, 25* (4), 336–343.

Strupp, H. H., & Hadley, S. W. (1977). A tripartite model of mental health and therapeutic outcomes: With special reference to negative effects in psychotherapy. *American Psychologist, 32,* 187–196.

Sullivan, H. S. (1970). *The psychiatric interview.* New York: Norton.

Tansey, M. J., & Burke, W. F. (1989). *Understanding countertransference: From projective identification to empathy.* Hillsdale, NJ: The Analytic Press.

Thompson, A. (1990). *Guide to ethical practice in psychotherapy.* New York: Wiley.

Williams, M. H. (1998). Boundary violations: Do some contested standards fail to encompass commonplace procedures of humanistic, behavioral and eclectic psychotherapies? *Psychotherapy, 34,* 238–242.

Yalom, I. D. (1997). *Lying on the couch.* New York: Harper-Collins.

PART 3

Boundaries

Part 3 provides a critical look at the traditional boundaries of psychotherapy. Chapter 9 opens with Dineen's broad-based, incisive discussion of the overall context into which professionalism and boundary issues in psychotherapy exist. Given that dual relationships are but one facet of boundary extensions, it is important to appreciate the complete picture—with all the subtleties and complexities that Dineen lucidly explains. In chapter 10, Lazarus elucidates how his personal background encouraged a familial, informal model of therapeutic interaction and discouraged a formal and traditionalist approach with many clients. Fay discusses boundary issues in chapter 11—from the perspective of a practicing psychiatrist who shed the shackles of his initial restrictive training. He presents many vignettes that illustrate a wide array of what would be considered not only boundary crossings but also violations according to psychoanalytic precepts—often with telling effects. The need for such flexibility is most compelling with patients who have failed to respond to more traditional interventions.

CHAPTER 9

The Psychotherapist and the Quest for Power

How Boundaries Have Become an Obsession

Tana Dineen, PhD, CPsych. (ON), RPsych. (BC)

> Psychology may have seeped into virtually every facet of existence, but that does not mean that it has always been there.... Understanding the recent history of psychological experts is critical to understanding psychology's place in contemporary society. That history is based on an extraordinary quest for power.
>
> —Ellen Herman, *The Romance of American Psychology* (p. 5, 1995)

Long before it dawned on me that I might become a psychologist, I was intrigued by some of the men and women considered to be pioneers of the discipline. It was the seemingly insignificant details about their lives, the provocative thinking, and the unexpected comments that caught my interest. Sigmund Freud seemed less arrogant to me than he is generally portrayed, for I remember that he once responded to an inquiry about one of his theoretical notions: "Oh, that was just something I dreamed up on a rainy Sunday afternoon" (Kardiner, 1977, p. 75). And the following tale, said to have been Carl Jung's favorite story, has stuck with me throughout my career as a psychotherapist:

> The water of life, wishing to make itself known on the face of the earth, bubbled up in an artesian well and flowed without effort or limit. People came to drink of the magic water and were nourished by it, since it was so clean and pure and invigorating. But humankind was not content to leave things in this Edenic state. Gradually they began to fence the well, charge admission, claim ownership of the property around it, make elaborate laws as to who could come to the well, put locks on the gates. Soon the well was property of the powerful and the elite. The water was angry and offended; it stopped flowing and began to bubble up in another place. The people who owned the property around the first well were so engrossed in their power systems and ownership that they did not notice that the water had vanished. They continued selling the nonexistent water, and few people noticed that the true power was gone. But some dissatisfied people searched with great courage and found the new artesian well. Soon that well was under the control of the property owners, and the same fate overtook it. The spring took itself to yet another place—and this has been going on throughout recorded history. (Johnson, 1991, pp. vii–viii)

What first attracted me to psychology was a fascination with the complexity of human life and a respect for scientific inquiry. Being both curious and skeptical, I was naturally inclined to challenge ill-founded authority. So I entered, with hopeful enthusiasm, what I thought to be an unpretentious profession.

My first teacher, Donald Hebb, despite his academic status, was easily approachable. During my first year as an undergraduate, he talked often with me about the science of psychology, its possibilities—and its limitations. Hebb was fond of stating that psychology must be "more than common sense," explaining that he did not mean to imply that psychologists had access to some hidden fund of superior knowledge but rather that we must always be skeptical of anything deemed obvious. Over and over again, he emphasized that psychologists had an obligation to avoid being swept along by socially sanctified beliefs. The essence of the profession, as I came to view it, was a combination of critical thinking and humility.

After graduation, in 1969, I worked in the psychiatry department of a large general hospital developing a system to monitor and evaluate how clinicians were diagnosing and treating their patients. Very soon, I was reminded of Hebb's warning when I had my first glimpse of just how dangerous people can be when they act as if they have access to some superior knowledge that separates them from, and places them above, others. The psychiatrists were "the doctors," the patients were "the patients"; the roles were clearly and hierarchically defined. As I watched, I began to suspect that behind the haughty professional, "I'm the doctor" image was a dubious ability to either understand or help patients. Because everyone seemed to be taking the experts' opinions so seriously, I became concerned about the actual impact these psychiatrists were having on people's lives.

Over the next 5 years, my research delved into the manner in which psychiatrists went about deciding what was wrong with their patients and what therapy to provide. As I systematically examined their decision-making, it became evident that personal beliefs and subjective theories, especially about the causes of problems, influenced diagnoses and treatments more so than did any available information about specific patients, including observable symptoms and verifiable histories (Dineen, 1975). It was clear that diagnoses were generally more consistent with psychiatrists' beliefs than with patients' problems and that prescribed therapies could be traced, not to any legitimate knowledge but rather to what they believed in—whether it was medication, Primal Scream, Gestalt, some version of psychoanalysis or a behavioral technique.

These findings became part of a growing body of literature challenging the authority of the psychiatric profession (e.g., Neisser, 1973; Rosenhan, 1973). The contrast between psychology and psychiatry seemed clear at that time:

- psychiatry was powerful; psychology was weak.
- psychiatry lacked genuine expertise; psychology would develop it.
- psychiatry slotted people into categories; psychology respected individuality.

What it seemed to boil down to was that psychiatry was unworthy of the power entrusted to it and that, if given a chance, psychology could make things better. Believing that to be so, I began clinical work, first in a hospital setting, then for several years as treatment director in a large psychiatric facility before moving, in 1981, into private practice.

Thinking that, as psychologists, we were challenging psychiatry's position of authority, it didn't occur to me that we were actually trying to grab the power for ourselves. I tried to ignore the continual flow of beliefs being disguised as findings, the psychological fads being promoted as the latest discoveries, and the spread of "pop psychology."

However, I cringed as I listened to my colleagues translating human life into a myriad of abuses, addictions, and traumas, creating labels for them, and then promoting competing brands and preferred flavors of psychotherapy as the cures.

As I watched psychologists take on the characteristics we had so strongly criticized in psychiatrists, my respect for the profession waned. Psychology seemed intent on building fences and claiming territory, all in an effort to bolster the illusion that we, and we alone, were the legitimate dispensers of psychological wisdom and healing. Whether one accepted it or not, it became a requirement that we take on a professional role in which we viewed patients-clients in debilitating ways, constructing barriers that would separate "us" from "them."

During more than 20 years of clinical work I encountered some people who might be considered so distraught, disoriented, or disabled that some acknowledgment of vulnerability may have seemed appropriate. But virtually all of the patients I saw in my office were people whom I would refuse to identify in any way that would set them apart from the rest of us. I would consider it dishonest to declare them "sick," harmful to label them traumatized or damaged, and disrespectful to treat them as less competent, capable, or mature than people I might meet in other contexts. All relationships, including those that patients have with psychologists and psychiatrists, involve a distribution of power, but rarely is this fixed or absolute. In most cases, this power is less clear and more fluid than is implied by the simplistic notion that places the power always with the therapist.

In April of 1993, no longer able to ignore how dramatically the profession had shifted from science to faith and from humility to arrogance, I closed my clinical practice. It was a moral decision strongly influenced by my uneasiness with the boundaries that have come to encircle psychology and to make absolute and inescapable the supposed "power" of the psychotherapist.

THE NATURE OF BOUNDARIES

I intended to turn my back on the profession; instead, I forced myself to take a cold, hard look at what psychology had become. Quickly, I began to suspect that boundaries served to create an illusion of power.

The profession of psychology and its derivative practice of psychotherapy are relatively new concepts, yet both are now taken for granted as part of our everyday lives. As Philip Cushman (1995) notes: "Psychology is one of the most significant cultural artifacts of our times, reflecting and shaping the central themes of the last 150 years" (p. 4). Over a brief, meteoric history, psychology has established itself not only in the minds of millions of individuals but also in the psyche of Western society.

Along with knowledge and skills, the profession claims power. But the power it wields comes not from its expertise but rather from the State and the presumed positive influence its theories and therapies exert on peoples' lives. For as Pope and Vasquez (1998) write: "In licensing therapists, the states invest them with the power of state-recognized authority to influence drastically the lives of their clients" (p. 43).

Intangible and unproveable as this influence is, it has led to the professional and legal establishment of rules referred to as "boundaries," including rules about dual and multiple relationships, which bar psychologists and psychotherapists from any involvement in the lives of their patients beyond the office and "couch."

What I have come to understand about these boundaries is that:

- Like all man-made fences, they are artificial and arbitrary. They "fence in" and "fence out," serving to exclude certain groups, certain movements, and certain behaviors. They can be constructed, heightened or lowered, moved, or taken down at any time. (The confusion expressed in recent years by many psychologists regarding what is and is not allowed and what is or is not an ethical violation serves as a constant reminder, and a clear demonstration, of this artificial quality);
- While it is argued that boundaries exist for the purpose of protecting patients from exploitation due to the supposed power of the therapist, the real and much grander reason for building these fences is to establish practitioners, and the profession itself, as an elite and potent force;
- These fences are not built to control therapists' power but rather to establish and embellish the impression that the people who are qualified to assume the role of psychotherapist are so powerful as to be able to exert a dangerous, Svengali-like, influence.

In this chapter, I will focus on how the quest for power captivated the profession in such a way as to make these arbitrary fences, as illustrated in the popularized notions of "dual" and "multiple" relationships, an obsession. I will look at the social and historical context in which psychotherapy has thrived, the nature of psychotherapy (if such an entity, in fact, exists), the primary characteristics of the therapeutic relationship, and the dilemma faced by those psychotherapists who question the legitimacy of current boundaries.

For convenience, I use the term "psychology" to refer to the licensed profession, "psychologist" to refer to anyone who, like myself, is a licensed psychologist, and the term "psychotherapist" in referring to any member of the various other mental health professions which sell psychotherapeutic services.

While my comments will be limited to the topic of psychotherapy, it should be noted that the concerns expressed extend into virtually all areas of psychology. Questions such as whether academics are in such clear positions of power over their students as to be "untouchable" or whether industrial psychologists should be free to have lunch with corporate clients, while relevant to the issues raised, are outside the current focus.

THE SOCIAL CONTEXT OF PSYCHOTHERAPY

"We must admit that the rapid growth of psychology in America has been due to conditions of the soil as well as the vitality of the germ" (J. M. Cattell, Presidential Address to the American Psychological Association, 1895).

When Cattell spoke these words, society was still deeply immersed in "modern" philosophy, which held that truth was objective and universal. By the end of the 20th century, this view had given way to postmodern thinking that "affirms that whatever we accept as truth and even the way we envision truth are dependent on the community in which we participate" (Grenz, 1995, p. 8). In other words, "there is no absolute truth: rather truth is relative to the community in which we participate" (p. 8). One postmodernist, Richard Rorty (1991), contends that once the notion of objective truth is gone, we must choose between either self-defeating relativism or ethnocentrism. We should, he argues, "grasp the ethnocentric horn of the dilemma" and "privilege our own group" (pp. 24, 29). Put in more cynical terms, truth is, and retrospectively, always has been, what works best for those establishing the truth. As Foucault (1979) concluded from his broad analyses of political and social power, whoever determines that truth holds the power. From prisons to advertising agencies, from schools and clinics to the media, truth became a matter of persuasion.

It was during these changing times that the practice of psychotherapy emerged as a profession and as Sarason (1981) points out, it was as much "shaped" by events and culture as it was a "shaper" of this new society. In many ways, it secured its social influence role by adapting its theories and practices to this 'zeitgeist'; the intellectual, political, and cultural climate of the era.

To understand the current obsession with boundaries, it is necessary to consider the social forces that influenced, restricted, and directed the practice of psychotherapy. At times, the predominant influences were war, immigration, and racism; at other times, industrialism and capitalism. And more recently, Cushman (1995) notes that "Permeated by the philosophy of self-contained individualism," psychotherapy "exists within the framework of consumerism, speaks the language of self-liberation, and thereby unknowingly reproduces some of the ills it is responsible for healing" (p. 6). He contends that psychotherapy has metamorphosed to "treat the unfortunate personal effects of the empty self (characterized by a pervasive sense of personal emptiness and committed to values of consumerism), without disrupting the economic arrangements of consumerism" (p. 6).

Earlier, in *Manufacturing Victims* (Dineen, 2001), I identified some aspects of the postmodern zeitgeist which merit brief consideration here:

1. Psychologism
2. Victimism
3. Professionalism
4. Feminism

PSYCHOLOGISM: THE PSYCHOLOGIZING OF POPULAR THINKING

In 1991 Christopher Lasch observed that "In the second half of the twentieth century therapeutic concepts and jargon have penetrated so deeply into American culture—most recently in the guise of a broad-gauged campaign to raise people's 'self-esteem' that it has become almost impossible to remember how the world appeared to those not yet initiated into the mysteries of mental health" (p. 219).

Despite psychology's beginning as an empirical science and its continued effort to craft that image, much of psychotherapy rests on unproven (and unprovable) theories. Cautions that have been raised within the profession have been conveniently ignored as the American public has adopted a psychologized way of thinking. The result of this love affair, as historian Ellen Herman (1995) points out in her aptly titled book, *The Romance of American Psychology*, is that "Psychological insight is the creed of our time" (p. 1). From talk shows to televised news reports to the front page of our papers, psychological notions are continuously presented to explain everything from tragedy to success, pain to prosperity, fame to depravity. People have acquired an unquestioning faith in psychotherapists, believing that they have a deep understanding of these issues as well as the skills to change lives.

Psychologists respond by providing explanations and solutions. Early on, John Watson, the "father of behaviorism," claimed that he could manipulate children for either genius and success, or "doltishness" and failure.[1] So effective was his persuasion that, in 1915, *Good Housekeeping* declared that "the amateur mother of yesterday" would be replaced by the behaviorally trained "professional mother of tomorrow." J. M. Cattell, R. M. Yerkes, and Frederick Winslow Taylor found their niche, applying psychometric skills to weed out mentally incompetent and disruptive characters in the military and in factories—an approach later applied to immigrants and blacks.[2] Commenting on this, Walter Lippman (1922) wrote of the power-hungry intelligence testers who yearn to "occupy a position of power that no intellectual has held since the collapse of theocracy" (p. 10), but his warning went unheeded. Elton (George) Mayo and Carl Rogers began offering employers strategies for resolving worker unrest and ways to increase productivity.[3] Regardless of the harmful effects or questionable benefits of these, and countless other psychological services, America became a "psychological society" (Gross, 1978), relying on psychotherapists not only to interpret what people say, feel, and do, and to explain their words, moods, and actions, but to guide them onward and upward.

Psychology was heralded as the source not only of 'cure' but of 'growth.' As therapists Erving and Miriam Polster put it: "Therapy is

---

[1] *Psychological Care of the Infant and Child.* (1928). "There is a sensible way of treating children: Treat them as though they were young adults. Never hug or kiss them, never let them sit on your lap. If you must, kiss them once on the forehead when they say good-night. Shake hands with them in the morning. Let them learn to overcome difficulties from the moment of birth."

[2] For example, psychologists advanced the notion that the ills of the nation could be treated in the same ways as the problems of the individual by treating "a sick nation." Such an orientation was expressed by Myrdal who, in considering the problem of race relations in the United States, suggested that every facet of black culture "*is a distorted development, or a pathological condition, of the general American culture.*" (Myrdal, G. *An American Dilemma.* p. 928 [emphasis is in the original])

[3] Although Mayo's research was severely flawed and later judged invalid, the well-known and often misunderstood "Hawthorne Effect" became the precursor of a new method of human control: "the power of human relations," the human-relations movement.

too good to be limited to the sick" (London, 1974, pp. 63–68). Virtually everyone donned psychologically-tinted glasses and spoke in a psychological language that distorted life and portrayed psychotherapists as powerful healers. So, psychology has, as Nichols Rose (1996) observes, "Given birth to a range of psychotherapies that aspire to enable humans to live as free individuals through subordinating themselves to a form of therapeutic authority" (p. 17). He continues, "freedom, that is to say, is enacted only at the price of relying upon experts of the soul"—the new psychologized *TruthMakers* of the 21st century.

PROFESSIONALISM—TURF OWNERSHIP

As psychology persistently inserted itself into our modern reality, the strategy of professionalization, of capturing and monopolizing market sectors, became progressively more urgent.

When G. Stanley Hall and six colleagues founded the American Psychological Association (APA) in 1892, it was their intention that it should advance the field of psychological research. Only 4 years later, Lightner Witmer at the University of Pennsylvania was suggesting to APA that psychologists should be involved in the professional training of students in areas of vocational, educational, correctional, hygienic, industrial, and social guidance. Initially, his proposal met with resistance from those who, as scientists, considered it both inappropriate and premature.

Despite these concerns, Witmer had cast the stone and psychology was on its way to becoming a profession that applied its supposed 'expertise.' Within a few years, Hall would tell Freud, during his 1909 visit to America, that he had come at a good "psychological moment"; at a time when, "with mobility of place, profession and status, and a new instability of values, old ways of looking at the world no longer applied. The individual is thrown back on himself and is more receptive to theories such as psychoanalysis which search for meaning in his dreams, wishes, fears, and confusion" (Turkle, 1978, pp. 30–31).

What psychology offered was a way of addressing these concerns that appealed to the public. Psychology, of course was not without competitors; medicine and religion had a long history of attending to such needs. The practical solution was to follow the example of medicine, which had already enacted laws restricting medical licensure to scientifically trained practitioners with penalties for even fraternizing with the unlicensed practitioner—an early form of boundary violation.

It is generally assumed that professional licensing exists to protect the public, but, in fact, its greater service is to the privileged group in society who possess the credentials. Rollo May (1992) shortly before his death reflected on the early days of psychological licensing. He describes the mid-1950s as the "dangerous years" when the American Medical Association threatened to outlaw nonmedical psychotherapists. May recalls that eventually he and his colleagues decided that "The best step for us as psychologists would be to clarify all the different branches of psychotherapy (p. xxiii)" and to organize a conference on the training, practice, and safeguards of psychotherapy. "From that moment on, the fact that psychotherapy was conducted by psychologists . . . was then accepted in the various legislatures around the country" (p. xxiv). May goes on to describe a conversation he had at that time with Carl Rogers: "Expecting his (Rogers') enthusiastic help, I was taken aback by his stating the he was not sure whether it would be good or not to have psychologists licensed. . . . During the following years, I kept thinking of Carl Rogers' doubts about our campaign for licensing. I think he foresaw that we psychologists could be as rigid as any other group, and this certainly has been demonstrated . . . " (p. xxiv).

As psychology's prominence grew, wrapped in the garb of a healing profession, it assumed an arrogant sense of self-importance. The brief experiment during the early 1970s, when psychotherapy was seen as an interaction between equals, quickly evaporated, giving way to the present medicalized, hierarchical form. The fence that was created dividing therapists and patients not only serves to separate psychologists from those they want to help, it also creates a "one-up" position in which power is usurped by psychologists. As Robyn Dawes (1986) notes: "It is impossible to consider oneself "one-up" without considering the other person involved in the relationship "one-down." That means treating the other as if he or she were not a fully autonomous moral being" (p. 2).

VICTIMISM—PATHOLOGY FOR EVERYONE

If these new *TruthMakers* were to appear powerful, what better way to do it than to make others appear weak by declaring "them" troubled, injured, damaged, sick—powerless.

From the outset of traditional psychiatry (and psychology) in America with Benjamin Rush, the approach has been to label personal and social problems as illnesses. Although Rush, whose portrait adorns the seal of the American Psychiatric Association, is considered to be the Father of American Psychiatry, some consider him, instead, to be the "Father of the Medicalization of Deviance" (Conrad & Schneider, 1980, p. 49). Exchanging a medical ideology for the earlier theological perspective, he perceived "the world in terms of sickness and health" (Szasz, 1970, p. 140), defining such behaviors as drinking, smoking, lying, and murder as medical problems.

For instance, one of the problems that Rush confronted was slavery. He claimed to abhor slavery both as a Christian and as an avowed supporter of the Declaration of Independence that held "that all men are created equal." But he had to deal with the realities of Negro slavery based on the view that blacks were racially inferior. To solve this moral dilemma, he reasoned that God did not create the Negro as black, nor were they black by nature, but rather, their blackness was a sign of a disease that he labeled "Negritude."

While this diagnosis and many others have come and gone in the intervening centuries, psychologists continue to invent pathologies according to the political and social climate of the day. In recent decades, most have been derived from a victim motif that explains away disappointments and difficulties as caused by trauma, abuse, and stress. People have been influenced to take on fabricated victim identities, prompting them to turn to psychotherapy for relief.

These individuals have been led to believe that they can be helped, as Gross (1978) puts it, "*Only* if they learn the mysteries of psychology which can unlock the Unconscious. Like the primitive witch doctor, the modern psychologist promises to do this in exchange for power and money" (p. 44). Charles Sykes (1992) notes that "The therapists (have) transformed age-old human dilemmas into psychological problems and claimed that they (and they alone) had the treatment. . . . The result was an explosion of inadequacy" (p. 34).

A further effect has been to accentuate the one-up/one-down relationship between psychologists and patients.

FEMINISM—DECONSTRUCTION OF THE PATRIARCHY

The 20th century served as the backdrop for women to set right the historical imbalances between the sexes and to overcome demeaning stereotypes and customs. Early feminism and the initial women's liberation movement were committed to an egalitarian view of the sexes, emphasizing fewer boundaries and a more equal power sharing. Later forms of feminism, referred to now as "radical," rejected "the principle of equal treatment either because legal standards are inherently 'male' or because one cannot treat oppressor and oppressed as equals" (Young as cited in Carnell, 2000, para. 4).

Psychology, rather than maintaining its objective and empirical perspective, quickly accommodated to the demands of this radical movement, particularly with regard to issues of violence. Accepting biased and generally unreliable data (Dineen, 1998), the APA endorsed the notion that aggression was a male characteristic. The APA task force on male violence against women, the members of which were described as "experts in different aspects of female-directed violence" declared that "one in every three women will experience at least one physical assault by an intimate partner during adulthood" and "34 to 59 percent of women are sexually assaulted by their husbands" (APA, 1994). Violence was defined as a gender issue: men were inherently violent and there was "no safe haven" for women.

Over recent decades, psychology has succumbed to the pressures exerted on it by radical feminism, allowing this political force to reshape the practice of psychotherapy. Tossing aside such psychotherapeutic principles as introspection and self-examination, Rachel Perkins writes, "Understanding one's experience as personal, private and psychological . . . is considered dangerous to the goals of feminism" (Satel, 1998, p. 14). In the same vein, Laura Brown (1997), a prominent "feminist practitioner," identifies feminist psychotherapy as an "opportunity to help patients see the relationship between their behaviors and the patriarchal society in which we are all embedded." Brown describes her work as the "private practice of subversion" and considers the job of a feminist therapist to be "the subversion of patriarchy in the client, the therapist, and the therapy process" (p. 453).

Not surprisingly, given that psychotherapy itself is seen as an expression of the patriarchy, much concern has been raised regarding the power differential in the therapist-patient relationship. Feminists have tried to neutralize it, by encouraging, within the therapeutic relationship, such initiatives as woman-to-woman mutual self-disclosure. These initiatives have, of course, served to confuse and confound the very nature of psychotherapy and to construct a political image of the female therapist as safe, caring, and friendly and a contrasting one of the male therapist as dangerous, self-focused, and predatory. Such imagery has served to support the assumption that virtually any type of dual relationship can reflect an underlying erotic intent, leading therapist and patient down some slippery slope into a sexual relationship that is inevitably harmful to the patient.

The overall effect has been to sexualize the issue of boundaries. Despite all the claims to the contrary, psychology continues to widen the power imbalance between men and women, portraying women as victims: weak and powerless, in need of both public and professional protection. The champions of this cause are not always women; often, in fact, they are men who, in earlier decades, would have been considered arrogantly paternalistic. Peter Rutter (1989), for example, writes, "A man in the position of trust and authority (as a therapist, doctor, clergy, teacher, and other) becomes unavoidably a parent figure and is charged with the ethical responsibility of the parent role" (p. 101). When this image of women as childlike is melded with the belief in therapists' power, it results in a preoccupation with gender, sexuality, and sexual abuse. "Violations of these boundaries are," as Rutter continues, "psychologically speaking, not only rapes but also acts of incest" (pp. 23–24). Women, he contends, have no power because those who "behave seductively in forbidden-zone relationships are blindly playing out the part of the masculine myth that wants them to behave seductively" (p. 79).

THE OBSESSION WITH BOUNDARIES AND POWER

If, at the beginning of the 20th century, America was ripe for psychology, by the end of the century, the ground had been prepared for seeding the notion of professional power, planting the abstract concept of dual relationships, and erecting boundaries.

While postmodernism provided the stimulus, the analyses of Foucault and Lacan were abstruse. Psychotherapy, on the other hand, steeped in theories about transference and heavily influenced by radical feminism, was particularly susceptible to moral panic about the potential harm of a power imbalance. The perception of patients as weak and vulnerable victims, and often female, and therapists as knowledgeable and powerful, and frequently male, invited an ideology of power. Replacing the objective standards of empiricism were the "subjective narratives," which simply put is: "If you say it's true, it is true!" This benchmark is applied not only to the reported histories of patients but also to the perception of boundaries, dual relationships, and the balance of power.

PSYCHOTHERAPY

> Psychotherapy is a service, a business, an industry, yet the mystique of psychotherapy endures beyond all reason.
> —Robert Langs (p. 5, 1989)

Talking sensibly about boundaries in and around psychotherapy requires that we first ask: "What is psychotherapy?"

"Psychotherapy," as Cushman (1995) points out, "has had many faces and utilized many ideologies during its stay in North America" (p. 2). Though the term was rarely uttered in the first decade of the 20th century (Caplan, 1998), and practitioners were scarce, by the final decade the word had come into common usage and hundreds of thousands were choosing psychotherapy as a career.

Despite the fact that virtually everyone uses the word and millions purchase the service yearly, "psychotherapy" defies any consistent definition, having shifted from mesmerism and moral treatment to "mental hygiene" and psychoanalysis and, more recently, to such varied and contrasting forms as Humanistic Therapy, Thought Field Therapy, and Cognitive Behavior Therapy. In 1978 Szasz highlighted this fundamental problem when he wrote of "the promiscuous use of the term" (p. 208).

Bolstering this semantic confusion is the notion that "There is no consistent evidence," as Orlinsky and Howard (1986) assert, "that any specific form of therapy produces better results than any other, whether it be individual or group therapy or family counselling, or short- compared to long-term treatment" (p. 321). Seligman (1998) echoes this conclusion, noting that "When one treatment is compared to another treatment specificity tends to disappear or becomes quite a small effect. . . . The fact is that almost no psychotherapy technique that I can think of shows specific effects when compared to another form of psychotherapy or drug, adequately administered" (p. 2).

Cognitive-behavior and interpersonal therapists reject this view, claiming that their approaches include "empirically supported methods" for the treatment of specific conditions, such as panic disorders, obsessive compulsive disorders, depression, and various persistent phobias. While they express concern that other clinicians are ignoring research findings in order to justify calling whatever they do "effective psychotherapy," their critics retort that their "promotions are more science fiction than science" (Miller, Duncan, & Hubble, 2001) and offer studies that suggest the importance of relationship factors on cognitive behavioral therapy outcomes (Keijsers, Schaap, & Hoogduin, 2000).

So, the problem remains that if we can't agree on its definition nor whether it really matters what it is, then why is psychotherapy seen as a potent treatment? In part, according to Leonard Bickman (1999), it is because "We (have been) seduced into believing this by the procedures we ourselves put into place for assuring effective services" (p. 968). These criteria—training, qualifications, experience, licensure—have all been held to affect therapy outcome and yet all are professional "myths" unsupported by evidence (Dawes, 1994). These same factors are, of course, seen as contributing to a power imbalance in the psychotherapeutic relationship—suggesting that we are being seduced into this belief in a similar mythological fashion.

If neither the specific therapy nor the professional qualifications explain it, then what is it that leads to the perceived positive effects? Apart from those relatively few conditions for which established treatments of choice seem to exist, research suggests that most of the change clinicians and their patients report is related to "nonspecific effects": time, patient expectation, implicit suggestion, and the therapeutic relationship. For instance, in reviewing the factors that accounted for significant patient progress, Lambert (1986) found that "spontaneous remission" (improvement without treatment) accounted for 40%, 15% of the change resulted from placebo effects (patient expectation), while a further 30% improved as the result of common relational factors such as trust, empathy, insight, and warmth. Only 15% of the overall improvement was attributable to any specific psychological intervention or technique. Based on this, as I concluded elsewhere (Dineen, 2001), one might expect that "Eighty-five percent of clients would improve with the help of a good friend and 40 percent without even that" (p. 117).

The research literature that generally supports this idea has led to the popular assumption that the "power" to help (or to harm) is somehow embedded in what is called the therapeutic relationship. The impression has been created that this "therapeutic alliance" is unique, deserving of the term "professional" and inherently powerful. But what are the characteristics that make this relationship so special, so unusual, and so powerful that it must be fenced in? The answer one frequently hears is that the "magic" can be attributed to such human factors such as trust and caring.

THE THERAPEUTIC RELATIONSHIP AND THE PRETENSE OF POWER

British psychologist David Smail (1999) began a presentation recently by listing the following: "kind, sensitive, intelligent, cultured in the arts and humanities, intuitively perceptive, supportive without being obtrusive, attentive rather than talkative." Only as he continued, "attractive, faithful, loves children, clean, and an excellent cook," did it become clear that he was listing not the characteristics of a "a good therapist" but rather those of "a good wife." While acknowledging that specifying good wifeliness was particularly patronizing and offensive, Smail had succeeded in making the point that, within the profession, there is held a predominant image of "a good therapist."

It is this stereotype that makes it appear reasonable when Pope and Vasquez (1998) assert, in *Ethics in Psychotherapy and Counseling*, that "The concept of trust is crucial for understanding the context in which clients approach and enter into a working relationship with psychotherapists" (p. 41). But when they go on to declare that the patient's trust in "therapy is similar to surgery" in that surgical patients allow themselves to be "opened up" by the surgeon while "therapy patients undergo a process of psychological opening up," one should question what they are saying, especially because they: (a) assume that all psychotherapy is similar to psychoanalysis, and (b) draw on Freud's (1968) comparison of psychoanalysis and surgery in his lecture on "The Analytic Therapy," when he commented that psychoanalytic suggestion works "surgically" (p. 458) and that "psychoanalytic treatment is comparable to a surgical operation . . . " (p. 467).

Of course not all psychotherapists are psychoanalysts, and even if they were, the analogy does not hold up, because in neither case did Freud's metaphorical expression have anything to do with Pope and Vasquez's contention that special powers exist in the therapeutic relationship. In the first reference, Freud sought to clarify the difference between hypnotic suggestion (at least as Freud saw hypnosis), which he viewed as "working cosmetically," and psychoanalytic observation, which he considered to be effective at a deeper level. In the latter reference, addressing the external resistances or impediments to analysis and offering surgery as a contrast, Freud spoke with envy of the surgeon who does not have to deal with the interference of the patient's family. "A surgeon is accustomed to making . . . preliminary arrangements—a suitable room, a good light, expert assistance, exclusion of the relatives," he writes. "Now ask yourself how many surgical operations would be successful if they had to be conducted in the presence of the patient's entire family poking their noses into the scene of the operation and shrieking aloud at every cut. In psychoanalytic treatment the intervention of the relatives is a positive danger and, moreover, one I do not know how to deal with" (Freud, 1968, p. 467). Contrary to Pope's belief in the therapist's power, Freud saw, with annoyance and frustration, that his power was drastically limited.

Szasz, commenting on this contemporary misinterpretation of psychotherapy as a medical treatment, observes:

> Because the therapeutic relationship is an intimate human relationship . . .
> psychotherapy could not be more different from physical therapies in medi-
> cine. The proper treatment of diabetes does not depend, and ought not to
> depend, on the doctor's personality. It's a matter of medical science. On the
> other hand, the proper treatment of a person in distress seeking help is a
> matter of values and personal styles—on the parts of both therapist and
> patient. (Wyatt, 2000, Psychotherapy, Szasz Style section, para. 2)

It seems that the inappropriate medicalization of the concept of
psychotherapy, especially when carried to the extreme level of equating
it with surgery, results in a manipulated, artificial image of therapists
based on an illusory sense of power rather than on any specific skills,
any genuinely human qualities, or any specialized body of knowledge.

Arons and Siegel (1995) describe the consequences for the therapist,
when they write, "When we [psychologists] sit in our consultation rooms,
we often try to present *a carefully sculpted image* to our patients. . . . At
times, we are much like the Wizard of Oz, trying to make an impressive
presentation while hoping that the curtain we hide behind won't be
pulled aside to reveal more vulnerable parts of ourselves" (p. 125).

A study of 421 psychologists reveals that psychologists prefer the
pretense, wishing to be seen as "irrepressibly superior"—dependable,
capable, conscientious, intelligent, friendly, honest, adaptable, responsible, reasonable, and considerate (Sharaf & Levinson, 1967). One female
therapist adds, "My clients aren't particularly open-minded. I fear their
rejection. Many wouldn't like me if they really knew me, and that
wouldn't be very good for my practice." This masquerade has become
a cornerstone of postmodern psychotherapy.

Along with truthfulness, another essential aspect that has been sacrificed is confidentiality. Although the psychotherapeutic relationship
would seem legitimately to have more to do with privacy than with
power, no longer can it honestly be said that what patients say to their
therapists—their fears, fantasies and self-accusations—are secrets safely
uttered (Bollas & Sundelson, 1995). Szasz accurately portrays the current situation when he says

> What is truly ugly about psychotherapy today is that many patients labor
> under the false belief that what they say to the therapist is confidential, and
> that therapists do not tell patients, up front, that if they utter certain thoughts
> and words, the therapist will report them to the appropriate authorities, they
> may be deprived of liberty, of their job, of their good names, and so forth.
> (Wyatt, 2000, Psychotherapy, Szasz Style section, para. 34)

Although therapists may protest that this responsibility is forced upon
them by the State, it is only done so with the cooperation of psychology.

So what are we left with? A profession that claims to:

- free society, especially women, from a perceived patriarchy while constructing a new version of inequality
- empower "victims" while all the while perpetuating a sense of weakness, vulnerability, and dependence
- promote the ideal of freedom and individuality while shaping both therapists and patients to conform to prescribed roles
- uphold confidentiality while failing to protect privacy
- be powerful while concealing insecurities

It is no wonder that psychology is obsessed with boundaries for, in many ways, that's all there is—*the Clothes have no Emperor*—there is appearance without substance.

But these boundaries, while they may be artificial, have a profound effect on the way we practice. Childress and Siegler (1999) identify five possible metaphors and models of the doctor-patient relationships. The first metaphor, *paternal or parental,* assigns moral authority and discretion to doctors because their competence, skills, and ability place them in a position to help patients regain good health. The second model, *partnership,* is based on the language of collegiality, collaboration, association, and co-adventureship. The third, *rational contractors,* specifies that professionals and their patients be related to each other by a series of contracts that share responsibility, preserve both equality and autonomy under less-than-ideal circumstances, and protect the integrity of various parties. The fourth, *friendship,* holds that doctors are limited, special-purpose friends in relation to their patients. And finally, a fifth model views the professional as a *technician.*

Any one of these models might apply to the therapeutic situation, depending on who the therapist and patient are and the nature of the service being provided. But our professional associations and licensing boards, cutting every therapist and every patient from the same cloth, ignore and confuse these choices. APA, for example, would have the public believe that "psychotherapy is a partnership"[4] while, at the same time, imposing on us boundaries that make a partnership impossible and a paternalistic relationship mandatory. By imposing simplistic, auto-

---

[4]"Psychotherapy is a partnership between an individual and a professional such as a psychologist who is licensed and trained to help people understand their feelings and assist them with changing their behavior." Retrieved from the APA web site: http://helping.apa.org/therapy/psychotherapy.html

cratic, nonnegotiable limits, psychology removes any possibility for therapists and patients to entertain any fully human and responsible relationship.

THE DILEMMA

> A choice that confronts every one at every moment is this: Shall we permit our fellows to know us as we now are, or shall we remain enigmas, wishing to be seen as persons we are not?
>
> —Jourard (1971, p. vii)

Recently, a colleague contacted me writing, "I am a clinical psychologist with 23 years of experience . . . and I am currently in a most serious dilemma in terms of my private practice. . . . I always perceived myself to be someone who would do his utmost not to influence my clients . . . however I may not have been always so noble . . . it is very difficult to be self-vigilant, to listen honestly to their needs attentively, follow my morals including keeping silent of my skepticism with Psychology, and also securing an income from people suffering." And he continued, " . . . in my private practice, clients come to seek my services with a great deal of expectations that are so deeply entrenched in their minds . . . and, despite my best intentions, I cave in to their many and varied therapeutic expectations, albeit unreal, and end up working with them at the 'mythical level' . . . I am considering ending my private practice slowly, but my family believes I should be able to sort this out with time and dedication . . . "

"Ah, there's the rub"—how to practice with ethics in a profession that pursues power and artificially imposes boundaries that exaggerate the therapists' authority and the patients' vulnerability. How to maintain a viable practice and still be honest about expectations, skills, and ability.

Given the current social and political climate and the restraints that stifle the individuality of psychologists and patients, I have doubts that there is an easy way to resolve his "most serious dilemma."

Since 1996, when I began to express my concerns publicly, many psychologists have contacted me, describing similar levels of disillusionment and moral turmoil. Some have remained in touch while most, after a time, disappeared. Though I could be wrong, I assume that they managed to sort it out in some pragmatic fashion.

The simplest and, arguably, the most practical resolution is to just obey the rules, behave predictably and responsibly, and uphold the image. After all, one can argue that being a psychotherapist is a job, which, like any other job, involves rules and regulations with which one may, at times, disagree but still has to go along with. That's a view that family, friends, and virtually every psychologist I know would consider sensible and justifiable even if it requires implicit acceptance that one's professional position is one-down in relation to the various licensing and governing boards, and recognition that one's patients are in what is effectively a two-down position, subject both to the mythological therapist power and to the statutory power of the boards.

While a few concerned colleagues are openly challenging "the code of ethics" and its rigid rules on dual relationships—some calling the code itself unethical—there are no doubt many more who are silently disagreeing and who are choosing, on occasion, to "bend the rules" regarding boundaries. Those living in rural, military, deaf, spiritual, or other small communities may simply find it unbearable, if not impossible, to avoid dual relationships. Those whose psychotherapeutic orientation would deem it not only appropriate, but beneficial, to interact with patients outside the office may very well decide to go for a walk, golf, or embark on a charity effort with a patient. Countless others might ignore the rules simply because they seem silly, insulting, or intolerably degrading to specific individuals who are, or have been, their patients. These are the people who might decide to visit a dying former patient in the hospital, offering not services but friendship, or who, without thinking, might offer a stranded patient a ride or, on reflection, might agree to be operated on by a patient—just because that person happens to be the best surgeon in town.

"Breaking the rules" more often than not has nothing whatever to do with abusing, coercing, or manipulating patients and everything to do with acknowledging them as fellow human beings. It also has to do with risk taking because, in reality, it involves shifting power in the direction of the patient, who can at any time and for any reason lodge a complaint, claim to be a victim, or cast the psychologist in an evil light.

Very few of us would be inclined to seriously consider another option but since I've opted for it, it seems appropriate that I end on it. A Canadian civil libertarian, Alan Borovoy (1991), calls this alternative "uncivil obedience," and he describes it as "raising hell without breaking the law" (jacket). Acknowledging that Martin Luther King, Jr. taught us how to pleasantly disobey the law, Borovoy suggests that we can protest, also, by unpleasantly obeying the law. "There are ways," he notes, "of being miserable to government without violating the law" (Bindman, 1997, para. 14).

Since I found it impossible to practice honestly and ethically given the mythical image of the psychologist as a powerful expert, as well as the bureaucratically imposed rules and standards, I stopped doing psychotherapy. Remaining a psychologist, maintaining my licenses and my memberships, and always being careful to conform to the rules, I became openly critical of the profession. On one occasion, an annoyed psychologist, after hearing one of my interviews on a national television program, lodged a complaint against me with my licensing board, as a "danger to the television-watching public." A year and a half later, after thoroughly investigating me, the board was forced to concede that I had done nothing wrong and to acknowledge my role as a "social critic."

While the route I took is one virtually everyone would consider too radical, there are other forms of uncivil obedience that might serve to bring attention to the issues and discomfort to those who enforce the dubiously "ethical" codes.

One way is to define and delimit any psychotherapy provided to a focused dialogue between two independent and responsible adults. This is how, for 45 years, Thomas Szasz practised psychotherapy. Long ago, he and Hollender (1956) presented a forceful argument for describing psychotherapy as an adult-adult partnership. Their understanding of the practice was based on a rejection of all efforts to view it within a medical model and an acknowledgment that there exists approximately equal power between therapist and patient. Operating in this style, confidentiality is an essential requirement and not only is no coercive (nonconsensual) treatment allowed, but the psychotherapist is not sanctioned to act as advocate or overseer when it came to matters outside of the therapeutic conversation. Actions, such as making referrals to doctors or lawyers, providing reports to insurance companies, or giving testimony in court, would contravene these principles.

Contrastingly, one might consider advising patients of the existing rules as currently imposed by regulatory boards and require them to sign an informed consent. Such a form might indicate that by entering into a therapist/patient relationship, they understand that they are:

- not guaranteed privacy—all situations in which the right to confidentiality does not hold should be specified
- considered less powerful than the therapist-parent and, like a child who might be influenced by a parent, viewed as incompetent to make independent decisions

- forbidden to have any other mutual and consensual relationship beyond the therapeutic one, either business or personal, with their therapist now or at any time in the future

I can imagine how some of my former patients would have reacted. Many, especially those who were high-status professionals, wealthy individuals, or celebrities, I'm sure, would have refused to sign. Sometimes I wonder what might have happened had these people become so outraged that they bombarded the institutions, licensing board, professional associations, and governments with their own human rights complaints.

When I faced this dilemma myself almost a decade ago, I handled it in my own way. My choice was consistent with who I am and with the skepticism I have harbored since the very beginning of my career. I would never suggest to another psychologist that he or she should follow my example.

Though a few may choose to step outside of the boundaries and some may choose to ignore them, most of us will choose to obey the rules. But we need not do that obediently. We can question authority, both our own and that imposed by others. And, perhaps, if enough of us do, psychology will be, as my earliest teacher insisted it should be, "more than common sense."

REFERENCES

American Psychological Association. (1994). *No safe haven, the report of the APA task force on male violence against women.* Washington, DC: Author. Retrieved January 17, 1995, from www.apa.org (No longer available.)

Arons, G., & Siegel, R. D. (1995). Unexpected encounters: The Wizard of OZ exposed. In M. B. Sussman (Ed.), *A perilous calling: The hazards of psychotherapy practice.* New York: Wiley Interscience.

Bickman, L. (1999). Practice makes perfect and other myths about mental health services. *American Psychologist, 54* (11), 965–978.

Bindman, S. (1997). Breaking the law for a cause: Activists disagree on conditions that justify civil disobedience. *The Ottawa Citizen,* April, 15. Retrieved September 19, 2001, from www.ottawacitizen.com/national/970415/980770.html

Bollas, C., & Sundelson, D. (1995). *The new informants: The betrayal of confidentiality in psychoanalysis and psychotherapy.* Northvale, NJ: Jason Aronson.

Borovoy, A. A. (1991). *Uncivil obedience: The tactics and tales of a democratic agitator.* Toronto: Lester Publishing.

Brown, L. (1997). The private practice of subversion: Psychology as Tikkun Olam. *American Psychologist, 52* (4), 449–462.

Caplan, E. (1998). *Mind games: American culture and the birth of psychotherapy.* Berkeley, CA: University of California Press.

Carnell, B. (2000). Men are from Earth, Women are from Earth?: A review of Cathy Young's "Ceasefire." Retrieved June 15, 2001, from www.equityfeminism.com/bookstore/ceasefire.html

Cattell, J. M. (1896). Presidential address to the American Psychological Association, 1895. *Psychological Review, 3,* 134–148.

Childress, J. F., & Siegler, M. (1999). Metaphors and models of doctor-patient relationships: Their implications for autonomy. In E. W. Kluge (Ed.), *Biomedical ethics* (2nd ed.). Scarborough, Ontario: Prentice Hall Allyn and Bacon Canada.

Conrad, P., & Schneider, J. W. (1980). *Deviance and medicalization: From badness to sickness.* Toronto: The C. V. Mosby Company.

Cushman, P. (1995). *Constructing the self, constructing America: A cultural history of psychotherapy.* Reading, MA: Addison-Wesley.

Dawes, R. M. (1986). *The philosophy of responsibility and autonomy versus that of being one-up.* Presented at the annual convention of APA. Washington, DC, August 24.

Dawes, R. M. (1994). *House of cards: Psychology and psychotherapy built on myth.* New York: The Free Press.

Dineen, T. (1975). *Diagnostic decision making in psychiatry.* Unpublished doctoral thesis. University of Saskatchewan, Saskatoon.

Dineen, T. (1998). *Manufacturing victims: What the psychology industry is doing to people* (2nd ed.). Montreal: Robert Davies Multimedia. (Originally published in 1996.)

Dineen, T. (2001). *Manufacturing victims: What the psychology industry is doing to people* (3rd ed.). Montreal: Robert Davies Multimedia. (Originally published in 1996, revised in 1998 and 2001).

Foucault, M. (1979) *Discipline and punishment: The birth of the prison* (A. Sheridan, Trans.). New York: Vintage.

Freud, S. (1968). *A general introduction to psychoanalysis.* Authorized English translation of the revised edition by Joan Riviere. New York: Washington Square. (Originally published in 1924.)

Grenz, S. J. (1995). *A primer on postmodernism.* Grand Rapids: Cambridge University Press.

Gross, M. L. (1978). *The psychological society: The impact—and the failure—of psychiatry, psychotherapy, psychoanalysis and the psychological revolution.* New York: Random House.

Herman, E. (1995). *The romance of American psychology: Political culture in the age of experts.* Berkeley, CA: University of California Press.

Johnson, R. A. (1991). *Owning your own shadow.* San Francisco: Harper.

Jourard, S. M. (1971) *The transparent self.* New York: Van Nostrand Reinhold. (Originally published in 1964.)

Kardiner, A. (1977). *My analysis with Freud.* New York: Norton.

Keijsers, G. P. J., Schaap, C. P. D. R., & Hoogduin, C. A. L. (2000). The impact of interpersonal patient and therapist behavior on outcome in cognitive-behavioral therapy: A review of empirical studies. *Behavior Modification, 24* (2), 264–297.

Lacan, J. (1982). *Ecrits* (A. Sheridan, Trans.). New York: W. W. Norton.

Lambert, M. J. (1986). Some implications of psychotherapy outcome research for eclectic psychotherapy. *International Journal of Eclectic Psychotherapy, 5* (1), 16–44.

Langs, R. (1989). *Rating your psychotherapist.* New York: Ballantine Books.

Lasch, C. (1991). *The culture of narcissism: American life in an age of diminishing expectations.* New York: W. W. Norton. (Originally published in 1979.)

Lippman, W. (1922, November 29). A future for the tests. *New Republic, 33,* 9.

London, P. (1974). The psychotherapy boom: From the long couch for the sick to the push button for the bored. *Psychology Today, June,* 63–68.

May, R. (1992). Foreword. In D. K. Freedheim (Ed.), *History of psychotherapy: A century of change.* Washington, DC: American Psychological Association.

Miller, S. D., Duncan, B. L., & Hubble, M. A. (2001). What really matters in the much ballyhooed cognitive-behavior therapy?! The relationship. Retrieved July 10, 2001, from http://talkingcure.com/Latest.htm

Neisser, U. (1973). Reversibility of psychiatric diagnoses. *Science, 180,* 1116.

Orlinsky, D. E., & Howard, K. I. (1986). Process outcome in psychotherapy. In S. L. Garfield & A. E. Bergin (Eds.), *Handbook of psychotherapy and behavior change* (3rd ed., pp. 311–384). New York: John Wiley.

Polster, E., & Polster, M. (1974). *Gestalt therapy integrated.* New York: Random House.

Pope, K. S., & Vasquez, M. J. T. (1998). *Ethics in psychotherapy and counseling: A practical guide* (2nd ed.). San Francisco: Jossey-Bass.

Rorty, R. (1991). *Solidarity or objectivity: Objectivity, relativism, and truth.* Cambridge: Cambridge University Press.

Rose, N. (1996). *Inventing our selves: Psychology, power and personhood.* Cambridge, England: Cambridge University Press.

Rosenhan, D. L. (1973). On being sane in unsane places. *Science, 179,* 250–257.

Rutter, P. (1989). *Sex in the forbidden zone: When men in power—therapists, doctors, clergy, teachers, and others—betray women's trust.* New York: Fawcett Crest.

Sarason, S. B. (1981). *Psychology misdirected.* New York: The Free Press.

Satel, S. (1998). The patriarchy made me do it. *Psychiatric Times, May,* 14.

Seligman, M. E. P. (1998). Why therapy works. *APA Monitor, 29* (12), 2.

Sharaf, M. P., & Levinson, D. (1967). The quest for omnipotence in professional training. *International Journal of Psychiatry, 4* (5), 426–442.

Smail, D. (1999). *The impossibility of specifying "good" psychotherapy.* A presentation made to The Universities Psychotherapy Association. University of Surrey.

Sykes, C. J. (1992). *A nation of victims: The decay of the American character.* New York: St. Martin's Press.

Szasz, T. S. (1970). *The manufacture of madness: A comparative study of the inquisition and the mental health movement.* New York: Harper & Row.

Szasz, T. S. (1978). *The myth of psychotherapy: Mental healing as religion, rhetoric, and repression.* Garden City, NJ: Anchor Press/Doubleday.

Szasz, T. S., & Hollender M. H. (1956). A contribution to the philosophy of medicine: The basic models of the doctor patient relationship. *Archives of Internal Medicine, 97,* 585–592.

Turkle, S. (1978). *Psychoanalytic politics: Freud's French Revolution.* New York: Basic Books.

Watson, J. B. (1928). *Psychological care of the infant and child.* (Reprinted 1976). New York: Arno Press.

Wyatt, R. C. (2000). *An interview with Thomas Szasz.* Retrieved June 15, 2001, from http://www.psychotherapistresources.com/current/totm/szasz.html

CHAPTER 10

How Do You Like These Boundaries?

Arnold A. Lazarus, PhD, ABPP

It may appear unseemly to cast a critical light on a facet of the Association that is granting me a significant award. But what better forum to expound on ideas about which I feel strongly, and to an audience that might give due credence to my observations? Elsewhere (Lazarus, 1994a, 1994b) I have emphasized my displeasure with and concerns about several ethical proscriptions, but in this talk, I will limit my criticisms mainly to the subject of dual relationships. The American Psychological Association first addressed the issue of prohibiting dual relations in 1958 (APA, 1958) and subsequently proscribed multiple-role relationships (APA, 1992). I will argue that these generalized interdictions are regrettable and may undermine clinical effectiveness. At the outset, it must be emphasized that what would be considered a dual relationship or another boundary crossing in psychoanalytic therapy may be an integral part of behavior therapy. For example, in the latter approach, dining with a client in a restaurant as a means of countering a fear of public scrutiny is (forgive the pun) standard fare.

The primary intent behind ethical principles and boundary regulations is to ensure that the welfare of clients will not be jeopardized and to provide them with protection from exploitation, discrimination, and

Reprinted by permission. Lazarus, A. A. (1998). How do you like these boundaries? *The Clinical Psychologist, 51,* 22–25.

harm. The foundation of an ethic of nonabuse rests on the fundamental principle of therapist accountability. We can probably all agree that noxious therapists eschew personal responsibility, tend to ignore conflicts of interest, take unfair advantage of clients, or deliberately mislead them. Clinicians who make threats, and use coercion or force, are also likely to have a detrimental impact. Perhaps physical and sexual intimacies with clients constitute the ultimate dual relationship, with resultant dangers to both parties. It makes sense to impose negative sanctions on therapists found guilty of the foregoing infractions, but to view the sharing of a meal with a patient, or the decision to attend a professional meeting with a patient who is a professional, in the same light as going to bed with him or her strikes me as misguided and unfortunate.

My own formative experiences belie the putative dangers that supposedly lurk behind those who provide clinical services to family members, friends, and associates. I was born and raised in Johannesburg, South Africa, and grew up in a devoted nuclear household with very close access to a large extended family. My mother had six siblings and my father came from a family of nine. I have almost four dozen first cousins. To seek services outside the family was almost unthinkable.

Would I rather buy a suit of clothes from a stranger or from one of several relatives who owned apparel stores? Would I buy a car from an outsider or from my cousin who ran a large automobile dealership? In the arena of professional services, the message was even more explicit. Family members look out for one another and care for and about one another. They provide personal, tender, and affectionate caring and offer genuine consanguine concern. Impartiality, neutrality, and objectivity were synonyms for distance and indifference. Caring required commitment, loyalty, and involvement. Thus, would I consult a stranger for medical or legal services, or turn to one of my devoted uncles? When I required a tonsillectomy and there was no ear, nose, and throat surgeon in the family, my uncle, the doctor, made the necessary referral and was present during the surgery. Even before I had completed my PhD, several family members had come to me for advice and psychological assistance.

I have helped many a friend and family member with issues ranging from marital spats to intense phobias. It made no difference whether a caring aunt or a total stranger was being treated for debilitating claustrophobic reactions via systematic desensitization and in vivo exposure. However, when my uncle, the doctor, inquired if I might attend to a female cousin who was unstable and deeply troubled, I demurred.

Given her bizarre perceptions, the most likely outcome would have been alienation from that wing of the family. This matter goes to the heart of my argument. Let us modify the edict, "Never treat family members or friends," to "It is advisable to be cautious about treating close associates who suffer from severe personality disorders or other significant psychopathology."

Upon emigrating to America in 1966, I was forced to rely on total strangers for advice, guidance, and especially, medical help. This was perhaps the most difficult adjustment for me. I sorely missed my family network. Of course, over the span of more than 3 decades, I have developed many close friendships. When I required surgery on two occasions over the past 10 years, I saw to it that a good friend wielded the scalpel in the first instance, and it was no coincidence that two former clients were members of my surgical team on the second occasion. How do you like those boundaries? Ethics committees have expelled psychologists from membership, and state licensing boards have revoked their licenses for having engaged in dual relationships. Ebert (1997) alluded to "unfair and inconsistent decisions . . . used by state licensing authorities" (p. 145) often with catastrophic results. He also stressed that "dual-relationship rules must not impede a psychologist's ability to perform optimum work with a client" (p. 138). Sanctions have been imposed on psychologists for such acts as going to lunch or dinner with a client, sharing meals during therapy, exchanging gifts, inviting a patient to one's home for social events, or playing racquetball.

I was recently retained by defendants' attorneys as an expert witness in two separate legal cases—in different states. The one, a male psychiatrist, was accused by a female patient of transgressing boundaries and providing substandard clinical care, and the other legal matter involved a male psychologist whose female client accused him of several nonsexual boundary violations. After perusing the various depositions and interrogatories, I agreed to render my opinions. (In a third case, also involving a male psychologist and a female client, I refused to testify on behalf of the defendant because his deposition led me to believe that the therapist was probably guilty of the sexual and nonsexual transgressions of which he was accused.) I have also been approached to give testimony on behalf of a female psychologist against whom the APA has launched an attack because she treated a couple with whom she had been friendly. This so-called infraction had occurred some years earlier, and the treatment went well. Nevertheless, about a year posttherapy, the couple decided to get a divorce. A custody battle then ensued and the wife lost her case, whereupon she brought a malpractice suit against the psychologist. When vindictive people make incriminating allegations, it would be comforting if the APA, our parent organization, offered us protection instead of adopting a prosecutorial stance. I hope we can put an end to what I regard as these deeply regrettable "witch-hunts." Ethics committees seem often to ignore the fact that therapists accused of malpractice may be completely innocent. These attitudes and practices bring to mind the horrors of the McCarthy era.

The psychiatrist to whom I have alluded was being sued by a patient who easily met the DSM–IV criteria for Borderline Personality Disorder. Her deposition was riddled with contradictions. Nevertheless, the plaintiff's expert witness recommended that the psychiatrist's license be revoked for having crossed over clinical boundaries—he had tutored the patient for college admission, and accepted gifts from her. Similarly, the expert witness who testified against the aforementioned male psychologist strongly recommended that he be severely censured for introducing "role confusions." The psychologist had asked the client to house-sit while he was on vacation, and he offered her a job in his psychotherapy center while she was still in treatment with him. (The intent behind this boundary crossing was to strengthen the client's self-confidence.) The case against the psychiatrist went to trial, and I emphasized to the jury that the defendant was facing every therapist's worst nightmare. "You go out of your way to help a patient," I explained, "and because you want to do your very best, you go above and beyond the call of duty. And then the patient turns around and sues you for malpractice." There was obviously a lot more to this case—I was under cross-examination for almost 4 hours—but the psychiatrist was acquitted on all charges. Regarding the case against the psychologist, I interviewed the plaintiff and inquired about previous complaints she had filed against other professionals. It became clear that she was a vindictive person, and she blatantly lied on several occasions. Her attorneys settled the case upon receiving my written report. I was informed that without my testimony, these professionals would most probably have been sent up the river!

Ebert (1997) remarked that "Some policies surrounding dual relationships could be considered as gender discrimination" (p. 143), although he did not elaborate. However, Miriam Greenspan's (1995) incisive essay underscores that whereas an ethic of nonabuse for professional relationships is clearly necessary, she is doubtful if the language of boundaries achieves this objective, and she argues that it conceals the political dimension of violence against women. She deplores what she terms "the distance model" and offers instead "a connection model of therapy." She states, "The imagery of relationships with hard borders between enclosed individuals does not make me feel safe. On the contrary, it brings up feelings of isolation, exclusion, and disconnection" (p. 52). She refers to the "boundaries police," and the increasingly rigid standards among review boards, professional organizations, boards of licensure, and malpractice insurers, which she considers by-products of a patriarchal model. "I worry that some of the most feminist and innovative aspects of my work are the most likely to be construed as unethical" (p. 52). She argues that the rigidification of boundaries may produce more, not less, power abuse in therapy. Elsewhere Greenspan (1994) states, "The standard of care itself conspires against the genuine meeting of persons that is the real sine qua non of healing. It keeps Patient and Professional separate even when they don't wish to be. It makes authenticity feel like a bad and dangerous thing" (pp. 199–200).

My position is easily misconstrued. I am not suggesting a generalized, laissez-faire context of business dealings, indiscriminate picnicking, partying, and socializing with clients. What I am advocating is a case-by-case, selective process of deciding when and when not to enter into a secondary relationship. The therapist is to be fully accountable and must ponder issues such as potential risks of harming the patient, possible conflicts of interest, whether or not a dual relationship will impair the therapist's judgment, if the patient's rights or autonomy will be infringed upon, and whether the therapist will gain a personal advantage over the client. When I wrote that "At times, I have learned more at different sides of a tennis net or across a dining room table than might ever have come to light in my consulting room" (Lazarus, 1994, p. 257), eight critics took me seriously to task [*Ethics & Behavior,* 1994, *4* (3)]. As I stated in my rejoinder to these critics, in terms of risk-benefit ratios, they dwelled mostly on potential costs and dangers, whereas I pointed to the advantages that may accrue when certain artificial boundaries are transcended. In essence, to date, no organization, including the American Psychological Association, has given us clear-cut and truly sensible guidelines vis-à-vis the essential dos and don'ts.

It seems to me that we need to employ carefully reasoned, case-by-case, nondogmatic evaluations of boundary questions. Individual client differences should be emphasized rather than subjugated to rigid standards. It should not prove too difficult to achieve consensus on clearly unacceptable behaviors (e.g., engaging in sexual relationships with clients, exploiting and manipulating clients for personal gain, deliberately jeopardizing the welfare of clients, breaching confidentiality, or obtaining financial gain beyond the agreed-upon fee for service—such as writing oneself into the will of an older client). Most would also rightly frown on a therapist who enters into a business relationship with an ongoing client. But a large number of gray areas exist. B. S. Held (1997, personal communication) pointed out that two dubious assumptions underlie the rigid boundary proscriptions that many advocate: (a) therapists are not uniformly competent, therefore we need the codified ethical boundaries we now have, and (b) clients are pathological and/ or powerless, therefore they need the codified ethical boundaries we now have. Corey, Corey, and Callahan (1997) emphasize that "Not all multiple relationships can be avoided, nor are they necessarily always harmful" (p. 231). Instead of embracing a right-wrong dichotomy, they advise therapists to consider very carefully the circumstances in which they may decide to stretch the boundaries. I applaud their emphasis on learning "how to manage boundaries, how to prevent boundary crossings from turning into boundary violations, and how to develop safeguards that will prevent exploitation of clients" (p. 231).

REFERENCES

American Psychological Association. (1958). Ethical standards of psychologists. *American Psychologist, 13,* 268–271.

American Psychological Association. (1992). Ethical principles of psychologists and code of conduct. *American Psychologist, 47,* 1597–1611.

Corey, G., Corey, M. S., & Callahan, P. (1997). *Issues and ethics in the helping professions* (5th ed.). Pacific Grove, CA: Brooks/Cole.

Ebert, B. W. (1997). Dual-relationship prohibitions: A concept whose time never should have come. *Applied & Preventive Psychology, 6,* 137–156.

Greenspan, M. (1994). On professionalism. In C. Heyward (Ed.), *When boundaries betray us* (pp. 193–205). San Francisco: Harper Collins.

Greenspan, M. (1995). Out of bounds. *Common Boundary, July/August,* 51–54.

Lazarus, A. A. (1994a). How certain boundaries and ethics diminish therapeutic effectiveness. *Ethics & Behavior, 4,* 255–261.

Lazarus, A. A. (1994b). The illusion of the therapist's power and the patient's fragility. *Ethics & Behavior, 4,* 299–306.

CHAPTER 11

The Case Against Boundaries in Psychotherapy

Allen Fay, MD

In the 1960s, when I was a psychiatric resident, there was rampant unaccountability in the psychotherapy professions, for both therapeutic results and therapist conduct. With regard to the latter, therapists could have sex with patients almost with impunity. As a reaction to this deplorable situation, trends have developed to deal with the problems in ways that approach the opposite extreme. A number of prominent psychiatrists, psychologists, social workers, and counsellors have taken a strict and narrow view of professional ethics that would sharply restrict therapists' behavior with patients. Whereas this trend potentially has value in heightening awareness and accountability and correcting the abuses of the past, it also has adverse and potentially dangerous consequences. In a way, what is now insisted upon in some quarters is preposterous, if not impossible.

The chapter title, "The Case Against Boundaries in Psychotherapy," might seem absurd because of the obvious existence of limits in all relationships. The basic difference as I see it between the pro and antiboundary positions is in the orientation to the patient-therapist relationship. In the former case, predetermined boundaries are applied to all patient-therapist dyads, whereas in the latter, the possibility for levels of (nonsexual) intimacy is left open. Limits evolve rather than exist by decree. In this sense, there is a case for boundaries, and a case against boundaries. In my opinion the case against boundaries is more compelling. Before attempting to make the case, I want to express the opinion that boundary and even strict boundary proponents are motivated by a sincere desire to prevent exploitation of patients and are correct in their assessment of the seriousness of ethical problems in psychotherapy. Ethics committees in particular have a difficult task striking a balance between recommending guidelines of conduct on the one hand and limiting therapists' freedom to act in their patients' best interest on the other. In fact, the official statements of ethics committees tend to be more moderate than the views of some of the most prolific writers in the field. I believe that the pendulum has swung too far in the restrictive direction and that the prevailing view in the literature and in some official circles must be challenged vigorously. The issue is not simply where the pendulum is, but the fundamental fabric of the arguments used to justify the current position. I believe that neither the logic nor the data support some of the draconian views that have been put forth and in some cases implemented. *There is no question that ethics in the professions is a critical area of concern and that vigilance is required, but vigilance about the right issues—not about behavior that in some instances is used to exploit, but about exploitation itself.*

The subject of ethics in psychotherapy is enormously important. It is, in fact, one of the pillars of effective therapy and essential in distinguishing a profession from a commercial venture. The opportunity to render health care service, and psychotherapy in particular, is a privilege and a sacred trust, no matter how diverse the methods of rendering the services are. Although I was always interested in ethics as a branch of philosophy, I started paying more attention to the literature in professional ethics in the mid-1990s in response to several events. The first was a change in the annual application form for renewal of professional liability coverage. For decades, a few simple questions had been asked, such as "Has your professional license been revoked?" "Have your hospital privileges ever been suspended?" "Have you ever been convicted of a felony?" The applicant checked off a few boxes and that was that. One of the changes was the addition of the question, "Have you ever had any social, romantic, or sexual relationships with any current or former patients?" It was the word "social" that troubled me. I had the same reaction as if the question had read "Have you ever been involved in driving at night, driving while intoxicated, or vehicular homicide?" I have occasionally attended patients' social functions, had a meal with a patient, played tennis with a patient, and I have had ongoing social relationships with a few former patients.

Second, an article in the *Journal of the American Medical Association* entitled "Professional Boundaries in the Physician-Patient Relationship" by Gabbard and Nadelson (1995) caught my attention. Although dealing with some important issues, the authors made a few points that I felt were clinically wrong and logically flawed (Fay, 1995). One of the more troubling statements dealt with therapist self-disclosure. "Even if revealing personal issues to a patient does not lead to more extreme boundary violations, self-disclosure is itself a boundary problem because it is a misuse of the patient to satisfy one's own needs for comfort and sympathy" (p. 1348).

Another event was A. Lazarus's sharing a manuscript with me in which he strongly challenged the growing influence and the arguments of strong boundary proponents and expressed concern about potentially serious adverse consequences for clinicians and patients (1994). I had met Lazarus in the early 1970s and was frankly astounded at his openness with patients. I had read Jourard when I was a resident but had no idea of the potential clinical value of therapist self-disclosure until observing Lazarus and reading some of the literature on modeling. I had been trained in a formal orthodox psychodynamic residency program and was approaching the end of my second analysis. Although I sometimes applied unorthodox solutions to patients' problems and tried to expand my knowledge base and technical repertoire, the psychiatric world was relatively insulated from the major "alternative" therapies. This was so, even though people like Wolpe, Beck, Minuchin, Whitaker, Moreno, and Berne were physicians. I attended weekly seminars given by Lazarus and he would invite me to sit in on some of his sessions with patients. His part-time practice was conducted in an office in his house and if a session ended just before lunch, he would invite the patient to join us. His wife and children were always present, and all manner of topics were discussed, from world events, to the kids' school, to anything the patient might contribute. Jokes were exchanged, a few even salacious. I was curious about the impact on patients. Would he have a high dropout rate? A high suicide rate? Psychotic decompensations? Patients appearing unannounced on his doorstep at all hours of the night? Frequent litigation? His patients seemed to do at least as well as those of other practitioners, and sooner. He was totally himself, defects and all, and was full of creative insights and suggestions for patients. He gave them relevant books, articles, and tapes to use in conjunction with the sessions. Time was of little interest to him. The sessions were an hour long, and it would mean nothing to him to go over the hour if something was happening that made it seem useful. Nor was he good at charging. His fees were considerably lower than would be justified by his reputation. Students and colleagues were not charged. (He didn't have independent wealth but lived comfortably on his university salary, patient income, lecture fees, and royalties.)

Returning to the 1990s, a female patient who had had several prior experiences in psychotherapy brought in the following excerpt from Carter Heyward's (1993) book, *When Boundaries Betray Us,* and expressed appreciation for my being a nonboundary-oriented therapist:

> Conscientious healing professionals are trying to be genuinely ethical— nonabusive—in our work. It is important that, in this morally critical moment in which abuse, that is the misuse of power, is flagrant and systemic, those of us who work as healers . . . understand how badly abusive we can be by withholding intimacy and authentically emotional connection from those who seek our help. For "abuse" is not simply a matter of touching people wrongly. It is, as basically, a failure to make right-relation, a refusal to touch people rightly. We as professionals—indeed, we as people on this planet—are as likely to destroy one another and ourselves by holding tightly to prescribed role definitions as we are by active intrusion and violation. (p. 10)

The case for relatively strict boundaries in psychotherapy has been made by many writers (e.g., Epstein, 1994; Gutheil & Gabbard, 1993). Among the areas of concern, which such advocates regard as crossings or violations, in addition to the almost universally and I believe justly condemned behavior of sex with patients are: socializing with current or former patients; financial dealings with current or former patients (loans, monetary gifts, joint ventures, investment tips); mutual first name form of address; nonsexual physical contact besides a handshake; treating friends or relatives; treating relatives or friends of current or former patients; treating someone who is also a student or supervisee; asking for or accepting favors from patients (an occasional small gift is acceptable); failure to maintain consistent place where services are rendered, schedule of appointments, duration of session, and fees; therapist self-disclosure; and contact between sessions except for emergencies. I will present a number of arguments that question the conceptual framework as well as the implementation of the policies promoted by staunch boundary advocates. Many of these dictates fly in the face of common practice, various theoretical orientations, and the principles of logic. Although I will argue that much of the language and substance of boundary policy is heavily and inappropriately influenced by psycho-

dynamic thinking, many competent and ethical psychodynamic therapists disregard at least some of the above injunctions. In addition there
are a number of moderate voices that do not merely pay lip service to
impartiality but bring a genuinely balanced perspective to the complexity and the contextual aspects of potential problems associated with
therapists' professional conduct (e.g., Bersoff, 1999; J. Lazarus, 1994).

THE ARGUMENTS

There are two broad views in opposition to boundaries, the categorical
or qualitative, and the dimensional or quantitative. The categorical
posits that the very concept of boundaries is inimical to a human interactive process and precludes genuineness, authenticity, and therefore
an optimal therapeutic alliance. The dimensional, or quantitative, view
accepts the boundary concept but questions where the barrier should
be placed and how flexible it should be (e.g., small gifts are all right,
large aren't; occasional therapist personal disclosures are, but not sexual
disclosures; maintain strict boundaries with borderline, psychotic and
anti-social patients, but not others). The following encompasses what
I consider to be some of the basic arguments against and concerns
about the prevalent boundary positions. These points are not entirely
discrete; there is a degree of overlap among them.

Humanists tend to argue that the very notion of boundaries embraces
the distance model and poses a barrier to intimacy. Greenspan (1995)
states, "I am a great believer in the art of therapist self-disclosure as a
way of deconstructing the isolation and shame that people experience
in an individualistic and emotion-fearing culture. When strict boundaries are used as the litmus test of professional ethical behavior, this
art—and therapist authenticity in general—can appear dangerous" (p.
53). This view stands in sharp contrast to that, for example, of Epstein
and Simon (1990) who underscore that throughout the course of treatment, maintaining boundaries is a continual struggle for any conscientious psychotherapist.

Anonymity and neutrality inhibit the patient's growth and the therapist's effectiveness. A boundary represents a limit, a set of conditions,
a barrier between people, and while there are no unconditional adult
relationships, an orientation that starts from a position of intimacy and
openness to any approach that could help patients is apt to be more
facilitative than an orientation that starts with "anonymity," contracts,
and boundaries. Once you are oriented toward boundaries, you are

inevitably going to be looking for "crossings," which then will sometimes lead to "violations," which are tantamount to abuse. It is a fundamental question *where a therapist stands on the patient-therapist distance spectrum.* I think that we need more emphasis on closeness rather than distance, on intimacy rather than boundaries or barriers to intimacy. I believe that the argument that intimacy is fostered by the therapist's anonymity is spurious.

Therapy without preconditions and restrictions allows the therapist to do whatever might be necessary to help patients. Ethics is not in the boundaries; it is more comprehensively in the way you treat a suffering or struggling human being—your ability and willingness to act in a caring, empathic, competent and nonexploitive manner. When residents sound sanitized or distant or neutral in their interactions with patients, I ask, "Is that how a human being talks?" or "How do you think you might feel if you were on the receiving end of that communication?"

It is well-known, as documented particularly by Goffman (1961), that one of the characteristics of institutions in general, and psychiatric institutions in particular, is the sharp boundaries between staff and patients. In general the higher your position in the administrative structure, the farther removed you are from the patients and the less you know about them. When I was a resident, it was recognized that if you needed sensitive information about an inpatient, you were more likely to get it from the staff members who were lower in the administrative hierarchy and more real to the patients than from the doctors or nurses. Vital information was often provided by nurses aides, who tended to be more open and informal with patients than the rest of the staff, who made more of patients' resistance to being helped than therapists' resistance to intimacy and novel treatments (Lazarus & Fay, 1982).

The purpose of ethical guidelines is to discourage behavior that is or may be inimical to the welfare of patients, but restrictions on behavior that is not inherently toxic or exploitive will curtail therapeutic possibilities. What does a therapist do if his or her policies and procedures are not working with a given patient? It seems self-evident that if an approach is not working, it is important to try something else. If an impasse might be broken and a successful outcome would be more likely if the therapist were on a first-name basis with a patient or moved the venue of therapy to a cafeteria, would it be justified? Is it not obvious that sometimes the adherence to prescribed standards of conduct could actually be depriving patients of treatment options that are essential for them? A major error on the part of many boundary-oriented thinkers is that *much of what they consider to be violating a boundary is actually the application of a technique in another model of therapy.* One of the problems in our field is that when an approach doesn't work, we tend to apply what strategic therapists call first order solutions—more of the same, instead of thinking outside of the box. In my view it is better to be solution- (result) oriented than method oriented. A central tenet of strict bound- ary proponents is the importance of defining and maintaining the therapeutic frame (e.g., Gruenberg, 2001), whereas strategic therapists suggest that this practice is often the very problem in nonresponsive patients (e.g., Watzlawick, Weakland, & Fisch, 1974).

There is a difference between what is unethical and what an individual or a group believes to be unethical. I used to serve as a member of a committee with someone who frequently opined that a position with which he disagreed was "unethical." It is important in my view to avoid the Humpty Dumpty fallacy, expressed in the often-quoted line from Lewis Caroll's *Through The Looking Glass,* " . . . when I use a word, it means just what I choose it to mean—neither more nor less."

Many psychoanalysts in good faith and with benevolent motive, com- ing from an orientation that places great emphasis on sexuality and transference, ask patients about their masturbation fantasies and about their sexual feelings toward the therapist. In the absence of sexual problems, I regard such questions as intrusive, and were I boundary- oriented, I would declare them to be "boundary violations."

The field of psychotherapy, for better or worse, is not monolithic. It is my contention that the assertion "Behavior X is a boundary violation" is meaningless without specifying the labeler and his or her definition. One of the most serious problems with the prevailing boundary position is that it reflects a marked psychodynamic bias. It often makes a critical difference when a patient receives more from the therapist than is agreed upon, for example, going over the time in a particular session. If the patient is bearing his or her soul and feels that we care, is it gratifying an infantile neurotic wish if we go over time? Or does it have to reflect our need for approval, our grandiose rescue fantasies, or masochism? Many of these notions are based on the psychodynamic idea that is desirable to frustrate patients and on the universality of resistance and the centrality of transference. This leads to the error of universalizing the applicability of the model rather than embracing an eclectic approach that will address as fully as possible the patient's legitimate need to be helped. Therefore it stands to reason that a code of ethics would allow for not only diverse but even mutually exclusive views of what are permissible and impermissible behaviors.

At about the time I was starting to work on this chapter I participated in a case discussion at the New York Academy of Medicine with a psychoanalyst. Because the large majority of the audience was psychodynamically oriented, by way of introduction I said that some of my suggested interventions might sound unusual, even bizarre or unethical, unless one were conversant with learning theory and techniques derived from the specific learning models. As an example, I mentioned that recently a resident and I had taken a patient, his sister, and their elderly parents into the clinic bathroom where we all put our hands in the toilet bowl. I explained that if one is familiar with the techniques of flooding, response prevention, participant modeling, prompting, and shaping, the approach is not only rational but standard practice—indeed, the nonpharmacological therapy of choice for Obsessive Compulsive Disorder.

Because the concept of transference is central to the psychoanalytic model, an analyst who knowingly compromises or vitiates the model, for example, by revealing personal details about his or her life, would be acting unethically. On the other hand, the attempt to characterize therapist self-disclosure as unethical is probably the single most egregious error made by the boundary advocates. It results from a profound misunderstanding of learning-based therapy and an ignorance of the power of the technique to enhance the therapy relationship, promote higher patient self-esteem, and facilitate the acquisition and disinhibition of adaptive behavior through the modeling effect. To cite but one example of the strong psychodynamic bias in the writings of boundary advocates, the following is taken from the *Ethics Primer of the American Psychiatric Association* (2001), which is being distributed without charge to all psychiatric residents: "Even psychiatrists not practicing analysis recognized that telling patients about themselves sometimes had the effect of burdening the patient with the doctor's own problems. This tended to add a separate component to the professional relationship, an additional element of the patient becoming a caregiver" (pp. 4–5). An example is then provided of a psychiatrist who discloses to the patient that he also had difficulty getting along with his father. "The patient may hear this in a way that suggests that the doctor is even more flawed than the patient feels himself to be, thus decreasing the rapport" (Gruenberg, 2001, p. 5). It is difficult to imagine that a clinician experienced in therapeutic self-disclosure would find this example credible. Of course the patient *may* hear anything, and there certainly are emotionally needy therapists, but it seems unlikely that he would think the therapist *more* flawed on the basis of the statement in the example. If the patient did hear it in the suggested way, is that necessarily untoward? Therapists skilled at self-disclosure often deliberately attempt to show the patient that they themselves are defective and in some instances, even more defective than the patient. Finally, it is assumed that rapport would be decreased, another tenuous assumption that runs counter to humanistic, behavioral, strategic, and transactional models of therapy. As with most psychotherapy techniques, the precise disclosure, the rationale, how it is conveyed, and individual patient response characteristics are important. With regard to patient misinterpretation, relationships in general involve misattributions that are corrected with further experience and testing. An integral part of therapy is to correct misperceptions and misattributions about people and events in the world. If a patient thought that the therapist might be using him emotionally, or making an inappropriate overture, and then there was no follow-up, subsequent opportunities were ignored, and the therapeutic rationale was evident, even greater levels of trust would be fostered. It seems to me that the more the patients know the real person of the therapist, the more likely it is that trust will develop—trust not merely to avoid exploiting them, but to take active steps to help them. Telling a patient that I occasionally take a beta blocker before giving a lecture and how effective it is has more immediacy than if I quote the literature or clinical experience with other patients. In this instance I have knowledge of the field, clinical experience, and personal experience. It destigmatizes the patient and promotes higher self-esteem and greater intimacy. I have not had evidence that patients' respect for me or my credibility has been compromised by self-disclosure.

Gutheil and Gabbard (1993) provide another example of misunderstanding and bias: "However, when a therapist begins to indulge in even the mildest forms of self-disclosure, it is an indication for careful self-scrutiny regarding the motivations for departure from the usual therapeutic stance" (p. 190). "Usual therapeutic stance" means "rigid psychodynamic stance." The "mildest form of self-disclosure" does not deviate significantly from the way that most nonpsychodynamic therapists and many psychodynamic therapists practice. The authors' strong psychodynamic orientation is further reflected in other quotes from the same paper on boundaries. "Almost all patients who enter into a psychotherapeutic process struggle with the unconscious wish to view the therapist as the ideal parent who, unlike the real parents will gratify all their childhood wishes" (p. 191). After conceding that "Therapists may occasionally use a neutral example from their own lives to illustrate a point," Gutheil and Gabbard go on to say, "the therapist's revelations, however, of personal fantasies or dreams; of social, sexual, or financial details; of specific vacation plans; or of expected births or deaths in the family is usually burdening the patient with information" (p. 194). No evidence is given to support this assertion. There is, in fact, evidence to the contrary, that is, that therapist self-disclosure is facilitative in the therapy process (Barrett & Berman, 2001; Knox, Hess, Peterson, & Hill, 1997). A recent review of the subject concludes with the following statement: "The therapist's intentional self-disclosure is an essential, valuable therapeutic tool that deepens the therapeutic conversation and relationship and leads to unexpected, growth-fostering opportunities" (Bridges, 2001, p. 29).

Borys and Pope (1989) in a study of therapists' attitudes and practices with respect to boundaries, concluded that because psychodynamic therapists are more concerned about and more observant of traditional boundaries, they have a "greater awareness of the importance of clear, nonexploitive and therapeutically oriented roles, boundaries, and tasks, as well as of the subtle but far-reaching consequences of violating these norms. . . . Furthermore, psychodynamic training, with its attention to the needs, motives and desires of the therapist, may better enable its practitioners to recognize and avoid exploitive relationships that advance the welfare or pleasure of the therapist at the expense of the client" (p. 290). Thus, the difference in responses between psychodynamic and other therapists is attributed not to a legitimate difference in philosophy but to a difference in the quality of their training. I think the evidence is compelling that we must construct standards of conduct that transcend any particular theoretical model in order to legitimize pluralism in the field and help as many patients as possible. Whether a behavior is or is not unethical depends on several factors that are often ignored but in my view are critical to a rational determination.

To reiterate, it is a fallacy to declare behavior per se unethical. This argument may be summarized in one short sentence: Context is everything. The operative ethical issues are exploitation and harm, not behavior itself. The attempt to interdict therapist behavior independent of therapist motivation (to help or exploit), therapist competence, therapeutic rationale (desensitization, behavioral practice, disrupting an interpersonal game transaction, modeling), patient satisfaction, effects on the patient-therapist relationship, and outcome places a heavy burden on advocates of such interdiction.

There are several accepted definitions of the term "ethics." One refers to a general or universal standard of moral conduct; another refers to the standards of conduct of a group or culture; and a third involves the individual's concept of right or wrong. The rigid boundary advocates say the problem is mainly in the behavior and not in the situation. I think the problem is not in the behavior, except when violating the universal definition of ethics involving exploitation, for example, encouraging or pressuring a patient to do something that is purely for the therapist's benefit and to the patient's detriment. The practice of categorizing, judging, or demonizing practitioners who don't act in a specified way is not healthy for the profession. Encouraging evidence-based practice and discouraging exploitation is important, but imposing bias-driven policies is in no one's interest. With rare exceptions, anyone who makes ethical pronouncements about a therapist's behavior without knowing the therapist, the patient, or the context is either extraordinarily gifted or grandiose. Some writers on the subject of professional ethics have difficulty distinguishing the behavior from the context and the consequences. What I think is worse is that without knowing the therapist, the patient, or the particular model of therapy that is being practiced, they make a determination for both about what is appropriate or inappropriate, ethical or unethical, therapeutic or destructive. To decide in advance that there is a problem or an unacceptable risk of a problem does not deal with the realities and the exigencies of life, relationships, or therapy.

When boundary proponents acknowledge the therapeutic possibility or even necessity of crossing their designated boundaries, such instances are deemed exceptions that should be carefully documented. We are talking about two categories of therapist responses. The first is the class of responses that *is* standard, but in a nonpsychodynamic framework, for example, in vivo exposure. The second category refers to novel responses that are generally linked to a theoretical model, but are idiographic—designed for the particular patient. Unfortunately, in the current climate there can be a hundred favorable outcomes with novel interventions, but one untoward incident, whether or not it is related to the intervention, can spell ruin for the practitioner.

Many boundary proponents have appropriated the almost hackneyed phrase in the Hippocratic Oath, "first do no harm." This in my opinion is an example of taking part of a message out of context and then concretizing it, treating it as if it were literally true. The primary message is "Whatever house I may enter, I will come for the benefit of the sick." The rest of the sentence is " . . . and will abstain from every voluntary act of mischief and corruption . . . "

There is no such thing as a medical intervention and perhaps not any human action that is not associated with risk. The ethical imperative is to act competently and in the best interest of the patient and not to exploit him or her. With rare exceptions, *a rational recommendation cannot be made about the ethical status of an action without knowing not only the potential risks, but also the potential benefits, the risks of not taking the action and the benefits of refraining from the behavior.* I believe that the strict boundary position is clearly defective in this regard. The potential harm of the boundary posture is stagnation, prolonged suffering, and great expense for the identified patient and his or her social network. When crossing some traditional boundaries in the quest of being more helpful, it is best to inquire, "Are *these* risks justified?" You cannot "do no harm." We can actually *do* harm in the attempt to avoid harm. You can prevent or deter intentional harm and negligent harm. You can be careful not to take unnecessary risks. But you cannot "do no harm." You cannot even "first do no harm" because you would be eliminating some of the most promising therapeutic modalities. The potential harm in imposing boundaries on patients is grossly underweighted as are the potential benefits of ignoring or crossing those boundaries. In my view, the *ethical duty to help* by any available, feasible, and lawful means is central to the Hippocratic legacy.

The notorious "slippery slope" argument, which is an extension of the predicate logic solecism, has been discussed in several chapters. It proposes that because therapists who have sex with patients usually start with "boundary crossings," such as using first names—then proceed to personal disclosures, a shared meal, and touching—therapists who are on a first-name basis or who self-disclose are at risk. The argument defies the laws of logic (Fay, 1995), and the notion that sexual behavior is more likely following such therapist activity is unsupported by the data, according to Schoener (2001), who specializes in the rehabilitation of therapist sexual offenders.

VIGNETTES: A PERSONAL ODYSSEY

The following clinical vignettes are meant to illustrate many of the points made earlier. They are taken mainly from my own private practice abut also from the experiences during my residency training, from my personal life, from my supervisory work with residents, and from the experience of colleagues. The particular cases were selected to demonstrate as starkly as possible the contrast with strict boundary views. Although a few of the presentations are more extensive, most are fragmentary, describing a single interaction. Most of the therapeutic interventions had a rationale in well-recognized psychological principles, but the form in which they were expressed reflects idiographic and in some cases sui generis characteristics. Several of the responses might have occurred once or twice in a professional lifetime.

It is clear that although a few of my interactions with patients were unusual, many are common in psychotherapy practice but are not talked about as much as I think they should be. It is possible to criticize almost any therapist action, but were there a response that was beyond criticism, that is, absolutely safe for the patient and the therapist, it probably wouldn't be helpful to many of the patients who were prior therapy failures.

On the day I started my residency training, I was on the elevator with one of the senior residents who asked whether I was nervous. I acknowledged that I was, and she said all I had to do was remember not to answer any questions that patients might ask, and not to say anything about myself, and I would be fine. This actually proved somewhat reassuring, although I didn't have the presence of mind to wonder how this formula would be helpful to patients. This advice is in sharp contrast to my own suggestions when residents feel bewildered about what to do. I ask how they would respond to a friend with the same problem and recommend starting there. I believe that the major difference between therapy and a friendship is not so much in how the therapist acts but in what the therapist can reasonably expect from the other person.

My first patient was a 16-year-old boy who had a severe school truancy problem and a great deal of paranoid thinking. After many weeks of being in the hospital, he disappeared and everybody was concerned about him. Because I knew that when truant from school he used to go to Kennedy Airport (then called Idlewild), I decided to drive to the airport and look for him. I found him and brought him back to the hospital. This clearly illustrates the off-location and "session in the car" boundary issue. In addition, for those who might be interested, he was homosexual. Twenty years later, I was having lunch in a restaurant and as I was leaving, a voice called out to me, and although I hadn't seen him in all those years, I recognized him immediately. We had a brief conversation and I was struck by how intact he seemed.

Private Practice

A woman in her early 20s was known to me because her parents were close friends of friends of mine. When visiting her parents' home one day with my wife, I was introduced to her and couldn't help noticing how depressed she seemed. I had heard that she had not responded to a couple of years of psychotherapy and pharmacotherapy with several psychiatrists. Her family subsequently asked me to see her. She had most of the classical stigmata of depressive illness, although she was not actively suicidal. In addition she met the DSM criteria for agoraphobia. It became obvious that she had already received state-of-the-art pharmacological interventions. When I asked what her interests were or had been before she became depressed, she said, "Nothing." She couldn't think of anything that interested her, until her parents mentioned that she used to love horseback riding. I then arranged to have some of our sessions in Central Park. Since I had no idea how to ride a horse, I jogged on the bridle path while she walked the horse at the same pace. Her parents were overweight and I suggested that they join us, which they often did. In the office we had some family sessions and some individual sessions. On the occasions when a man on horseback would come from the other direction on the track I would say to her, "Smile!" At first she would manage the weakest response. However, with repeated prompting and reinforcement, the smile became more robust. We worked on assertiveness and attempted to enhance her social interactions. The treatment went on for many months in this fashion. Then, with her consent, I asked a friend of mine who had a business if he could give her a part-time job, which would allow her to work at home most of the time. This was effected and occasionally she would come to the office for short periods of time. I had recently been separated from my wife, a fact known to her because her family knew it. (If other patients would inquire if I was married or how my wife was, I would tell them.) I had two tickets for a Carnegie Hall concert, and one day, at the end of a session, with some hesitation, I said the following to her: "This is not in the 'dirty old man' category of communications, but I have two tickets to a concert for tonight. Would you like to go? It might be an opportunity for you to get out." Boundary-oriented people will regard this as outrageous but it was motivated entirely by therapeutic considerations. She agreed, and since her family's apartment was between my office and the concert hall, I picked her up in a cab. I did not go up to her apartment, as a date might, but buzzed up and she came down. She was always very anxious about any excursion outside of the apartment. Several times during the concert I asked how she was doing and she said that she was managing. Over a period of about a year and a half she made what her family considered to be a remarkable recovery. She felt well, she was working part-time, and dating. I cannot prove that she ultimately would not have recovered spontaneously without my unusual methods or even without any therapy, but I believe that the various interventions outside of the traditional therapeutic framework were necessary. With regard to the concert outing, it would have been impossible, regardless of the therapeutic potential, had I *not* known her family. I was invited to and attended her wedding a couple of years later. After more than a decade she was still well and had three children.

A patient approaching retirement age announced that she had lost 75% of her net worth in the 2000 stock market crash. The identical thing had happened to me and I shared that fact with her. It was enormously comforting, and my relative equanimity about it, I think, was helpful to her. In the next session she was viewing it realistically as a disappointment she could handle.

I have treated a number of patients for paruresis (inhibited micturition in public bathrooms). The approach to such problems is pretty straightforward in uncomplicated cases. One of the interventions that I use is sharing the fact that I had this problem myself for many years. Most people with this problem have similar cognitions and respond within a few sessions to a basic exposure approach, some cognitive work, and a few paradoxical exercises. In general, patients feel less defective when they know the therapist can relate directly to the experience.

Chronic cocaine abuse is admittedly one of the most difficult problems to treat in the present state of our knowledge. The daughter of a patient of mine, after many unsuccessful attempts at treatment, started seeing a psychiatrist who specializes in treating such patients and openly acknowledges that he himself had a major problem with cocaine in the past. He apparently has a high success rate and was more helpful to my patient's daughter than anyone else had been in the past. If a therapist's conduct were to be evaluated strictly on the basis of behavior and without regard to context, this psychiatrist's license could be revoked.

A patient whom I had known for a few years and who worked in the theatre said that if I ever wanted tickets that were difficult to get, I should let him know because he had ready access to the major shows. He was a stable, high-functioning person, we had a good relationship, he had done very well in therapy for chronic, low-grade depression, and it was clear that he had the access he said he had. As it turned out, guests were going to be visiting me from out of town in a few weeks. I asked how inconvenient it would be for him to get tickets, and he said that it wouldn't be inconvenient at all. It would involve one simple phone call and he would be delighted to do it. The tickets were left at the box office and, of course, I paid for them. Several years later there was a show I was eager to see for which there was a 1-year wait for tickets, and even though he had a direct connection with the show, I didn't ask. Had he offered, I would have accepted. I am quite certain (one can never be positive) that my asking would not have compromised his treatment in any way, but the prospect did not pass the comfort test for me.

A couple of writers have invited me to book parties on the occasion of the publication of their work, which they had been discussing in many prior sessions. It seemed reasonable that I go, and I did. The major drawback for me has been responding to a stranger's question "How do you know Vivian?" when the patient hasn't revealed that she is my patient. It is advisable to discuss this type of issue with the patient beforehand.

I was treating a woman with a lifelong history of depression. She is a talented musician, and when she was particularly depressed and questioning the purpose of living, I would sometimes call her and play a selection of magnificent classical music from a CD. Although she knew a great deal of piano literature, I enriched her repertoire by introducing her to baroque opera and renaissance music. This would often lift her spirits to a degree and also give her a better sense of the meaning of life, sustaining her until the next day or longer. I believe that this benefited her beyond the short-term effect. When I took a medical leave, I had her see a colleague who was very experienced in the cognitive-behavior therapy orientation. After I returned she continued with both of us. My colleague and I have had dinner at her home on several occasions, he with his wife and children, and I with the woman in my life at the time. She was so fond of one of my friends that they occasionally talked without my participation. Her son worked on Wall Street, and she regaled me with stories of his brilliance in investing and mentioned some of the stocks he was buying. She volunteered that it would be fine if I bought them. I bought one of them, and over a period of months, lost about $10,000. That represents a lot of session time, but I doubt if there is anyone who knows me or knows the patient or who studied our interactions who could say that either my feelings or my behavior toward this patient changed in any way. It is true she felt bad that the money was lost (she subsequently lost many times that when he had a cold streak), but I told her with absolute sincerity that she had done this with the best of intentions, that I always take full responsibility for any investment decisions I make, that stock losses occur frequently, and that I wasn't the least bit concerned about it. If anything, the relationship was strengthened by the incident rather than compromised by it. I think that when there is an opportunity for a therapist to have a negative reaction to a patient—and doesn't—the relationship is enhanced, in the same way as when the therapist has the opportunity to seduce or otherwise exploit a patient and doesn't, that relationship is also strengthened.

Many years ago, a prominent psychoanalyst referred his adolescent daughter to me. Her session was in the morning before school started. When she didn't show up for the third appointment I called the home. Her father answered the phone, and I asked for the patient, who was not home. I certainly could have and perhaps should have asked him to give her the message to call me, but since he had referred her, she was a minor living in his house, and he knew that she was seeing me, I said that I was concerned because she hadn't shown up. He was horrified, declaring that it was unethical for me to disclose that fact to him. I never saw her again.

One of my recent supervisees confided to me that she went to a pharmacy with a female patient to have her buy condoms because the patient was having unprotected sex and the resident over several sessions had not been able to persuade her to do otherwise. I felt this crossing of the "place" and the "autonomy" boundary was appropriate and maybe lifesaving.

A man in his 30s who had spent half of his life in therapy was in a profession he "hated." He wanted to try his hand at something else. When he lost his job, he decided to become a writer. He did almost nothing about it for weeks, which fueled his feelings of being unaccomplished. Although in the year we had worked together considerable progress had been made in his romantic life and in his control of anger, his frustration and dissatisfaction with his lack of self-discipline were marked. We had talked about the possibility of his writing for some time before his dismissal, but procrastination was a problem. After a few weeks, he was doing little about his professed interest. We had discussed the problem from several perspectives and I had suggested a few approaches, which he was not pursuing. During one of our sessions, I disclosed that I also had been procrastinating on a writing project and was planning to spend the coming Friday working on it in the medical school library. I asked if he thought it would be helpful if we worked together. He accepted the offer and was very productive for about 2 1/2 hours. He started writing more thereafter, though hardly prolifically. Two months later, he was still writing more than he had been, but continued to procrastinate and feel unproductive. Another stint in the library for 2 consecutive 8-hour days was valuable for both of us. In my view, when an intervention is recommended specifically for the patient's benefit, and concomitantly benefits the therapist, it is not a problem. I didn't make the recommendation because I needed him to help me. The patient himself observed that there were two helpful elements, working with someone else present, and working in a different location. The techniques were participant modeling and stimulus control. In his apartment there were many distractions, and he came to associate the apartment with failure, frustration, and self-denigration. At the end of the 2-day stint, he decided to look for another writer who might join him at a neighborhood library (generalization). Although the library experience was therapeutic, it was not therapy in the sense that I did my work and he did his, although at one point he asked me to listen to a plot outline he had constructed (reinforcement). There was of course no charge.

One of the questions raised by some of the vignettes is whether it is necessary to have many problems, such as procrastination, social anxiety, divorces, paruresis and God knows what else in order to help patients? In my view it is necessary not to be perfect and it is particularly desirable not to be perfect in the eyes of your patients. It can be most helpful to use the resources you have, your talents (maybe knowledge of some area of interest to the patient), *and* your limitations.

WHAT TO DO ABOUT THE PROBLEM?

If boundaries are not the answer to ethical problems in the practice of psychotherapy, what is? Some of the suggestions listed below were discussed at the recent American Psychiatric Association Annual Meeting in 2001.

1. Better screening of applicants for psychotherapy programs. Grade point averages and Graduate Record Exam scores are still the main criteria for admission to most graduate programs. Evaluation of moral development through more extensive interviewing, formal assessment instruments, and possibly even criminal background checks might be helpful. One of the freshmen in my medical school class had been admitted on the basis of a forged transcript and was exposed when he became involved in other antisocial acts. It has always been my impression, in any case, that academic performance is not positively correlated with moral development.

2.   Better exposure to ethical issues for medical students, psychiatric residents, and psychotherapy trainees. Conduct classes devoted to professional ethics, emphasizing case histories and discussion in addition to or even instead of didactic lectures. Focus more on challenging problems and practical management than on risk avoidance.

3.   Requirement of annual continuing education credits in professional ethics for practitioners. Encourage therapists to take an Epstein and Simon-like self-assessment test (exploitation index, 1990), only without the psychodynamically biased questions.

4.   Publicize the importance of ethical practice to consumers, encouraging patients to ask their therapists or others about the meaning of or rationale for particular interventions. Caution them about exploitation, not arbitrary boundaries.

5.   Discuss ethical dilemmas and unusual interventions with colleagues. Many practitioners work alone, and experienced clinicians rarely see other professionals for supervision. Collegial interactions are stimulating and also help keep perspective.

CONCLUSION

It is my contention that what could be called the modern boundary movement began as a well-meaning attempt to restore the reputation of psychotherapy as an ethical calling but has become a runaway train propelled by psychodynamic ideologies, which have wielded enormous influence at the expense of more eclectic practitioners and their patients. Nonpsychodynamic approaches to boundary issues are marginalized if not delegitimized, in keeping with the continuing practice of using the term psychotherapy as synonymous with psychodynamic therapy. At a time when eclecticism, multimodalism, and integrationism have substantial support, program accreditation committees are requiring that trainees demonstrate proficiency in several modalities of treatment, and research data are supporting not only the power of the patient-therapist relationship, but the value of specific prescriptive approaches in effecting favorable outcomes for patients, some of the older views are untenable. Psychodynamic therapy is not the standard of care, and a code of ethics derived from that model cannot reasonably be imposed on the entire professional community. In addition, many patients fail to respond to standard interventions and are entitled to nonmainstream or novel treatments. Many influential writers on the subject of ethics and boundaries have ignored findings from other orientations, common clinical experience, research data, and principles of logic. Risk-benefit characteristics have been grossly distorted, therapist behavior that is incompatible with psychodynamic orthodoxy is ethically disparaged and pathologized, regardless of the benefit or potential benefit to patients. Normal human responses to patients are also pathologized. The judgment of skilled, experienced clinicians is superseded by a biased set of ethical standards. The disproportionate emphasis on pathology over adaptive capacities of patients, a view of patients as inherently more disturbed, less competent, and universally resistant—always looking to gratify their infantile wishes and test limits—has always troubled me. In a profession characterized by pluralism, it is important to seek a more encompassing standard of conduct, as well as programs, to address the serious issues of exploitation and unnecessary risk. The duty to help the patient is as important as the duty not to wrong the patient.

REFERENCES

Barrett, M. S., & Berman, J. S. (2001). Is psychotherapy more effective when therapists disclose information about themselves? *Journal of Consulting and Clinical Psychology, 69,* 597–604.

Bersoff, D. N. (Ed.). (1999). *Ethical conflicts in psychology.* Washington, DC: American Psychological Association.

Borys, D. S., & Pope, K. S. (1989). Dual relationships between therapist and client: A national study of psychologists, psychiatrists, and social workers. *Professional Psychology: Research and Practice, 20,* 283–293.

Bridges, N. A. (2001). Therapist's self-disclosure: Expanding the comfort zone. *Psychotherapy, 38,* 21–30.

Epstein, R. S. (1994). *Keeping boundaries.* Washington, DC: American Psychiatric Press.

Epstein, R. S., & Simon, R. I. (1990). The exploitation index: An early warning indicator of boundary violations in psychotherapy. *Bulletin of the Menninger Clinic, 54,* 450–465.

Fay, A. (1995). Boundaries in the physician-patient relationship (Letter). *Journal of the American Medical Association, 274,* 1347–1348.

Gabbard, G. O., & Nadelson, C. (1995). Professional boundaries in the physician-patient relationship. *Journal of the American Medical Association, 273* (18), 1445–1449.

Goffman, E. (1961). *Asylums.* New York: Anchor.

Greenspan, M. (1995). Out of Bounds. *Common Boundary Magazine, July/August,* 51–56.

Gruenberg, P. B. (2001). Boundary violations. *Ethics primer of the American Psychiatric Association*. Washington, DC: American Psychiatric Association.

Gutheil, T. G., & Gabbard, G. O. (1993). The concept of boundaries in clinical practice: Theoretical and risk-management dimensions. *American Journal of Psychiatry, 150,* 188–196.

Heyward, C. (1993). *When boundaries betray us.* Cleveland: The Pilgrim Press.

Knox, S., Hess, S. A., Peterson, D. A., & Hill, C. E. (1997). A qualitative analysis of client perceptions of the effects of helpful therapist self-disclosure in long-term therapy. *Journal of Counseling Psychology, 44,* 274–283.

Lazarus, A. A. (1994). How certain boundaries and ethics diminish therapeutic effectiveness. *Ethics & Behavior, 4* (3), 255–306.

Lazarus, A. A., & Fay, A. (1982). Resistance or rationalization? A cognitive-behavioral perspective. In P. A. Wachtel (Ed.), *Resistance.* New York: Plenum Press.

Lazarus, J. A. (1994). Ethics. *American Psychiatric Association Review of Psychiatry, 13,* 319.

Schoener, G. R. (2001, May 8). Preventative and remedial boundaries training: Effective tools and methods. *154th American Psychiatric Association Annual Meeting.* New Orleans.

Watzlawick, P., Weakland, J. H., & Fisch, R. (1974). *Change: Principles of problem formation and problem resolution.* New York: Norton.

Laws, Boards, Ethics, and Other Forensic Matters

Part 4 covers the issues pertaining to legal, constitutional, and ethical matters and the complexities of dealing with ethics committees, civil lawsuits, and licensing boards. Chapter 12 commences with Ebert's scholarly legal challenge, on constitutional grounds, of the prohibition of any kind of dual relationships. Ebert asserts that the prohibition, besides being too vague and too broad, also violates therapists' and clients' constitutional rights of privacy and freedom of association. In chapter 13, Saunders exposes the irony that while licensing boards bear down on therapists who engage in dual relationships, they are engaged in unethical multiple roles as they serve as prosecutor, police, judge, jury, and (professional) executioner. He then gives a chilling report of several vindictive boards who ignored courts' decisions and pursued complaints against blameless therapists who had been found innocent by the courts. In chapter 14, Williams exposes the fallacious logic that all multiple relationships are unethical and how the demonization of dual relationships has constrained therapeutic effectiveness and harmed decent and honest therapists who face unjust accusations in front of misinformed boards and courts. In chapter

15 Lazarus discusses, among other things, posttreatment friendships, totalitarianism, and the defenseless psychologist. Chapter 16 explains the intricacies of board investigations and civil lawsuits against therapists, and Fleer exposes how well-meaning therapists can be harmed by vengeful clients and greedy attorneys. Chapter 16 discusses some legal benchmarks for social dual relationships as Scheflin outlines their positive effects on therapeutic alliance and trust.

CHAPTER 12

Dual-Relationship Prohibitions

A Concept Whose Time Never Should Have Come

Bruce W. Ebert, PhD, JD, ABPP

In 1977 the American Psychological Association (APA) created a prohibition against dual relationships that were exploitative (APA, 1977). The designation of dual relationships as an ethical problem first appeared in Principle eight (8) of the Ethical Standards of Psychologists in the category called Client Relationships (APA, 1958). Later (APA, 1977) the prohibition against entering dual relationships by a psychologist appeared in Principle six (6), called the Welfare of the Consumer. The exact same language of the 1977 Ethics Code appeared in the 1979 revision of the APA Code (APA, 1979). The primary reason to label exploitative dual relationships as unethical, in my opinion, was to attempt to prevent therapists from engaging in sexual relations with their clients. Initially the term was introduced to attempt to prohibit psychologists from providing clinical services to friends, family members, associates, and others such that the client's welfare may be jeopard-

Reprinted by permission. Ebert, B. W. (1997). Dual relationship prohibitions: A concept whose time never should have come. *Applied & Preventive Psychology, 6*, 137–156.

ized by the clinical relationship (APA, 1958). The actual and direct prohibition against sexual contact with a client followed the term "dual relationship" by 19 years. The first actual prohibition against sexual relations with a client appeared in the Ethical Standards of Psychologists in 1977 (APA, 1977). There was no reference to dual relationships in the first ethical code promulgated by the American Psychological Association (1953). Although the ethical principle of competence was recognized in Principle 1.3 in the 1953 ethical principles (APA, 1953), the notation of dual or multiple relationships took an additional 5 years to make its way into the APA Ethics Code. There were antecedent principles to prohibitions on dual and multiple relationships, however. These involved relationships that presented a conflict of interest or caused harm to a client. Consider Principle 2.22–2: "The misuse of the clinical or consulting relationship for profit, for power or prestige, or for personal gratifications not consonant with the concern for the welfare of the client, is unethical" (APA, 1953, p. 51). Also consider Principle 2.21–1, which provided:

> A cardinal obligation of the clinical or consulting psychologist is to respect the integrity and protect the welfare of the person with whom he is working. Vigilant regard for this principle should characterize all of the work of the psychologist and pervade all his personal relationships. (APA, 1953, p. 49)

From these principles of 1953 came prohibitions of dual relationships (APA, 1958), followed eventually by prohibitions of multiple-role relationships (APA, 1992). But the forgotten aspect of these prohibitions is that only those multiple-role relationships that are harmful to or against the interests of the client are prohibited. Only those types of role relationships that cause or are likely to cause harm should be prohibited. In addition, the rule was designed to prohibit therapists from taking advantage of their clients through nonsexual dual relationships.

Dual relationships refer to circumstances in which there are multiple-role relationships extant between the therapist and the client, such as when the therapist is sexually involved with a client.

During the past few years, there have been numerous articles written on the subject of dual relationships. These articles have provided significant advances in the conceptual understanding of dual-relationship issues. Some authors have focused on state licensing board actions regarding dual relationships (Bader, 1994; Gottlieb, Sell, & Schoenfield, 1988), some have explored general ethical issues (Youngren & Skorka, 1992), whereas others have identified unique problems such as avoiding dual relationships in a rural area (Jennings, 1992). Some have argued that the prohibitions against dual relationships have gone too far (Clarkson, 1994). It is clear that dual relationships are prevalent and present a significant problem for mental health professionals (Borys & Pope, 1989).

There is a need for an analytical model to use in evaluating dual or multiple-role relationships that balances constitutional rights of both clients and therapists and serves to protect consumers of psychological services. The rules surrounding dual relationships must be constitutionally sound, protect the interests of the client, but not be overly restrictive to psychologists. Dual-relationship rules must not impede a psychologist's ability to perform optimum work with a client.

In 1981, the APA Revised Code of Ethics included the prohibitions against some types of dual relationships under Principle 6: Welfare of the Consumer (APA, 1981). The American Psychological Association (1992) promulgated a new set of ethical standards and rules of conduct. Principle E provides: "Psychologists are sensitive to the real and ascribed differences between themselves and others, and they do not exploit or mislead other people during or after professional relationships" (p. 1600). Standard 1.17 was written to address the problem of multiple-role relationships (APA, 1992). The purpose of including prohibitions against dual relationships under Principle 6, Principle E, and Standard 1.17 was twofold: to emphasize protection of consumers who use psychological services from abuses resulting from the theoretical inequality of power that exists in the psychotherapist-patient relationship and to guide psychologists who may have psychological blindspots that may cause them to make errors in judgment. Principle 6 of the APA Code of Ethics provided:

> Psychologists respect the integrity and protect the welfare of the people and groups with whom they work. When conflicts of interest arise between clients and psychologists' employing institutions, psychologists clarify the nature and direction of their loyalties and responsibilities and keep all parties informed of their commitments. Psychologists fully inform consumers as to the purpose and nature of an evaluative, treatment, educational, or training procedure, and they freely acknowledge that clients, students, or participants in research have freedom of choice with regard to participation. (APA, 1981, p. 636)

The Preamble to both the 1981 and 1992 codes contains general consumer-protection language creating an ethical obligation for psychologists not to engage in behavior that would adversely affect the client and to act in ways that promote the best interests of the client

(APA, 1981, 1992). It is both a prohibition and an interpersonal guide. The Preamble of both codes creates a duty to be aware of actual conflicts of interest as well as potential conflicts. Once a conflict is recognized there is a duty to fully disclose, the idea being that full disclosure provides the client with information such that an informed choice can be made regarding whether to proceed with psychological services.

Parts of Principle E and Standard 1.17 (APA, 1992) deal with exploitation, undue influence, and control of client behavior by a psychologist operating from a position of power. They are designed to prevent a psychologist from using the influential position as therapist to take advantage of a client, resulting in client harm and therapist gain at the expense of the client. It should be noted that not all dual relationships are prohibited, nor was there an intent to prohibit all such relationships. Further, not all dual relationships are necessarily bad and not all can be avoided. In fact one type of dual relationship, billing clients, is often to the detriment of the client and is considered acceptable. No one has suggested that billing clients or allowing them to make payments is unethical, although the practice creates a dual relationship (e.g., therapist-client; debtor-creditor). Further, collection efforts by therapists may be quite detrimental to the client. Despite the great potential for harm when a client's bill is sent to a collection agent or filing a lawsuit against him or her for nonpayment, the profession has avoided discussion of this type of dual relationship, thereby communicating tacit approval for it.

The plain language of the new APA Code does not call for prohibitions of all dual relationships. Many authors have argued for a broad interpretation of the Principles and Standards that prohibit dual relationships (Pope & Vasquez, 1991). Their influence has been felt in a wide range of settings from disciplinary actions by regulatory boards to ethics committee decisions. Not only are dual-relationship prohibitions applied to cases in which the therapist engages in sexual contact or enters a business relationship with a client, but they now apply to cases far beyond what was conceived by the original authors of the prohibition or beyond what is an appropriate ethical standard. There appears to be a misunderstanding of the reasons for the prohibition. Although APA's newly proposed ethical principles are better than those in the past, they do not resolve many of the problems of determining which dual/multiple relationships are unethical. The new Code includes dual-relationship prohibitions under Principles 1.14 et seq. The relevant provisions in addition to Standard 1.17 are shown in Table 12.1 along with a depiction of the evolution of the concept of dual relationship.

TABLE 12.1 APA Ethics Codes @ 1953, '58, '77, '81, and '92, by the APA. Reprinted or adapted with permission.

**1953 ETHICS CODE

Principle 2.22-2:

"The misuse of the clinical or consulting relationship for profit, for power or prestige, or for personal gratifications not consonant with the concern for the welfare of the client is unethical" (APA, 1953 at page 51).

Principle 2.21-1 which provided:

"A cardinal obligation of the clinical or consulting psychologist is to respect the integrity and protect the welfare of the person with whom he is working. Vigilant regard for this principle should characterize all of the work of the psychologist and pervade all his personal relationships" (APA, 1953 at page 49).

1958 ETHICS CODE

Principle 8: Client Relationship

8(c) Psychologists do not normally enter into a clinical relationship with members of their own family, intimate friends, close associates, students, or others whose welfare might be jeopardized by such a dual relationship.

1977 ETHICS CODE

Principle 6: Welfare of the Consumer

Psychologists respect the integrity and protect the welfare of the people and groups with whom they work. When there is a conflict of interest between the client and the psychologist's employing institution, psychologists clarify the nature and direction of their loyalties and responsibilities and keep all parties informed of their commitments. Psychologists fully inform consumers as to the purpose and nature of an evaluative, treatment, educational or training procedure, and they freely acknowledge that clients, students or participants in research have freedom of choice with regard to participation.

a. Psychologists are continually cognizant of their own needs and of their inherently powerful position vis-à-vis clients, in order to avoid exploiting their trust and dependency. Psychologists make every effort to avoid dual relationships with clients and/ or relationships which might impair their professional judgment or increase the risk of client exploitation. Examples of such dual relationships include treating employees, supervisees, close friends or relatives. Sexual intimacies with clients are unethical.

b. Where demands of an organization on psychologists go beyond reasonable conditions of employment, psychologists recognize possible conflicts of interest that may arise. When such conflicts occur, psychologists clarify the nature of the conflict and inform all parties of the nature and direction of the loyalties and responsibilities involved.

(continued)

TABLE 12.1   *(continued)*

c. When acting as a supervisor, trainer, researcher, or employer, psychologists accord informed choice, confidentiality, due process, and protection from physical and mental harm to their subordinates in such relationships.

d. Financial arrangements in professional practice are in accord with professional standards that safeguard the best interests of the client and that are clearly understood by the client in advance of billing. Psychologists are responsible for assisting clients in finding needed services in those instances where payment of the usual fee would be a hardship. No commission, rebate, or other form of remuneration may be given or received for referral of clients for professional services, whether by an individual or by an agency. Psychologists willingly contribute a portion of their services to work for which they receive little or no financial return.

e. The psychologist attempts to terminate a clinical or consulting relationship when it is reasonably clear that the consumer is not benefitting from it. Psychologists who find that their services are being used by employers in a way that is not beneficial to the participants or to employees who may be affected, or to significant others, have the responsibility to make their observations known to the responsible persons and to propose modification or termination of the engagement.

1981 ETHICS CODE

Principle 6: Welfare of the Consumer

Psychologists respect the integrity and protect the welfare of the people and groups with whom they work. When conflict of interest arises between the client and the psychologists' employing institutions, psychologists clarify the nature and direction of their loyalties and responsibilities and keep all parties informed of their commitments. Psychologists fully inform consumers as to the purpose and nature of an evaluative, treatment, educational or training procedure, and they freely acknowledge that clients, students or participants in research have freedom of choice with regard to participation.

a. Psychologists are continually cognizant of their own needs and of their potentially influential position vis-à-vis persons such as clients, students and subordinates. They avoid exploiting the trust and dependency of such persons. Psychologists make every effort to avoid dual relationships that could impair their professional judgment or increase the risk of exploitation. Examples of such dual relationships include, but are not limited to, research with and treatment of employees, students, supervisees, close friends or relatives. Sexual intimacies with clients are unethical.

b. When a psychologist agrees to provide services to a client at the request of a third party, the psychologist assumes the responsibility of clarifying the nature of the relationships to all parties concerned.

c. Where the demands of an organization require psychologists to violate these Ethical Principles, psychologists clarify the nature of the conflict between the demands and these principles. They inform all parties of psychologists' ethical responsibilities and take appropriate action.

TABLE 12.1 *(continued)*

d. Psychologists make advance financial arrangements that safeguard the best interest of and are clearly understood by their clients. They neither give nor receive any remuneration for referring clients for professional services. They contribute a portion of their services to work for which they receive little or no financial return.

c. Psychologists terminate a clinical or consulting relationship when it is reasonably clear that the consumer is not benefitting from it. They offer to help the consumer locate alternative sources of assistance.

1992 ETHICS CODE

1.15 Misuse of Psychologists' Influence

Because psychologists' scientific and professional judgments and actions may affect the lives of others, they are alert to and guard against personal, financial, social, organizational, or political factors that might lead to misuse of their influence.

1.17 Multiple Relationships

(a) In many communities and situations, it may not be feasible or reasonable for psychologists to avoid social or other nonprofessional contacts with persons such as patients, clients, students, supervisees, or research participants. Psychologists must always be sensitive to the potential harmful effects of other contacts on their work and on those persons with whom they deal. A psychologist refrains from entering into or promising another personal, scientific, professional, financial, or other relationship with such persons if it appears likely that such a relationship reasonably might impair the psychologist's objectivity or otherwise interfere with the psychologist's effectively performing his or her functions as a psychologist, or might harm or exploit the other party.

(b) Likewise, whenever feasible, a psychologist refrains from taking on professional or scientific obligations when pre-existing relationships would create a risk of such harm.

(c) If a psychologist finds that, due to unforeseen factors, a potentially harmful multiple relationship has arisen, the psychologist attempts to resolve it with due regard for the best interest of the affected person and maximal compliance with the Ethics Code.

1.19 Exploitative Relationships

(a) Psychologists do not exploit persons over whom they have supervisory, evaluative, or other authority, such as students, supervisees, employees, research participants, and clients or patients. (See also Standards 4.05–4.07 regarding sexual involvement with clients or patients.)

(b) Psychologists do not engage in sexual relationships with students or supervisees in training over whom the psychologist has evaluative or direct authority, because such relationships are so likely to impair judgment or be exploitative.

Specific prohibitions are present in the Code to prohibit sexual conduct with current psychotherapy patients (APA Standard 4.5). In addition, psychologists may not provide therapy to people with whom a prior sexual relationship existed (Standard 4.06). Because there is some divergence of opinion regarding sex with former patients, two options are presented in the new APA Code (Standard 4.07). The 2-year rule is offered for consideration in the new code (see Standard 4.07, APA, 1992). The rule in Standard 4.07(a) of the new APA Code (1992) provides that "Psychologists do not engage in sexual intimacies with a former therapy patient or client for at least two years after cessation or termination of professional services" (p. 1605). The interesting aspect of this proposed rule is that it is in conflict with some state statutes. For example, in California a patient may sue a therapist under Section 43.93(b) (2) of the California Civil Code (1994) if sexual contact occurs within a 2-year period from the end of treatment. The therapist is guilty of a misdemeanor if sexual contact occurs during the existence of the therapeutic relationship but is guilty of no crime if sexual contact occurs the day after, provided therapy was not terminated to engage in the sexual conduct. Similarly, in Florida, Chapter 491.0112 (Florida Civil Code, 1994) classifies sex as sexual misconduct if it occurs within the therapeutic relationship, or after, if therapy is terminated for the purpose of having sexual contact with the patient. Many states have passed similar laws.

A particularly positive step in ethical decision-making was taken by the American Psychological Association in the development of language regarding sexual intimacies with former patients. In Standard 4.07(b), several analytical factors are proposed to be used in determining whether a psychologist is acting ethically in engaging in sexual contact with a former patient 2 years after cessation of treatment.

One psychologist has identified a critical issue in reducing the harm of multiple-role relationships as that of maintaining therapeutic boundaries (Borys, 1994). It is impossible to avoid dual or multiple-role relationships with clients. This is especially true in rural settings. Suppose you engage in treatment of "Bart" to help control his oppositional, defiant behavior. You have treated him for six sessions and have developed a client-therapist relationship. After work one night, you stop at a grocery store nearby to pick up some soda, celery, corn, chicken, and a bottle of deodorant. You take your purchases to the counter and you suddenly notice that Bart is the clerk who is ringing up the purchase. You buy the food and proceed home. You now have a dual relationship: therapist-client as well as buyer-seller or customer-sales clerk. Are you unethical if you buy the food and proceed home? What happens if you buy the food this time and return with full knowledge that Bart is an employee of the store? The new APA Code attempts to deal with this problem by adding the section listed above (Standard 1.17c). Minimal or socially remote relationships are considered unlikely to violate the standard involving multiple-role relationships (APA, 1992). Unfortunately, the Code does not define minor or remote relationships.

There are many examples of dual relationships that probably cannot be avoided. Most of these are harmless dual relationships. But without specificity in ethics codes or specific interpretive cases covering most circumstances, it is difficult to know which remote or minimal relationships are problematic and which are benign. There is no current methodology of analysis to be applied to resolve multiple-role-relationship problems that can assist a practitioner in making appropriate ethical decisions. Absent such methodology, psychologists are subject to hindsight scrutiny without well-defined guiding principles.

Ethics committees act to sanction psychologists or even to expel them from membership. State licensing boards can act to remove a psychologist's license. Given the recently developed national disciplinary data bank of the Association of State and Provincial Psychology Boards, the effect of such an action can be catastrophic. Most often, state licensing boards look to the APA Ethics Committee and APA standards for guidance as to how to judge dual-relationship issues. Pope (1991) is leading the way in expanding the concepts of nonsexual dual relationships as unethical. In his book he cited several examples of dual relationships that he believes are unethical. These include: (a) treatment of a records clerk working in the same facility as the therapist, (b) socializing with a client by spending weekends at a client's beach house in which the psychologist brings his wife, (c) selling cats to clients (selling products to clients), (d) trading services between a lawyer and a psychologist, and (e) providing therapy in exchange for the client painting the therapist's house.

Pope (1991) provided a clear and accurate description of the problems with dual relationships. These include: (a) erosion/distortion of therapy; (b) conflicts of interest; (c) adverse affects on the client's rights in court; (d) not to enter other relationships, such as business, equally; (e) if allowed, the therapy would change; (f) cognitive processes affecting therapeutic outcome become adversely affected. Borys (1992) described several types of nonsexual dual relationships that are likely to create problems. Problems arise because therapeutic boundaries are shattered by therapist behavior (Borys, 1994).

PRIOR ETHICS CASES

To fully understand the actual prohibition against dual or multiple-role relationships that are exploitative, it is critically important to know how the APA Ethics Committee has dealt with actual cases through the years. This leads to a better understanding of exactly what is prohibited and what is acceptable. It is not unlike examining legal cases to ascertain how a particular statute is interpreted by the courts.

In 1982 the APA Ethics Committee reported a dual-relationship case in which a complainant, who was a pastoral counselor, was upset that a counseling psychologist did not encourage the complainant's son to seek counseling with the complainant (APA, 1982). The committee commented on the actions of the complainant but did not comment on the nonsexual dual-relationship problem raised in the scenario.

The APA (1983) and Hall and Hare-Mustin (1983) published additional information regarding dual relationships. A psychologist was given a reprimand for treating a supervisee. Another case was closed against a psychologist, without action (after receiving a complaint from the husband of a secretary), because the psychologist had a sexual relationship with his secretary. The committee report did not address the problems of such conduct with respect to dual-relationship prohibitions. Another psychologist was censured for being the minister of a client's church and her marriage counselor. There was an allegation of sexual misconduct that was not sustained. Also in 1983 were notes of four cases in which sexual allegations were brought against a psychologist (APA, 1983). The APA found the first psychologist guilty of an ethics violation for having sex with a client during therapy. The psychologist was given a 5-year stipulated resignation and required to be under close supervision. The second psychologist terminated therapy after he became attracted to his patient. Thereafter he had a 1-year sexual relationship with her. He was found to have violated Principle 6(a). He was given a 1-year stipulated resignation. The third psychologist, who wrote a sexually explicit letter to an adolescent client, was found to have patently violated the dual-relationship prohibitions. This psychologist was expelled from membership. The fourth psychologist was accused of having sexual contact with several of his supervisees. This conduct was considered unethical. The psychologist agreed to a 6-year stipulated resignation.

The committee made no comments about dual relationships in its 1984 report (APA, 1984). The only reference to dual relationships occurred in the report of cases under investigation under the category "sexual intimacy with client, dual relationship, or exploitation and/or sexual harassment" (APA, 1984, p. 672). Likewise, in 1985, there was no elucidation of the rules and regulations on dual relationships in the committee's report.

In 1986 the APA Ethics Committee further attempted to clarify the meaning of the dual-relationship prohibitions of Principle 6 of the Code. Almost as an afterthought, APA (1986) wrote "Principle 6(a) of the Ethical Principles is clear that 'dual relationships' such as *social contact* with patients are to be avoided and that sexual intimacies with patients are unethical" (p. 695). For the first time, the APA Committee took the position that social contact with current patients may be unethical. They offered no definitive opinion regarding social and sexual relations with ex-patients. Without describing the types of social contact that were considered inappropriate, the committee concluded that contact with current patients was likely to be unethical. Unfortunately, they did not clarify whether some types of social contact may be appropriate or under what circumstances social contact with a current patient may be ethical. We must only guess at the specific prohibitions.

We do not know whether the committee believes that going to lunch with a patient after the last therapy session is unethical or whether being at the same large party with a patient is considered socializing. How about going to dinner with a patient and his wife? Is having your patient and her husband over to your house for a dinner with your spouse unethical? What if you discover your patient plays on the same softball league as you do? Is it socializing to play on the opposing team?

Should going to lunch with a patient be in the same category as using cocaine with that same patient? These questions remain unanswered. Although it is easy to use common sense and reason to conclude it would be an unethical dual relationship to use illegal drugs with your client, it is more difficult to apply common sense to other situations. The absence of an analytical model leaves these questions subject to inquisitional-type justice when such problems are brought to the attention of ethics committees. Further, there is no guidance for the professional psychologist struggling with the question of what is appropriate behavior.

The APA (1986) addressed the issue of bartering. The committee rules that "bartering (or exchange) of services, for example, having a patient perform bookkeeping services for his or her therapist is, per se, a 'dual relationship' and therefore, unethical" (p. 696). The committee's logic seemed to be that if a relationship is "per se" a dual relationship, then it is unethical. Because bartering for services involves multiple-role relationships, and those multiple-role relationships may create a conflict of interest for the therapist or substantially blur the therapeutic boundaries, it was considered unethical, per se. The American Psychological Association (1992), however, in Standard 1.18, relaxed the rules on bartering. Standard 1.18 provides "A psychologist may participate in bartering only if (1) it is not clinically contraindicated, and (2) the relationship is not exploitative" (p. 1602).

In 1987 the committee addressed the problem of dual relationships again. It did so in the form of vignettes in which a faculty member of a school was also a therapist for a student. They described the multiple-role relationship as therapist-patient and professor-student. Another scenario was offered in which an advanced graduate student was a group therapist for other graduate students. In this case the roles are therapist-patient and student-student. The committee concluded that therapy would be jeopardized and there would be contamination in the role relationships to the detriment of all. Thus, the treatment was unethical only "(a) in the absence of suitable alternatives, and (b) with full awareness of the potential risks that may await both parties" (APA, 1987b, p. 734).

The committee made an attempt to offer some factors to be used in analyzing an ethical dilemma regarding students. Unfortunately, these factors do not apply to many types of dual-relationship problems, such as sexual contact between patient and therapist or entering a joint business venture with a patient. Apparently, the committee believed the problem was not thoroughly addressed in previous Ethics Reports. The Committee wrote about it in its 1988 report (APA, 1988). The thrust of the report was on sexual intimacies with patients.

The committee reported state licensing board cases in which state courts have upheld disciplinary action against therapists who have sex with their patients (APA, 1988). The report addressed nonsexual dual relationships, particularly those of providing therapy to students, friends, and/or employees. The writer of the article concluded that all of the above "would be found to be unethical" (p. 568). The new APA Ethics Code is much more clear on the issue of sexual contact with a student (Standard 1.19, APA, 1992). The committee reinforced its concerns about bartering but did not expressly distinguish bartering for services versus goods, particularly where the fair market value can be established by a reliable independent means. Nevertheless, bartering for services has been consistently judged to be unethical.

In 1991 the committee gave little insight into the continuing problem of defining and analyzing dual-relationship problems. As an afterthought, one sentence was included about nonsexual dual relationships. Business involvement, personal involvement, and financial exploitation were mentioned as "exploitative dual relationships" (APA, 1991a, p. 752).

The confusion continued when the committee reported on its efforts in 1991. There were two references made in the text about dual relationships. In its commentary, the committee wrote that not all cases in the category of Sexual Intimacy involved sexual misconduct. It reported that "some involve other types of exploitive dual relationships, such as inappropriate business or personal involvement or financial exploitation" (APA, 1991a, p. 752).

The committee divided the category of dual relationship cases into sexual misconduct, sexual harassment, and nonsexual dual relationships in 1993 (APA, 1993). There were no illustrative cases on dual relationships from 1992 to 1996 in the Report of the APA Ethics Committee.

Finally, the APA *Casebook on Ethical Principles of Psychologists* provides the only other real notice to psychologists regarding interpretation of the Ethics Code (APA, 1987a). The case examples cited in the book include a psychologist who is involved in a sexual relationship with a patient and one who treats a student who she is directly supervising at the graduate level. Another case cited was a faculty member who offered a psychotherapy group as a course in group process and participated in discussions and evaluations of students. One case involved a psychologist who evaluated a patient, referred her to another therapist, then later dated her after she saw him in his office for a follow-up at a later time.

The last example involves a case in which a psychologist first attended business workshops with a person during which time they had a few drinks together; 2 years later the psychologist provided therapy to the man and his spouse. The spouse later complained that the psychologist was biased. The psychologist was found to have violated the prohibition against dual relationships in Principle 6 of the Ethics Code (APA, 1981). Because cases are not published in a legal reporter type service, no other guidance is available for the psychologist to use to guide his or her behavior. There is a substantial amount of ambiguity extant in the rules regarding dual relationships.

SUMMARY OF DUAL-RELATIONSHIP PROHIBITIONS

By tracing the decisions and comments by the APA over the past 10 years and examining the thinking of experts who have published in the area of ethics, we know the following dual relationships are unethical: (a) sexual contact with a patient; (b) treatment of close friends, family members, relatives, and/or employees; (c) treatment of students (unethical most of the time); (d) bartering whereby services are exchanged for services (unethical some of the time); (e) entering into a business relationship with a patient; (f) entering into a business relationship with an ex-patient (may be unethical); (g) a minister/pastor who is also a psychologist who provides counseling to a church member (will likely be judged as unethical conduct).

AREAS SUBJECT TO CONFUSION

The following areas are subject to confusion: (a) socializing with a patient may or may not be unethical; (b) socializing with an ex-patient is probably not prohibited; (c) bartering with a patient whereby goods offered by the patient are given in exchange for psychotherapy may not be unethical; (d) sexual contact with an ex-patient may not always be judged to be unethical; (e) treatment of a former student may be allowed; (f) developing a friendship with an ex-patient may not always be prohibited; (g) treatment of an individual employed in a facility where the psychologist works may be ethical and may be unethical; (h) buying goods from a patient may be unethical; (i) treatment of a current student may be ethical; (j) performing an evaluation and treatment on the same client may or may not be ethical, depending on when each is performed; (k) attending professional meetings with a patient who is a professional may be unethical; (l) psychologists who have consenting sexual relationships with their employees may be unethical; (m) socializing with students may be unethical; (n) psychologists who date each other and work in the same setting may be unethical; (o) exchanging gifts with a patient may be unethical; (p) charging money for supervision in which the hours will be used for licensure purposes may be unethical except that in some states payment is required; (q) having a social relationship with a supervisee may be unethical; (r) hiring a former student or supervisee may be unethical. The scenarios listed above all involve dual relationships. These are but a few of the examples of problem areas not fully addressed by the Ethics Code and/or the ethics decisions by the Committee.

PROBLEMS WITH DUAL-RELATIONSHIP RULES

Many of the problems with prohibitions against dual relationships have been described. There is inadequate publication of cases in which psychologists have been sanctioned for engaging in nonsexual dual relationships, and there is no publication of ethics decisions by APA and/ or state associations that would serve as both precedent and guidance for the psychologists. Borys (1992) suggested that those who are expected to adhere to ethics codes are left guessing regarding what is acceptable practice and are often in the position to be judged arbitrarily and capriciously by ethics committees.

In creating standards for psychologists, associations should strive to model the appropriate behavior particularly in how complaints are processed. As Bandura (1969) has pointed out for years, modeling is a powerful learning device. It is also humane and honorable. If those who create ethics standards and those who judge them are honorable and seek true justice, then those who are expected to adhere to ethical standards will be more likely to do so. But justice is not easy, a point repeatedly emphasized for those who work in the judicial system.

There are major problems with dual-relationship prohibitions. Because they are poorly defined and there is limited publication of decisions regarding nonsexual dual relationships, they are vague in the constitutional sense. Second, they tend to be overly broad in that, as written, the prohibitions tend to restrict constitutionally protected rights while also restricting nonconstitutionally protected rights. Third, they are often interpreted literally as prohibitions against all dual relationships when that was never the intent of APA, nor is it appropriately used. Fourth, the prohibitions interfere with the constitutionally protected right to privacy. This substantive due-process right guaranteed under the 14th Amendment of the Constitution has been one often used by APA to support its position on nondiscrimination and pro-choice. Fifth, the First Amendment Right to Association is unacceptably restricted. Some policies surrounding dual relationship could be considered as gender discrimination. Finally, the way in which decisions have been handed down, the confusion regarding accepted practices, and the lack of publication of cases as well as the lack of an analytical model to be applied to ethics decisions, have created a system without adequate procedural due process. One solution is to reject the concept of unethical dual relationships and replace it with a conflict-of-interest standard.

All psychologists, and particularly those employed by the association representing them, should act in ways that are constitutionally sound (see U.S. Constitution Amendments I–X, XIV). They should promote constitutional principles, particularly those related to human rights as set forth in United Nations and European documents on human rights (United Nations, 194p, Universal Declaration of Human Rights, 1948:

U.N.G.A. Res. 217 [A] [III] Un. Doc. A/810). The American Psychological Association has taken this stance, especially in cases involving discrimination against gay people, promoting the right of choice for women, as well as protecting the rights of the mentally ill. But our own house must be in order. We must not support constitutional principles only when they are consistent with our views on a particular subject. The following problems exist with dual-relationships prohibitions.

DUAL-RELATIONSHIP PROHIBITIONS AND VAGUENESS

Vagueness is a constitutional doctrine whereby a rule or law must be clear enough to be understood before an individual may be held accountable for a violation of such a rule. It is a rule applicable in prohibitions against exploitative dual relationships in that a mental health professional should know what is unethical before he/she is found to have acted unethically. There is a legitimate issue of vagueness in interpreting some parts of the APA Ethics Code. Although it is clear that a psychologist may not engage in sexual relations with a client it is unclear whether any type of socialization is considered unethical. Many of the areas of confusion noted on pages 142 and 143 are unresolved, thereby raising vagueness issues. A law will not stand or pass constitutional muster if it is vague (*Grayned v. City of Rockford*, 1972). The 14th Amendment of the Constitution has been interpreted to prohibit enforcement of vague laws. In order for 14th-Amendment protection to apply to individuals, there must be some form of state action (*Connally v. General Construction Co.*, 1926; *Mahler v. Ebby*, 1924; *U.S. v. L. Cohen Grocery Co.*, 1921; *Yu Cong Eng v. Trinidad*, 1926; also see *Edmonson v. Leesville*, 1948). It is arguable whether they employ the requisite state action when associations' ethics committees decide cases, but at least one case has found sufficient state action to apply judicial review to an ethics committee decision (*Budwin v. APA*, 1994).

Vagueness will be found in a rule or statute if "its prohibitions are not clearly defined" (*Grayned v. City of Rockford*, 1972, p. 108). Once the statute or rule is determined to be vague, it will generally be considered void. It is void because a vague rule is considered apposite to the principles of due process. An individual who is charged with a violation is in a difficult position if required to conform to a rule in which the meaning is subject to broad interpretation or reasonable divergence of thought as to what it means.

The Supreme Court has concluded that "Life, liberty and property could not, furthermore, be taken by virtue of a statute whose terms were so vague, indefinite and uncertain that one cannot determine their meaning" (*Lanzetta v. New Jersey*, 1939, p. 458).

Most would agree that the right to practice a profession in good standing involves a liberty interest (*Gibson v. Berryhill*, 1973; *Hampton v. Mow Sun Wong*, 1976; *Schware v. Board of Bar Examiners of New Mexico*, 1957). The rules surrounding the practice of psychology must be well defined and not so broad as to be able to catch all potential offenders, especially without adequate notice that the acts engaged in are prohibited. Consider the opinion of the Supreme Court in *U.S. v. Reese* (1875) in which they concluded it was dangerous if any legislature used a net large enough to catch all possible offenders and leave it to the court to step aside and say who could be rightfully detained, and who should remain at large.

The Constitution prohibits a regulation or law from being so vague as to apply to virtually any situation in order to pull an unknowing individual into a judicial system, for the court to then make a determination whether the conduct of the individual meets or does not meet some arbitrary standard. The vagueness rule is designed to prevent "arbitrary and discriminatory enforcement" (*Grayned v. City of Rockford*, 1972, p. 108) and thus requires explicit standards. This goes to the heart of fundamental fairness and is necessary if the rule will be sufficient to withstand a constitutional test (see *Ashton v. Kentucky*, 1966; *Gregory v. Chicago*, 1969; *Kunz v. New York*, 1951; also *Grayned*, 1972, supra note 56 at pp. 108, 109). The doctrine is often called Unconstitutional Uncertainty (see *Collings, Unconstitutional Uncertainty—An Appraisal*, 1955). A statute or law must provide notice to those who will come under its scrutiny. Justice Brennan, in *Paris Adult Theatre I et al. v. Slaton, District Attorney, et al.* (1973) concluded "First, a vague statute fails to provide adequate notice to persons who are engaged in the type of conduct that the statute could be thought to proscribe" (p. 86). The problem with such a rule is that it "invites arbitrary and erratic enforcement of the law" (p. 88).

The *Lanzetta* Court made this point quite clear, stating:

> And a statute which either forbids or requires the doing of an act in terms so vague that men of common intelligence must necessarily guess at its meaning and differ as to its application without notice on, violates the first essential of due process of law. (*Lanzetta v. New Jersey*, 1939, p. 453)

One should not be required to guess at the meaning of a rule; it should be clear and understandable. The greater the ambiguity in a rule, the more likely it will be found "repugnant to the due process clause of the Fourteenth Amendment" (*Lanzetta v. New Jersey*, 1939, p. 458). Notice is an essential element of due process. A rule that does not give adequate notice to those who are subjected to its enforcement is unconstitutional (*Cramp v. Board of Public Instruction*, 1961; *Gentile v. State Bar of Nevada*, 1991; *International Harvester Co. v. Kentucky*, 1914; *Papachristou v. City of Jacksonville*, 1972; *U.S. v. Harris*, 1954). Without notice as to exactly what is proscribed, the accused does not receive fundamental fairness in the process. Those who review complaints are not guided by specific codes or rules (see *Smith, Sheriff v. Goguen*, 1973; and *Connally v. General Construction Co.*, 1926). There have been no Supreme Court cases on vagueness and licensing laws. There is a recent state court case dealing with the issue. In *Toussant v. State Board of Examiners* (1991), the Supreme Court of South Carolina held the licensing law prohibiting unprofessional conduct was not unduly vague. One court examined the 1989 APA Ethics Code with respect to vagueness issues. In *White v. North Carolina State Board of Examiners of Practicing Psychologists* (1990), the State Court of Appeals in North Carolina found the preamble provisions of the APA Ethics Code to be vague in the constitutional sense. Hence the court prohibited the state psychology board from enforcing any discipline on a psychologist based on a perceived violation of the ethics code. The court cited *In re Wilkins* (1978) approvingly when they adopted the test to determine whether an ethics code provision was constitutional. They concluded, "the test is whether a reasonably intelligent member of the profession would understand that the conduct in question is forbidden" (p. 152; also see In Re Wilkins, 1978, p. 829).

The very best language to provide guidance on the issue of notice and vagueness appears in the case of *In Re Hawkins* (1973). The court wrote:

> It is reasonable to assume . . . that as one goes to the outer edges of the concepts of "unprofessional," "dishonorable," or "professional and ethical standards" with reference to the practice of medicine, as in the practice of law or other learned professions, he reaches an area in which there is no room or differences of opinion among the most honorable and respected practitioners. There is, we are satisfied, no sharply defined drop off point between ethical and professional . . . practice and that which is unethical and unprofessional. However, there is at and around the central core of these concepts much conduct which so clearly constitutes improper practice that few, if any, members of the profession would seriously claim to be unaware that such conduct is not consistent with these same concepts. (p. 548)

Those words, written in 1973, are applicable to today's ethical problems in psychology. Using this standard, it is clear that sexual contact with clients, or entering a business relationship with a client, or exploiting an older client by writing oneself into his or her will would be universally considered an ethical violation. However, the areas of confusion mentioned earlier in this chapter provide a few examples of the lack of notice to psychologists about which activities are ethical and which are not. Psychologists who face real-life problems involving dual relationships are left with little guidance and therefore little notice about what can or cannot be done. This problem is further complicated by the environment in which a psychologist works. Those who are employed in rural settings constantly face dual and multiple-role relationships with their clients. It would be fundamentally unfair to discipline psychologists working in a rural setting for being involved in multiple-role relationships depending on the nature of such relationships. No one would condone sexual contact with a client simply because it occurred in a rural setting. But would everyone universally conclude a client who provides baby-sitting services for therapist for a reasonable fee in a rural setting as unethical all the time unless there is direct evidence of exploitation? Would a psychologist who works in a community mental health center with seriously disturbed patients be labeled as unethical for assisting them in participating in an on-site agency work project such as a community kitchen?

Although the strictest rules of vagueness apply to rules that prohibit speech, other First Amendment protections are generally included (see *Hynes v. Mayor and Council of Borough of Oradell et al.*, 1976). The rules surrounding dual relationships do prohibit activities protected by the First Amendment, particularly the Right of Association.

As was presented earlier in this article, some prohibitions are clear, such as the restriction of therapist-patient sex, whereas others are unclear. This includes socializing with clients or ex-clients, entering a business relationship with an ex-patient, as well as other examples mentioned earlier. The vagueness of the rules regarding dual relationships has led to Ethics Committee reports that seem to conclude the opposite, depending on who is on the committee. If Ethics Committee members cannot agree on the meaning of the rules, then how can the average psychologist use the rule as a guide to control conduct? As was cited earlier, no published case exists that finds social contact with a client unethical, but the Ethics Committee report in 1986 categorically concluded it was unethical, in a single, sweeping sentence (APA, 1986).

The problem is made worse by virtue of the fact that there are no analytical tools provided for psychologists to use to determine whether a particular relationship is in the category of unethical dual relationships. This has led to unfair and inconsistent decisions and has been used by state licensing authorities to find unethical behavior in situations in which the rules are unclear. Consider the cases of *In the Matter of the Accusation Against Marianne Maxwell,* Case No. D-4177, in which the Attorney General for the State of California concluded that going to lunch or dinner, exchanging gifts, going on ski trips, inviting her patient to her home for social events and jacuzzi, and encouraging or permitting a friendship with her patient and her husband were both examples of unethical dual relationships. Also consider *In the Matter of the Accusation Against George Selleck,* Case No. D-4183, in which playing racquetball, scheduling and going to breakfast, scheduling and going to lunch, as well as encouraging his patient to attend a basketball game in which he was coaching were all considered a breach of the prohibitions against dual relationships. Also *In the Matter of the Accusation Against Donald Gates,* Case No. D-3827, in which Gates treated a former student 3 months after she completed one class with him, the only class taken with him, was considered unethical. Probably more disturbing is the case of *Stipulation in the Matter of the Accusation Against Mark den Broeder,* Case No. D-4339, in which having dinner, sharing meals during therapy, and discussing business investments, licensing-exam worries, and personal struggles, as well as his impending divorce, were found to be violations. State authorities rely on the guidance of the APA and on the Ethics Code of the APA. In each of the above cases sexual misconduct was involved as well. The nonsexual dual relationships were found to be unethical per se, however.

OVERBREADTH

A related legal construct to vagueness is that of overbreadth. This refers to the case in which a rule designed to prohibit a nonprotected activity actually prohibits or adversely affects a protected or fundamental right, especially those that are protected by the First Amendment (see Lockhart et al., 1991; Tribe, 1988). An ethical prohibition should not be overly broad such that it affects conduct protected by the Constitution. The doctrine has been clarified such that there must be a substantial effect on protected activities (*Broderick v. Oklahoma,* 1973). If the meaning of a rule is unclear, then it will cause those who are subject to it to avoid many activities that are protected (*Baggett v. Bullitt,* 1964; *Grayned v. City of Rockford,* 1972; *Stromberg v. California,* 1931).

Many of the rules surrounding dual-relationship prohibitions are unconstitutionally overbroad. Like the vagueness problems discussed previously, the rules are so indefinite as to, at times, cause those who engage in constitutionally protected behavior to come under the scrutiny and discipline of ethics committees. They cause ethical psychologists to avoid appropriate interactions with clients, supervisees, and students. This is the adverse affect the rules have on protected behavior. Some limited contact could be helpful to the clients, students, and supervisees, provided the client is not exploited and consideration is given to therapeutic boundaries. I have often heard psychologists as well as my students conclude that all dual relationships must be avoided. Neither the American Psychological Association, writers in the field of ethics, nor any state licensing board has ever suggested all dual relationships are unethical.

THE RIGHT TO PRIVACY

Although nowhere expressly stated in the Constitution, the right to privacy has become one of our most fundamental rights. Ever since the landmark case of *Griswold v. Connecticut* (1965), this right has developed over the past 25 years and has been supported by APA in virtually all spheres. Expanding on footnote four of *U.S. v. Carolene Products* (1938), the *Griswold* Court concluded that certain zones of privacy existed and that the Constitution created a penumbra of rights under which a general right to privacy could be construed (318 U.S. 479 [1965]; also see *U.S. v. Carolene Products* (1938) footnote four which states "There may be a narrower scope of the presumption of constitutionality when legislation appears on its face to be within a specific prohibition of the Constitution such as those of the first ten amendments which are deemed equally specific when held to be embraced within the Fourteenth Amendment" (p. 152). This has been referred to as the right to personal autonomy; it is the right to be free from unwarranted government intrusion. The right of privacy as noted in *Eisenstadt v. Bard* (1972) applied to marital as well as nonmarital relationships. Justice Goldberg, in his concurring opinion in *Griswold* (1965), argued for a much broader right in his characterization of the Ninth Amendment as present to protect fundamental rights not expressly covered in the previous amendments from unwarranted government intrusion. In another major privacy case, the Supreme Court in *Roe v. Wade* (1973), found the right of privacy grounded in liberty, protected by the 14th

Amendment, and applicable to such personal matters as whether to bear a child or not. The liberty construct emerged in two prior Supreme Court cases: *Meyer v. Nebraska* (1923) and *Pierce v. Society of Sisters* (1925).

The right of privacy as it pertains to liberty is particularly strong in the area of family matters (*Moore v. City of Cleveland*, 1977). It also may apply to acts engaged in while in the privacy of one's home (see *Stanley v. Georgia*, 1969; the court has backed away from this case somewhat by construing it as applying to a First Amendment interest that was protected). One of the leading constitutional scholars in the nation argues for a broad interpretation of the right to privacy (see Tribe, 1988). Such a broad interpretation has not yet been accepted by the court.

The privacy interest has been addressed in psychotherapy. Other cases have found the right to privacy present in the psychotherapeutic relationship (In re Lifschutz, 1970).

The issue of privacy and sexual behavior has been addressed in two major cases. In *Paris Adult Theatre I et al. v. Slaton, District Attorney et al.* (1973), the court found there was no First-Amendment protection for obscene material, although the case involved viewing obscene material in a public theater. Justice Brennan, writing an impassioned dissent argued for broad protections and warned of the problems of not doing so. In *Bowers v. Hardwick* (1986), the court concluded there was no constitutional right to engage in homosexual sodomy, even in the privacy of one's own home and between consenting adults. This case was decided on a 5 to 4 vote. It has been sharply criticized since it was announced. The American Psychological Association has been critical of it. Recently one of the majority, Justice Powell, admitted he thought he voted the wrong way in the case (see Dorsen, 1990).

The point of this presentation is that where people's fundamental rights to privacy are at issue, regulations that affect those rights should be very carefully crafted. Some rules in the APA Ethics Codes, both old and new (1981, 1992) are not crafted carefully. They are broad, vague, and affect clients' and psychologists' fundamental rights. In some instances, as in sexual contact with a patient, a compelling interest exists that can be used to support regulations of such private matters. As the harm in question to the patient is less clear, then the interest in regulating such matters is more remote. The more remote the interest, the less the conduct should be regulated. Although there is direct and overwhelming evidence of harm to patients who have been involved in sexual relations, as well as business relations with psychologists, there is not empirical support for other types of conduct, such as having lunch, dinner, or even treating a former student. By showing consistent respect for the right of privacy, the APA will be able to continue its lead in advocating for fundamental rights for all, and will be a proper role model.

PROCEDURAL DUE PROCESS

Consequences of regulatory bodies, such as disciplinary action, will be altered or struck down when they lack procedural due process (see *Carey v. Piphus*, 1978). The principle behind this rule is that the Due Process Clause of the 14th Amendment serves to guarantee fairness in procedures to protect against wrongful deprivations of liberty, among other protected rights (*Zinermon v. Burch*, 1989). When the interest of liberty is involved, certain procedural protections are required (*Board of Regents v. Roth*, 1972). These protections are federally mandated and emanate from the Constitution (*Cleveland Board of Education v. Loudermill*, 1984; *Vitek v. Jones*, 1980). They apply when a liberty interest is involved (*Board of Regents v. Roth*, 1972). Further, the action of an association's ethics committee will be subject to review by the courts (*Budwin v. American Psychological Association*, 1994).

The requirements are relatively simple. An evidentiary hearing is required when a liberty interest is at stake (*Goldberg v. Kelly*, 1970). Due process also requires notice; this involves notice of the specific charges as well as notice of a hearing (*Addington v. Texas*, 1979). The requirement of a hearing is part of a basic due-process right, that of the opportunity to be heard (*Goldberg v. Kelly*, 1970). Other required safeguards involve the right to counsel, the right to examine and call witnesses, the right to have the charges heard before a neutral decision maker, as well as the right to have a decision based on a record with a statement of the reasons for the decision (see Nowack, Rotunda, & Young, 1986).

Not all deprivations require procedural due-process protection. The court has developed a balancing test to determine whether due-process protection is required (*Mathews v. Eldridge*, 1976). The test involves consideration of the interest at stake plus the risk of erroneous deprivation versus the interest of and burden on the government. Where the individual interest is fundamental and the risk of erroneous deprivation high, greater procedural safeguards will be required.

Ethics procedures developed by the APA and state associations are somewhat effective at ensuring procedural due-process protections are granted to the accused. One area of deficiency involves the notice and report of the findings. Because the rules surrounding dual relationships are vague and overly broad, proper notice is not given to psychologists except for those acts that are clearly proscribed. Hence, an accused may enter an ethics hearing without knowing exactly what conduct is the subject of the hearing and without the ability to properly prepare a defense. Because the written decisions generally do not include references to the record, it will be difficult to know exactly on what the findings were based. Further, there is only a limited right of appeal for ethics decisions.

The procedures used in handling ethics complaints deprive the accused of some fundamental protections because of the vagueness and overbreadth of the rules governing professional behavior. They have the effect of depriving the accused of constitutionally based rights. The current Ethics Code prohibits psychologists from engaging in conduct that diminishes the civil rights of others, especially those of the accused. We must lead the way to ensure human rights in all our actions. In doing so we become the model we psychologists should be for the rest of the people. There is a clear relationship between the vagueness problem discussed previously and the procedural due-process requirement of notice. Vagueness is a more generalizable requirement for rules and/or prohibitions whether they be laws, regulations, or ethical standards. The notice requirements in procedural due process refer to the fact that a person charged with a violation must be given actual notice of the nature of the charges in sufficient specificity so that the person can mount a proper defense.

RIGHT TO ASSOCIATION

The First Amendment to the United States Constitution has been interpreted, in recent times, to guarantee freedom of association (Tribe, 1988; also see *Cantwell v. Connecticut,* 1940; *Gitlow v. New York,* 1925; *Griswold v. Connecticut,* 1965). The freedom to associate with those of one's choosing and to do so in an intimate way is considered a very important fundamental freedom. Consider the following opinion of Justice Brennan in *Roberts v. United States Jaycees* (1984, p. 618):

> The Court has concluded that choices to enter into and maintain certain intimate human relationships must be secured against undue intrusion by the State because of the role of such relationships in safeguarding the individual

freedom that is central to our constitutional scheme. In this respect freedom of association receives protection as a fundamental element of personal liberty.

This right is still under development as a constitutional theory and in case law and includes the freedom to associate with others to express ideas and beliefs (*NAACP v. Alabama,* 1959). The freedom to associate is so important that "possible applications" of a rule will be considered and are sufficient to strike down the rule if protected activities are adversely affected (*NAACP v. Button,* 1963). In other words, both direct and subtle attacks on freedom to associate will not be tolerated (see *Healy v. James,* 1972).

Although there is no fundamental right to engage in social association, association pertaining to basic First-Amendment freedoms of assembly, free expression of ideas, and free expression of religion are protected (*City of Dallas v. Stanglin,* 1989). When a rule prohibits people from associating with those whom they choose, the First-Amendment protections will come into play (*Hisho v. King & Spalding,* 1984; see footnote four of Justice Powell's concurring opinion at p. 78). Further, when a First-Amendment right is involved, rules governing vagueness and overbreadth will be applied rigorously (*NAACP v. Button,* supra note 107 at pp. 432, 433).

Generally, the more intimate the association, the more protection is derived from the First Amendment (*Board of Directors of Rotary International v. Rotary Club of Duarte,* 1987; also see *Moore v. East Cleveland,* 1977). In *City of Dallas v. Stanglin* (1989), the Court concluded that less intimate associations, such as the right to patronize a dance hall, did not deserve First-Amendment protection, whereas closer and, in effect, more private associations deserved the strongest protection.

The rules surrounding dual relationships definitely affect the fundamental right to associate. They preclude psychologists from interacting with patients in many ways. They prohibit psychologists from treating certain classes of people. They even, in effect, prohibit psychologists from marrying patients, an act that is a fundamental right in and of itself (*Zablocki v. Redhail,* 1978; also see *Loving v. Virginia,* 1967). Although a state may develop rules that affect this fundamental right, it must have a compelling interest to do so and the rule or law must be narrowly tailored to support the interest (*Roberts v. United States Jaycees,* 1984).

Since the rules surrounding dual-relationship prohibitions are vague and ambiguous, they are not likely to pass constitutional muster. The prohibition against sexual contact with patients would likely pass constitutional muster because it is specific, clear, understandable, and has been enacted to support a compelling interest of the profession: protecting patients against abuse. Recently, the Supreme Court concluded the right of associations cannot be used to justify violating the rights of others (*Madsen v. Women's Health Center,* 1994). Other prohibited conduct may have a less negative effect on patients. In such cases, rules surrounding the conduct should be required to pass the strictest scrutiny.

When we as psychologists enact codes of conduct, we must never forget the human rights issues that are connected to our actions. We must also remember that our codes of conduct affect our patients. Our Ethics Code restricts the actions of patients by attempting to control the actions of psychologists. This is proper in areas where we are sure there is harm if extratherapeutic contact occurs or the conflict of interest is substantial; it is not proper in all other areas.

PROPOSED SOLUTIONS

Because many of my criticisms could apply to other provisions in the Ethics Code, my solutions will be general. It should also be noted that APA's 1992 Ethics Code is a vast improvement over the 1981 edition.

One of the first changes that should be made is that ethics decisions should be published in a legal reporter type service. The identities of the parties could be concealed, if necessary. Only those cases that shed some new light on an ethical issue in question should be published. A summary of these decisions should appear every 6 months in *The American Psychologist,* with a clear explanation and presentation of newly addressed issues. If new and specific prohibitions emerge, then a clear and concise statement of the rule should be written. This could be as simple as "treatment of students is a substantial conflict of interest and, therefore, is unethical." The new rules could be added to a book that is clearer than the current *Casebook on Ethical Standards of Psychologists* (APA, 1991b). Doing this would provide psychologists with part of the requisite notice of prohibitions of specific acts that are likely to create a substantial conflict of interest. Many who read this may comment that professional psychology and ethics committees would become too judicial in nature. But the ethics business is quasi-judicial in nature. Ethics committees are judicial in the way they hear cases and their decisions are as far reaching as court cases. In law the highest due-process procedures exist for an issue that involves fundamental rights. It is time to recognize this and make appropriate changes.

The second solution is to list the acts that are specifically prohibited by the Code. A list like the one that appears on page 181–182 of this chapter could be included in the Ethics Code. We know that certain acts are expressly prohibited, such as sexual contact with a patient as well as treatment of a close friend or family member.

The third and critically important solution is to develop and publish an analytical model to use in determining whether a substantial conflict of interest exists in a particular type of relationship or conduct. There have been two previous attempts to construct a decision-making model to analyze dual relationships (Gottlieb, 1993; Haas & Malouf, 1989). In Gottlieb's model, psychotherapists are asked to analyze dual relationships using three dimensions—power, duration, and termination. Gottlieb's model is a good start, as is that of Haas and Malouf. Both models are incomplete and do not take into account constitutional considerations, however. The model should be used by ethics committees to decide cases. A particularly good, albeit incomplete, model is that proposed by Haas and Malouf (1989). In their model, psychologists are required to ask themselves a series of questions to determine whether the client may be inhibited from making independent decisions or whether the psychologist might be restricted with respect to actions to be taken to help the client by the secondary role relationship. In addition, the psychologist must examine his/her motives to determine if they are in the best interests of the client. If not, then the secondary relationship should either be discontinued or the client should be referred to someone else. Psychologists are expected to keep in mind that dual relationships may exploit a client or interfere with a psychologist's ability to treat a client effectively when asking these questions. Finally, in the Haas and Malouf model there is a direct prohibition against engaging in sexual contact with a client. Further, they believe a psychologist should never engage in sexual contact with a former client. Hence their model has two prohibited areas of conduct: sex with a current or former client. Then the few questions must be asked to ascertain whether other dual relationships are acceptable or prohibited. The model is good but lacks the kind of detailed specificity that is needed in current practice.

In the Gottlieb model, there are seven assumptions that are to be applied when using his decision-making model (Gottlieb, 1993). They are the rules regarding dual relationships that are applicable to all professional relationships, all dual relationships cannot be avoided, there are risks with each additional role relationship that requires separate analysis to determine if a client may be harmed, not all dual relationships are exploitative per se, psychologists must be sensitive to problems with dual relationships, the model does not apply to cases where a secondary-role relationship exists but for one that is contemplated and all dimensions are examined from the standpoint of the consumer (Gottlieb, 1993). There are three dimensions in Gottlieb's model: power, duration, and termination. A relationship must be examined to determine the extent and nature of the power of the psychologist, the duration of clinical services to be provided to the client, and how definite termination will be. The three dimensions are used to pose a series of questions. If the answers are affirmative then the secondary relationship should be discontinued. Finally, consultation is always important, although the role of it is not totally clear in Gottlieb's model. A very important factor in Gottlieb's model is that any dilemma should be discussed with a client and informed consent obtained to proceed with a secondary relationship.

The Gottlieb and Haas and Malouf models provide excellent beginnings but they are incomplete. A detailed model such as that presented below is now necessary to guide psychologists and other mental health professionals to act appropriately in their dealings with clients.

That way there would be no gray areas for case scenarios to fall into. The model involves consideration of a set of factors or tests to determine whether a secondary relationship is likely to create a substantial conflict of interest. The following factors should be taken into consideration.

1. What is the nature of the therapeutic relationship? Is it short term versus long term; psychoanalytic versus biofeedback?
2. What is the nature of the professional relationship? Is it incidental, forensic, less intimate, such as in a one-time teacher-student relationship?
3. What is the nature of the secondary relationship? Is it in the prohibited class?
4. How close is the secondary relationship?
5. What are the risks of harm to the patient, including the nature of the risk and the type of harm?
6. Are there alternatives available to the therapist?
7. What is the severity of harm to the patient with the secondary relationship?
8. How long will the secondary relationship last?
9. What is the intensity of the secondary relationship?
10. Will the judgment of the therapist be impaired by the secondary relationship?

11. Can the therapist use his or her influence as therapist to gain a personal advantage with/over the client?

12. Will the freedom of the therapist to choose techniques/methods/plans in treatment be restricted?

13. Will the patient's responses/communications/disclosures be restricted in therapy?

14. What is the extent to which the patient's choice to return to therapy might be restricted?

15. Can the professional relationship between the therapist and the patient be maintained?

16. What is the likelihood of conflict of interest now or in the future?

17. What effect will the secondary relationship have on the public regarding their perception of the profession?

18. What is the specific interest pursued by the professional?

19. Will the interest pursued by the professional be in any way adverse to the client or receiver of professional services?

20. For those relationships not in the prohibited class, will the geographic or cultural contexts allow for the secondary relationship to exist?

21. Is the mental health professional psychologically stable to the extent necessary to interact with a consumer of services outside the confines of the professional setting?

Further, the analysis depicted in Figure 12.1A and 12.1B could be applied to factual circumstances in ethics cases and licensing boards in determining whether a psychologist's behavior was in conflict with the interests of the client.

Once the Ethics Committee applies the factors to the particular case, it can generate a well-reasoned decision. Most important, these factors provide psychologists with a tool to guide decisions whether to engage in a particular type of behavior with a client. The model would take away many of the excuses psychologists use to defend their actions. A systematic method of analysis of the behavior would lead to greater clarity for psychologists who must accurately determine whether a conflict of interest may exist as the result of a multiple-role relationship. Several questions should be asked (see Table 12.2). A systematic model for analysis of conflict of interest and multiple-role relationship problems is presented in Figure 12.1. The categories noted in Figure 12.1B are defined next.

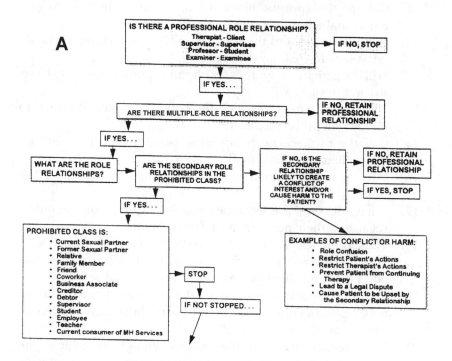

FIGURE 12.1A   Analytical model for multiple-role relationships.

Environment.   Where the secondary-role relationship occurs is quite important. If the contact occurs outside of the therapist's office or in a more private environment, one would expect more conflict for the client generally. Having lunch with a client in a crowded and open restaurant is different than having dinner in a quiet, romantic establishment.

Purpose of the Activity.   One must examine the therapist's motive to determine the objective analysis of such a motive. Is the therapist motivated by a nonprofessional need versus one designed to promote the client's best interests? Is the conduct solely or primarily designed to satisfy a well-documented therapeutic objective or a goal that is identified in the client's treatment plan? If the conduct is in the interest of the client it may be acceptable provided the determination of what is in the best interests of the client is made objectively.

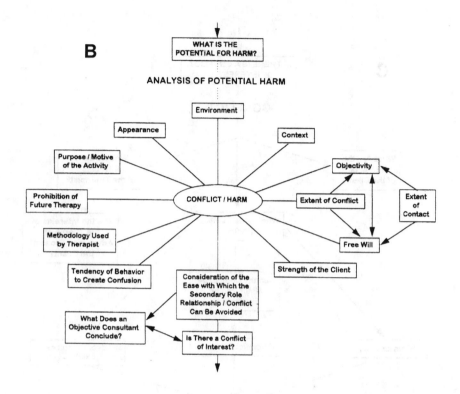

FIGURE 12.1B (continued)

The Extent of Contact.   This factor involves the extent of physical contact with the client. Does the contact involve a short handshake versus sexual intercourse? One is more cursory and accepted, whereas the other is intimate and extensive. The greater and more intimate the physical contact the more likely it will be harmful. Sexual behaviors involving activities such as intercourse, oral sexual contact, sexually oriented massages, long embraces, long kisses that are lip-to-lip and involve lengthy intimate contact are known to cause harm to the client and the therapeutic relationship. Other behavior, such as a short hug offered at the appropriate time—such as at the end of a difficult therapeutic session and with no sexual connotation—may be helpful to the client and the relationship.

Methodology Used by the Therapist.   Does the therapist use coercion, force, either actual or perceived threats to obtain a client's acquiescence

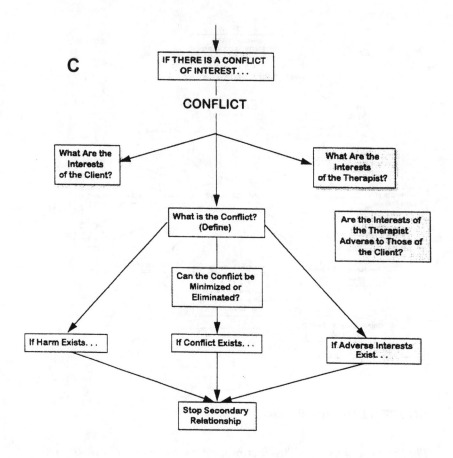

FIGURE 12.1C   (continued)

to the questionable conduct? Has the therapist engaged in behavior over time that is designed to magnify the power differential with the client? Does the therapist in any way threaten the client to force the client into the proposed conduct? Threats could take the form of reports to child-protective service agencies, employment, police, relatives, or others who may be able to use confidential information about a client adversely. Does the therapist agree to reduce the client's bill in exchange for the client's involvement in the secondary-role relationship?

Tendency of the Behavior to Create Confusion.   Does the behavior or secondary-role relationship create confusion for the client regarding

TABLE 12.2 Analytical Model for Multiple-Role Relationships

Question 1:	Is there a professional relationship or are you providing psychological services to person "X"?
Question 2:	Are there multiple-role relationships?
Question 3:	What are the role relationships?
Question 4:	Are the secondary-role relationships in the prohibited class?
Question 5:	If not in the prohibited class, is the secondary relationship likely to create a conflict of interest and/or cause harm to the patient?
Question 6:	How easy is it to avoid the secondary-role relationship/conflict of interest?
Question 7:	Has an independent and objective consultant approved of the secondary-role relationship or proposed conduct?
Question 8:	How will the role relationship or conduct reflect on the profession?

the therapeutic purpose of the primary-role relationship? Will the client have difficulties?

Appearance. This refers to the appearance of the activity with the client. If the behavior of the therapist appears to others to be against the interests of the client or to be harmful, it should be prohibited. If others considering seeking treatment may be disinclined to do so because they observe the behavior in question, the psychologist might consider refraining from the intended conduct.

Context. This calls for an analysis of the context in which the conduct of the psychologist occurred. If the conduct occurred in the context of a planned or structured therapeutic activity in the interests of the client, such as in a therapeutic recreational group visit to a bowling alley, or if it is more likely to be harmful to the client, such as an intimate dinner with no therapeutic purpose.

Prohibition of Future Therapy. If the conduct in question would have a chilling effect on the client's choice to pursue therapy with the psychologist in the future it is likely to be both harmful and pose a conflict of interest to the client. When therapeutic boundaries are maintained such that a client could easily come back for treatment at a later time, it is clearly in the client's interest to preserve such an option.

Objectivity. This calls for a determination as to whether the objectivity of the therapist as well as the client will be diminished by the activity in question. Such behavior as having a sexual relationship with a client clearly impairs the objectivity of both the therapist and the client. Impairment of activity must certainly be harmful to the client.

Free Will. This refers to the extent to which the free will of a client is impaired by the conduct in question. If the client's will is impeded in some way the conduct in question may be harmful, if it is not in the interests of the client. Arguably, the development of positive feelings by the client toward the therapist may adversely affect free will. If the conduct is still aimed at the best interest of the client, however, it may be helpful.

Strength of the Client. Rarely has this been considered in an analysis of the harm to the client. This factor calls for a consideration of the strength of the client. The client who is mentally healthy is clearly in a better position to make independent decisions about the secondary relationship. A client in a psychiatric hospital or one with a borderline personality disorder is not the kind of client who should be involved with nonsexual dual relationships with psychologists.

The final portion of the analysis must focus on the mental health of the professional. There is no justification for engaging in conduct that involves conflict of interest as well as multiple-role relationships that fall in the prohibited class. For those areas that are less clear, however, the mental health of the professional should factor into the equation. That is, the more mentally healthy the professional, the more latitude he or she should have in deciding on involvement in multiple-role relationships that are not necessarily harmful. The less mentally healthy the professional the less that person should stray from strict professional boundaries. Many mental health professionals engage in boundary violations when they are vulnerable, depressed, or when they are experiencing significant psychosocial stressors. Those who have certain types of personality disorders themselves may be more likely to engage in boundary violations. The depressed, vulnerable, personality disordered, and stressed should have less latitude than those who are not the least bit impaired. Again the latitude only applies to those situations in which the conduct in question is not in the prohibited class and may not be harmful or exploitative to the client. Some case examples will illustrate the use of the model.

Case Examples

Case #1: A psychologist is treating a 16-year-old patient for stress she experiences in school. The adolescent has a mild adjustment-disorder diagnosis. The adolescent and the psychologist live in a small town in Nevada with a population of 30,000. The psychologist keeps no confidential material at his home. He is mentally healthy and has kept very tight boundaries in the past. Given the managed care insurance plan for the patient as well as the nature of her problems the psychologist anticipates that she will only need six sessions of supportive therapy.

The psychologist is married and has a 7-year-old daughter. One of the stresses for the patient is a lack of money although she tries to baby-sit every weekend. The psychologist learns during the fourth session that his wife knows the patient incidentally. The patient becomes aware that the psychologist and his wife must be at a very important meeting on a Friday evening. She offers to baby-sit in exchange for her regular fee of $6.00 per hour. Now we will examine this situation in light of the model.

A professional relationship is in place. There are multiple-role relationships (therapist-patient; parent-baby-sitter). The secondary relationship is not in the prohibited class. Using the harm analysis, there is some concern raised because the secondary-role relationship will take place in the home of the psychologist. There is no confidential material there, however. The purpose of the activity will meet both the needs of the patient and the therapist. The activity is not clearly directed at promoting the best interests of the client exclusively. There will be limited contact, none of which will be physical. The therapist is using a short-term treatment model making it less likely for a powerful attachment to occur between himself and the patient. The behavior may create some minor confusion although the role of a baby-sitter is not completely opposite that of a therapeutic relationship. There is no evidence that the objectivity of the therapist may be adversely affected, nor will the free will of the client be injured in any way. Both the therapist and the patient are relatively healthy. Using the model there are some negatives that might make the activity unwise although it is probably not completely unethical.

Change some of the facts and there would be a different result. Make the environment urban, the patient seriously ill, the psychologist a sexual predator, and the therapy analytic, and every one of these changes would lead to the conclusion that the activity would create a conflict of interest.

Case #2: *A psychologist who is psychologically healthy is treating a 7-year-old female who is in a residential treatment center. The 7-year-old was physically abused by both her mother and her father, resulting in removal from the home and termination of their parental rights. The psychologist provides weekly treatment and the patient responds. The patient has a variety of symptoms including depression, anxiety, social withdrawal, poor school performance, difficulty concentrating, memory problems, and uncontrollable crying* *at times. She has no independent source of money and the residential treatment facility has a limited budget. The psychologist takes the girl to the local town one day and purchases several appropriate outfits for the child. In addition, the psychologist invited the child to her home for Thanksgiving dinner. An independent consultant concludes the behavior is appropriate.*

Using the model it is clear a professional relationship exists. There is also a secondary relationship. The secondary relationship is not in the prohibited class. The behavior in question is in the best interests of the client. There would be no likely adverse affect on future therapy as the therapeutic boundary in the primary relationship is not contaminated. There does not appear to be any adverse affect on objectivity. The appearance of the conduct would not discredit the profession in any way. Finally, the objective consultant concludes the conduct is appropriate. This scenario would be ethical using the model.

Case #3: A 28-year-old psychologist is working in a county inpatient psychiatric center. She is treating a 16-year-old patient who has been psychotic and who has an IQ of 85. She uses a long-term dynamic treatment method with the patient. She expresses her attraction for the patient in a session. Later she hugs him after each of her sessions. She continually asks him if he is attracted to her. After one session she gives him $100 as spending money. He is surprised and elated. He asks what he can do to pay her back. She looks seductively into his eyes and tells him she will think of something. The psychologist herself has been treated for a borderline personality disorder and discontinued treatment after a verbal altercation with her therapist.*

In this scenario there is both a professional relationship and a secondary relationship. The secondary relationship is not yet in the prohibited class. The patient and therapist both are psychologically impaired to the extent that the psychologist should not involve herself in any unusual secondary-role relationship. The conduct in question is likely to create role confusion because there are clear personal sexual overtones to therapy and the cash is an unusual gift to a patient who does not need the gift. The motive of the activity is suspect; it is not likely to be in the best interests of the patient. Further, the objectivity of the psychologist and the patient are likely to be impaired in this instance. The psychologist is using a long-term treatment model, which depends on the purity of the relationship across time. The conduct may ultimately impede progress in the future or lead the patient to want to discontinue treatment with the psychologist.

The appearance brings discredit on the profession. In this case no consultant was contacted. Clearly there is a major conflict of interest in the actions of the psychologist. The analysis in this case would lead to an unequivocal conclusion that the behavior is unethical and should be avoided.

Case #4: A 54-year-old patient has been in cognitive-behavioral therapy with a supportive therapy overtone for the past 1 1/2 years. She has decided to terminate therapy with the approval of the psychologist. After the last session the psychologist and the patient go to lunch in a very public setting as a celebration of the success of treatment.

This case involves a clear professional relationship with a secondary-role relationship that involves going to lunch with the patient. The conduct is not in the prohibited class, however. The context is one involving a time-limited contact to symbolize success in therapy. There is no extratherapeutic reason for the conduct. No objectivity is impaired in either the patient or the psychologist. Both are relatively healthy at this point. There is no adverse affect on the free will of either the patient or the psychologist. The patient will probably not be uncomfortable about pursuing future therapy with the psychologist as the result of going to lunch with him. It is unlikely that the lunch will create any confusion in the primary relationship. Under the model the conduct would be considered ethical.

Case #5: A 29-year-old psychological assistant of a psychologist needs to complete a therapy requirement in order to complete a graduate school requirement. He does not have any money to pay for therapy. He approaches his psychologist supervisor who agrees to provide therapy.

In this case there is a primary professional-role relationship. There is also a secondary-role relationship. Further, the secondary-role relationship is in the prohibited class. Hence, according to the model, the psychological assistant must be referred elsewhere for therapy.

To return to the solutions I have proposed to clarify ethical dilemmas, a fourth change that needs to be made is to establish a reverse trilevel scrutiny system to be applied to ethics decisions, as is used by the Supreme Court in deciding cases. In areas where fundamental rights are involved, the prohibitions should be established only where the profession has a compelling interest. Any rules that follow should be narrowly tailored to support that compelling interest. This is referred to as strict scrutiny. A compelling interest could be proffered to prohibit sex with patients or treatment of a business partner or relatives. In areas where there is a clear consensus that harm occurs both to the patient and the profession, such as in sexual contact between therapist and patient, a compelling interest exists for the profession and regulatory boards to construct strict rules. This could apply to such situations as entering into a business relationship with a current client or treatment of a family member. Other levels of review include moderate scrutiny and rational basis. A moderate level of scrutiny should be applied to the type of involvement between a therapist and former patient. Rational basis means that a professional should have a rational reason for interacting with a client outside the professional relationship. This reason could be cultural, geographic, supportive, therapeutic, or genuinely useful to advance the image of the profession. Some examples of this may include attending a wedding of a client, going to lunch with a client in a nonintimate setting, participating in a local organization designed to advance an ethnic or cultural purpose, or accepting goods in exchange for professional services.

Justice Kennedy, before he was elevated to the Supreme Court, developed a set of four tests to be used in deciding how closely to review a particular regulation or law. His test involves consideration of (a) the nature of the individual interest allegedly infringed, (b) the importance of the governmental interest furthered, (c) the degree of infringement, and (d) the sensitivity of the governmental agency to create more carefully tailored alternative means of achieving the goal (*Beller v. Middendorf*, 1980).

The more fundamental the interest or right, the more likely it is that a closely tailored rule is needed, provided the interest of the regulating body is sufficient. Other areas should be left to less control and more situational latitude. The factors listed above could be used to come to conclusions about the ethics of such behavior quite easily. The system described previously would eliminate the need for the dual-relationship concept.

A rule could be created that specifically addresses conflict of interest. The language could be as simple as: Engaging in multiple-role relationships with a professional client that would present a conflict of interest with the primary-role relationship is prohibited.

Another version could be: Willful involvement in multiple-role relationships with someone who is receiving professional services in which a conflict of interest exists or occurs is prohibited. Examples of such role relationships include but are not limited to providing psychological service to a family member, coworker, close friend, psychological assistant, supervisee, or sexual partner.

Being a psychologist is an honor; it comes with great responsibilities and obligations. Perceiving the role of a psychologist as a privilege and not an entitlement will go a long way toward guiding ethical decision making. It will assist us in generating rules that protect the consumers of psychological services as well as treating our colleagues humanely and with dignity. The Constitution is about rights, dignity, and respect for humankind. The drafting of the Constitution and its orderly interpretation prevents unwarranted invasion into and control over people's lives. It helps ensure that all will be treated equally and that no one will be persecuted for some political or other unnecessary reason. By abiding by its principles and modeling ourselves after what has been done in the past as well as improving on it, we will keep our profession honorable, model the respect for people so deserving and important, and continue to display our dignity by treating others with the highest level of respect. Let us never hide behind the concept of dual relationships to prevent us from feeding the hungry, providing clothing for the needy, housing the homeless, or giving money to the indigent.

REFERENCES

Addington v. Texas, 439 U.S. 908 (1979).

American Psychological Association. (1953). *Ethical standards of psychologists.* Washington, DC: Author.

American Psychological Association. (1958). Ethical standards of psychologists. *American Psychologist, 13,* 268–271.

American Psychological Association. (1977). *Ethical standards of psychologists.* Washington, DC: Author.

American Psychological Association. (1979). *Ethical standards of psychologists.* Washington, DC: Author.

American Psychological Association. (1981). APA ethical principles of psychologists. *American Psychologist, 36,* 633–638.

American Psychological Association, Committee on Professional Standards. (1982). APA casebook for providers of psychological services. *American Psychologist, 37,* 698–701.

American Psychological Association, Committee on Professional Standards. (1983). Casebook for providers of psychological services. *American Psychologist, 38,* 708–715.

American Psychological Association, Committee on Professional Standards. (1984). Casebook for providers of psychological services. *American Psychologist, 39,* 663–669.

American Psychological Association. (1986). Report of the ethics committee: 1985. *American Psychologist, 41,* 694–698.

American Psychological Association, Board of Professional Affairs, Committee on Professional Standards. (1987a). *Casebook on ethical principles of psychologists.* Washington, DC: Author.

American Psychological Association. (1987b). Report of the ethics committee. *American Psychologist, 42,* 730–735.

American Psychological Association, Ethics Committee. (1988). Trends in ethics cases, common pitfalls, and published references. *American Psychologist, 43,* 564–573.

American Psychological Association. (1991a). Report of the ethics committee, 1989 and 1990. *American Psychologist, 46,* 750–758.

American Psychological Association, Committee on Professional Standards. (1991b). Casebook on ethical principles of psychologists. *American Psychologist, 46.*

American Psychological Association. (1992). Ethical principles of psychologists and code of conduct. *American Psychologist, 47,* 1597–1611.

American Psychological Association. (1993). Report of the ethics committee, 1991 and 1992. *American Psychologist, 48,* 811–820.

American Psychological Association. (1994). Report of the ethics committee, 1993. *American Psychologist, 49,* 659–666.

American Psychological Association. (1995). Report of the ethics committee, 1994. *American Psychologist, 50,* 706–713.

Ashton v. Kentucky, 384 U.S. 195 (1966).

Bader, E. (1994). Relationships: Legal and ethical trends. *Transactional Analysis Journal, 24,* 64–66.

Baggett v. Bullitt, 377 U.S. 360 (1964).

Bandura, A. (1969). *Principles of behavior modification.* New York: Holt, Rinehart, & Winston.

Beller v. Middendorf, 632 F.2d 788 9th Circuit (1980).

Board of Directors of Rotary International v. Rotary Club of Duarte, 481 U.S. 535 (1987).

Board of Regents v. Roth, 408 U.S. 564 (1972).

Borys, D. S. (1992). Nonsexual dual relationships. In L. Vandecreek, S. Knapp, & T. L. Jackson (Eds.), *Innovations in clinical practice: A sourcebook* (Vol. 11, pp. 443–454). Sarasota, FL: Professional Resource Exchange.

Borys, D. (1994). Maintaining therapeutic boundaries: The motive is therapeutic effectiveness, not defensive practice. *Ethics and Behavior, 4,* 267–273.

Borys, D. S., & Pope, K. S. (1989). Dual relationships between therapist and client: A national study of psychologists, psychiatrists and social workers. *Professional Psychology: Research and Practice, 20,* 283–293.

Bowers v. Hardwick, 478 U.S. 186 (1986).

Broderick v. Oklahoma, 413 U.S. 601 (1973).

Budwin v. American Psychological Association, 29 Cal. Rptr. 2nd ed., 453 (1994).

California Civil Code. \ 43.93(b) (2) (1994).

Cantwell v. Connecticut, 310 U.S. 296 (1940).

Carey v. Piphus, 435 U.S. 247 (1978).

City of Dallas v. Stanglin, 490 U.S. 19 (1989).

Clarkson, P. (1994). In recognition of dual relationships. *Transactional Analysis Journal, 24* (1), 32–55.

Cleveland Board of Education v. Loudermill, 470 U.S. 532 (1984).

Collings, R. A., Jr. (1955). Unconstitutional Uncertainty—An Appraisal. *Cornell Law Quarterly, 40*, 195–237.

Connally v. General Construction Co., 269 U.S. 385 (1926).

Cramp v. Board of Public Instruction, 368 U.S. 278 (1961).

Dorsen, N. (1990, December 3). Civil liberty's unlikely ally. *National Law Journal, 13*(13) [Col 1].

Edmonson v. Leesville, 334 U.S. 1 (1948).

Eisenstadt v. Baird, 405 U.S. 438 (1972).

Florida Civil Code. (1994). Chapter 491.0112

Gentile v. State Bar of Nevada, 111 S. Ct. 2720; 501 U.S. 1030 (1991).

Gibson v. Berryhill, 411, U.S. 564 (1973).

Gitlow v. New York, 268 U.S. 652 (1925).

Goldberg v. Kelly, 397 U.S. 254 (1970).

Gottlieb, M. C. (1993). Avoiding dual relationships: A decision-making model. *Psychotherapy, 30* (1), 41–48.

Gottlieb, M. C., Sell, J. M., & Schoenfeld, L. S. (1988). Social/romantic relationships with present and former clients; state licensing board actions. *Professional Psychology: Research and Practice, 19*, 459–462.

Grayned v. City of Rockford, 408 U.S. 104 (1972).

Gregory v. Chicago, 394 U.S. 111 (1969).

Griswold v. Connecticut, 381 U.S. 479 (1965).

Haas, L. J., & Malouf, J. L. (1989). *Keeping up the good work: A practitioner's guide to mental health ethics.* Sarasota, FL: Professional Resource Exchange.

Hall, J. E., & Hare-Mustin, R. T. (1983). Sanctions and the diversity of ethical complaints against psychologists. *American Psychologist, 38*, 714–730.

Hampton v. Mow Sun Wong, 426 U.S. 88 (1976).

Healy v. James, 408 U.S. 169.181 (1972).

Hisho v. King & Spalding. 467 U.S. 69 (1984).

Hynes v. Mayor and Council of Borough of Oradell et al., 425 U.S. 610 (1976).

International Harvester Co. v. Kentucky, 234 U.S. 216 (1914).

In re Donald Gates, Case No. D-3827. (1991). Board of Psychology, State of California, Sacramento, CA.

In re George Selleck, Case No. D-4183. (1991). Board of Psychology, State of California, Sacramento, CA.

In re Marianne Maxwell, No. D-4177. (1991). Board of Psychology, State of California, Sacramento, CA.

In re Hawkins, 17 N.C. Appl. 378. 194 S.E. Rptr.2d 540. (1973).

In re Lifschutz. 85 Cal. Rptr. 829: 467 P.2d 557 (1970).

In re Wilkins, 294 N.C. 528. 242 S.E. Rptr 2d 829 (1978).

Jennings, F. L. (1992). Ethics in rural practice. *Psychotherapy in Private Practice, 10*, 85–104.

Kunz v. New York, 340 U.S. 290 (1951).

Lanzetta v. New Jersey, p. 458. 306 U.S. 451 (1939).

Lockhart et al. (1991). *Constitutional law.* St. Paul, MN: West.

Loving v. Virginia, 388 U.S. 1 (1967).

Madsen v. Women's Health Center, 114 S. Ct. 2516 (1994). No. 93–880.

Mahler v. Ebby, 264 U.S. 34 (1924).

Mathews v. Eldridge, 425 U.S. 319 (1976).

Meyer v. Nebraska, 262 U.S. 390 (1923).

Mills, D. H. (1984). Ethics education and adjudication within psychology. *American Psychologist, 39,* 669–676.

Moore v. City of Cleveland, 431 U.S. 494 (1977).

Moore v. East Cleveland, 431 U.S. 494 (1977).

National Association for the Advancement of Colored People v. Alabama, 357 U.S. 449 (1959).

National Association for the Advancement of Colored People v. Button, 371 U.S. 415 (1963).

Nowack, J. E., Rotunda, R. D., & Young, J. N. (1986). *Constitutional law.* St. Paul, MN: West.

Papachristou v. City of Jacksonville, 405 U.S. 156 (1972).

Paris Adult Theatre I et al. v. Slaton, District Attorney, et al. 413 U.S. 49 (1973).

Pierce v. Society of Sisters, 268 U.S. 510 (1925).

Pope, K. S. (1991). Dual roles and sexual intimacies in psychotherapy. *Ethics and Behavior, 1*(1), 21.

Pope, K. S., & Vasquez, M. J. T. (1991). *Ethics in psychotherapy.* New York: Random House.

Powell, L. F. (1990, December 3). Civil liberty's unlikely ally. *National Law Journal, 13*(13) [Col 1].

Roberts v. United States Jaycees, 468 U.S. 7609 (1984).

Roe v. Wade, 410 U.S. 113 (1973).

Schware v. Board of Bar Examiners of New Mexico, 353 U.S. 232 (1957).

Smith, Sheriff v. Goguen, 415 U.S. 566 (1973).

Stanley v. Georgia, 394 U.S. 557 (1969).

Stipulation in the Matter of the Accusation Against Mark den Broeder, Case No. D-4339.

Stromberg v. California, 361 U.S. 359 (1931).

Toussant v. State Board of Examiners, 400 S.E.2d 488 (1991).

Tribe, L. H. (1988). *American constitutional law* (2nd ed., pp. 1302–1435). Mineola, NY: Foundation Press.

United Nations. (1948). 194p, *Universal Declaration of Human Rights;* U.N.G.A. Res. 217 [A] [III] Un. Doc. A/810).

U.S. v. Carolene Products, 304 U.S. 144 (1938).

U.S. v. L. Cohen Grocery Co., 255 U.S. 81 (1921).

U.S. v. Harriss, 347 U.S. 612 (1954).

U.S. v. Reese, 92 U.S. 214 (1875).

Vitek v. Jones, 445 U.S. 480 (1980).

White v. North Carolina State Board of Examiners of Practicing Psychologists, 97 N.C. App 144, 388 S.E. Rptr. 2d 148 (1990).

Youngren, J. N., & Skorka, D. (1992). The nontherapeutic psychotherapy relationship. *Law and Psychology Review, 16,* 13–28.

Yu Cong Eng v. Trinidad, 271 U.S. 500 (1926).

Zablocki v. Redhail, 434 U.S. 374 (1978).

Zinermon v. Burch, 494 U.S. 114 (1989).

CHAPTER 13

Can Boards of Examiners Constitute the Ultimate, Harmful Multiple Relationship?

T. Richard Saunders, PhD, ABPP

Ethical Standard 1.17 of the *Ethical Principles of Psychologists and Code of Conduct* of the American Psychological Association (APA, 1992) provides as follows with respect to multiple relationships:

> (a) . . . A psychologist refrains from entering into or promising another personal, scientific, professional, financial, or other relationships with such persons if it appears likely that such a relationship reasonably might impair the psychologist's objectivity or otherwise interfere with the psychologist's effectively performing his or her functions as a psychologist, or might harm or exploit the other party.

The author is indebted to Morris Roseman, PhD, for a helpful reading of an earlier draft of this paper. Dr. Roseman was a founding member of the Maryland Board of Examiners after the original licensure act for psychologists was passed by the Maryland General Assembly in 1957. The author is also indebted to Norma Simon, PhD and to David Mouille, PhD for their insightful ideas about the roles and importance of boards of examiners and state psychological association ethics committees, respectively. However, none of the ideas in this paper should be attributed to these consultants.

(b) Likewise, whenever feasible, a psychologist refrains from taking on professional or scientific obligations when preexisting relationships would create a risk of such harm.

(c) If a psychologist finds that, due to unforeseen factors, a potentially harmful multiple relationship has arisen, the psychologist attempts to resolve it with due regard for the best interests of the affected person and maximal compliance with the Ethics Code. (APA, 1992, p. 5)

These are noble-sounding words. In behavior, what do they mean? Among the many criticisms leveled at the APA Ethics Code (1992) over the years, few are more devastating than the idea that behaviorally, it is filled with exhortatory rhetoric, vague allusions, and practically meaningless verbiage that cannot be fulfilled in reality (Bersoff, 1994; Saunders, 2001).

A careful reading of the above passages, and similar segments in the proposed 2002 Ethics Code (APA, 2001), leaves one wondering from a practical perspective, what specific behavior is under discussion? Moreover, what does "harmful" mean? To whom is the psychologist so obligated—the paying client, or anyone in the client's personal or business life? What is the level of "likelihood" of any such "harm" that is acceptable or unacceptable, and to whom? Do we include only the putative patient, or do we include the patient's family, or a circle of friends, neighbors, or coworkers? Furthermore, how does one compute the hypothetical "risk" mentioned in section (b) above? The term is used absolutely, so the inference apparently should be that any risk, no matter how remote, should be avoided.

In other words, what are the limits, what are the boundary conditions of this obligation to "refrain"? Obvious answers to these questions are the desire not to exploit vulnerable patients, sexually or financially. But if these are correct interpretations of the text, why does the text not simply say so?

However, for several years there has been growing awareness of an even greater danger to psychologists than its vague and behaviorally nonspecific Ethics Code. Many observers have recognized for years (Lazarus, 1998) and told APA officials about their awareness of the deficiencies in the Ethics Code and other related documents, such as the various "Guidelines" that APA has issued under a variety of conditions over the years (e.g., K. W. Melchior, personal communication, March 18, 1991).[1] A major part of the debacle has come not in the interpretation of the Ethics Code by psychologists in the ethics structure of APA, but in the fact that the Ethics Code as a public document is free to be utilized by anyone. Of course this means it can be exploited, in civil litigation, or in the formal, adjudicative role played by boards of examiners in the various states, 29 of which have formally adopted the Ethics Code as legally enforceable (Fleer, 2000).

Thus, despite the truth of the dictum that every state has its own unique statutory regulation mechanism for the field of psychology, there is still a persistent thread that flows from APA to the professional community, and goes from there to each state's regulatory apparatus. The burden of this chapter is to show, in general, that the relationships between statutory boards of examiners and their licensees are just the type of harmful multiple relationship envisioned, however poorly, by section 1.17 of the 1992 Code of Conduct (APA, 1992).

BOARDS OF EXAMINERS AND THEIR MULTIPLE ROLES: RISK OF HARM PAR EXCELLENCE

Although formal charges against psychologists, both before the APA Ethics Committee and before boards of examiners, are fairly rare, few prospects are more chilling to practitioners than the idea of being "investigated" by a professional ethics body, whatever its authority. Even if we grant that the overwhelming majority of adjudicated cases are resolved in favor of the accused psychologist, upwards of 90% in most jurisdictions and in APA ethics adjudication (S. Glass, personal communication, August 18, 2000), the filing of a formal complaint is the beginning of a possible nightmare for most practicing clinicians.

Consider for a moment the process that is involved, as outlined some time ago by attorney-psychologist Bryant Welch, former executive director of the APA Practice Directorate (Welch, 1998). The board of examiners generally has the authority to receive and process the complaint, presumably making the preliminary judgment as to whether the behavior alleged is in fact a violation of its ethics (usually the APA Code of Ethics), or is a violation of the Practice Act in the jurisdiction in question. Next, assuming that the preliminary question has been

---

[1]Kurt W. Melchior was a California attorney, formerly a member of the House of Delegates of the American Bar Association and a member of the Board of Governors of the State Bar of California. At the request of Drs. Arthur Bodin and Arthur L. Kovacs, Mr. Melchior wrote in 1984 a very extensive legal critique of the 7th Draft of the Standards for Providers of Psychological Services of the American Psychological Association. His critique largely echoes the statements of more recent psychologists on professional documents by psychologists. The author is indebted to Dr. Bodin for making the commentary available. A copy may be obtained by writing the author at 200 Forbes Street, Annapolis, Maryland 21401.

answered affirmatively, the board proceeds to investigate, which of course is a police function in criminal law. Frequently, the investigative body begins with the presumption that the complainant has told the truth (Malone, 1997) and, again presumably, is a credible witness. Depending upon the nature of the complaint, the board may also have the authority to extend the investigation to other matters not related to the original complaint (*sua sponte*, meaning on its own initiative). Often, individual board members or the board operating as a whole will structure the investigation, deciding whom to interview, which facts to obtain, and generally how to proceed.

If the facts seem to support the existence of a "professional crime," then the board acts to draw up charges, which of course is a prosecutorial function. Depending upon the jurisdiction, the board may also then sit in judgment of its own charges, or it may have the case heard by an administrative law judge (ALJ). ALJs are creatures of the executive branch of government, as is the board itself. The granting of licenses to practice psychology, like all licenses issued by the state, from dog tags to motor vehicle operator permits, are granted under the authority of the executive (governor) of each state. The board's case is presented by representatives of the state attorney general's office, who are usually assigned to or even selected by the board for this purpose. If the ALJ makes a determination with which the board disagrees, in most jurisdictions the board can simply set the decision aside on grounds that are typically defined by statute.

Finally, the board having determined whether the psychologist is guilty of the behavior in question decides on which of a range of statutorily defined punishments to assign, including temporary or permanent destruction of the psychologist's ability to practice and thereby make a living. This awesome authority is essentially unchecked by any right of appeal. Generally speaking, simple errors of fact or a variety of legal problems that would be grounds for a reversal in civil or criminal proceedings have no merit in administrative law. Several implicit assumptions, legally, determine this leniency by the judicial branch. First, the rationale offered is the presumption that the board is probably the best judge available of the professional issues in question. Second, the hearing officer (either an ALJ or the board itself) is usually presumed to be in the best position to judge such matters as the credibility of witnesses because it has heard testimony directly, which an appeals body cannot do. Thus, in most states, the only grounds for appeal is a major legal flaw in the board's handling of the case on a constitutional issue. Each of these is extremely rare.

Consider now in summary the multiple roles the board has played in its case-handling function. It combines the roles in criminal law played by prosecutor, police, judge, jury, and (professional) executioner. The presumed advantage to the state of this process is that it is simpler, closer to the facts, probably more professionally appropriate, and certainly a lot cheaper than comparable civil or criminal actions. Wherever there is great power, of course, there is great potential for abuse. In any event, there is no doubt that in the sense of the Multiple Relationships section (1.17) of the *Ethical Principles of Psychologists and Code of Conduct* (APA, 1992), the relationship between each licensee and each board of examiners is indeed multiple, and indeed very likely to be potentially harmful. The fact that the relationship is sanctioned in law does not in itself address whether this undiluted authority should exist, and if so, in what form.

Psychology opted decades ago for professional self-regulation in the form of licensure and before that, for certification (Rodgers, 2000). This opened the door for the potential abuse of power by the boards, a potential that can cut in either of two ways. A board that is too narrow in its pursuit of professional misconduct may allow unscrupulous practitioners to prey on the public (Thomas, 2000). A board that over-reaches its authority may undertake frivolous prosecution of psychologists, to the detriment not only of the individuals involved in any specific case, but to the detriment of the profession as a whole and, ultimately, of the collective public (Williams, 2001). In law, this detrimental effect is called "chilling," meaning that board decisions may have the result of suppressing essential or constructive practices in the field or eliminating otherwise reputable and skilled practitioners.

In other words, the success of self-regulation in psychology and by extension, in all professional fields, depends upon a sensible written act (licensing law), an effective set of rules and regulations enabling the act, and an effectively written code of professional conduct. Successful self-regulation also demands competent, effective leadership in the board and adequate financial and professional resources for that board to operate properly.

ANECDOTAL EVIDENCE OF PROBLEMS IN THE REGULATORY APPARATUS OF PSYCHOLOGY

For a number of years, there has been extensive and growing concern on the part of many psychologists about the ability of state licensing boards to regulate effectively in the existing political and social climate (Woody, 2000). For one thing, there have been repeated reports of abuse of power by individual boards of examiners (Billet-Ziskin, 1995; Fleer, 2000; Jones, 1995; Newton, 2000; Petersen, 1999; Sall, 1994; Saunders, 2001; Sherven, 1994; Striano, 1998).

This anecdotal evidence, which by the way is all that can exist in this field, suggests that at the least, individual psychologists have been attacked by their own colleagues sitting on boards, in ways that were manifestly unfair, discriminatory, and unconstitutional. In the case of Gary Sall, for example, the Washington State Board of Examiners was required in a civil suit to print a public, written apology to him, and to pay Dr. Sall $100,000 for damages in compensation for its malicious and unfounded attack on his professional competence and reputation. In an even more egregious case in California, a psychologist was forced to spend $450,000 to defend himself against allegations of unprofessional conduct, which included no less than three separate court-directed reversals of the California Board of Psychology actions, which attempted extralegally to reinstate charges that the court had been ordered dismissed on appeal (Saeman, 1997).

It is worth noting that the American Bar Association does not itself adjudicate complaints of unethical behavior against its members. Instead, it relies upon each state's highest court, under statute and precedents unique to each state, to regulate the practice of law. The Bar does, however, promulgate a Model Rules document (1997) that elaborately defines terms, specifies necessary behavior for attorneys, and in general does a superb job of stipulating what is and what is not acceptable professional behavior for its practicing attorneys.

Some authors in the field of professional ethics claim that the problem here is one of "accountability" of individual psychologists to the public, not of accountability of APA as an organization to its membership. Thus presumably, accountability only runs in one direction, and organizational accountability does not exist at all (e.g., Hjelt, 2000). Younggren (2000), a frequent presenter of "risk management" seminars for the APA Insurance Trust, underscores the foregoing points.

MARYLAND BOARD OF EXAMINERS
STRIKES BACK: H.B. 989

Regrettably, no amount of ethical clarity or sensitivity can overcome an unscrupulous, entrenched bureaucracy. Saunders (2001) outlined a very strained, difficult case in which the Maryland Board of Examiners was summarily reversed by an appeals court judge, in a case that also cost the psychologist defendant an excess of $100,000, over a 7-year period of costly, painful litigation. In that prosecution, the Maryland Board was said by the trial court to have exhibited behavior toward the defendant that was "more than unethical" in its pursuit of a complaint originating in a child maltreatment examination. Clearly, a misguided board mishandled this case to the point that the court directed that neither it nor the defendant would be allowed to discuss the matter in public in the future, while the same judge declared unconstitutionally vague the "dual relationships" section of the pre-1992 APA Ethics Code (1981). He hinted strongly in that decision that if the post-1992 Code had been before him, he would make the same ruling, issuing a lengthy discussion of legal "notice" that is required before such provisions can be enforced. In practice, what this means legally is that objections like those raised at the outset of this paper to 1.17 of the current APA Code of Conduct (1992)—especially insufficient behavioral referents—make it impossible for the conscientious practitioner to adhere to the Ethics Code. Therefore, it is legally unenforceable in Maryland and remains so until APA takes it upon itself to issue a revision that is specific and clear.

This leads us to the discussion of the aftermath of the aforementioned legal case. After the board's ignominious legal defeat, the Maryland Board of Examiners undertook to try to eliminate the possibility of further losses by crafting legislation aimed at forcing the board's own unique conception of its adjudicatory role on its licensees.

The provisions of Maryland House Bill 989, enacted and signed by the governor, effective October 1, 1999, approximately 2 years after the board lost on appeal the case outlined above, are a professional nightmare come true. The Maryland Psychological Association, the presumptive organizational oversight body for Maryland psychologists, ignored legal advice to oppose 989, thus allowing it to become law without objection. Readers should note that the following provisions are excerpts from the Maryland Health Occupations Article, mostly Sections 18. For example, 18.206.1 provides as follows:

> The board may disclose any information contained in a record of the board to any other health occupations regulatory board of this state or another state if the health occupations regulatory board of this state or another state requests the information in writing. (para. A)
>
> The board, its executive director, or administrator, or the office of the attorney general, may disclose to any licensing or disciplinary authority or other law

enforcement, prosecutorial, or judicial authority, any information in the investigatory files of the board. (para. B)

These sweeping provisions make available, with no demonstrated need to know, information from the raw investigative files of the Maryland Board of Examiners, without regard to the truthful or factual nature of the contents. There is no provision that would protect the accused psychologist from release, accidental or otherwise, of any such information, such as to the media, thus destroying the psychologist's career with no legal recourse available to the psychologist. These provisions appear to be most likely operative in the rare eventuality of a criminal allegation against a psychologist, such as for some form of assault, or fraud. These are clearly overkill.

All that is required is a simple provision to allow referral to the states attorney if there is a preliminary determination of a possible felony or misdemeanor. The provision for "judicial authority" potentially involves the board in civil litigation actions, in which a court could simply permit the subpoena of the board's files in a civil case. Although other provisions of Maryland law appear to prevent this, no test of the contradictory provisions has yet been made. Even if a case has been closed by the board, presumably any of its findings or investigative materials could be available for inspection in a kind of multiple jeopardy. This ensures that once an allegation is made, psychologists will then have to spend the rest of their lives endlessly refuting it. Not coincidentally, the confidentiality of the board's complainants would also be violated. No notice to complainants is required that their written or oral statements to the board are being released. Will complainants then also be made available for criminal or civil actions, in any state in the Union, in any matter whatsoever, with no determination of reasonable access?

Space constraints do not permit me to discuss the specific additional details of this horrendous legislation. Problematic Maryland psychologists are subject to reprimand, probation, suspension, or revocation of a license. Among other things, licensees are in jeopardy of the Fifth Amendment right to refuse to incriminate themselves. Furthermore, the board is authorized by H.B. 989 to levy fines up to $10,000 literally for anything, especially anything that can remotely be construed as violating an ill-defined "professional standard." Thus, the clinician's clothing, demeanor, speech, or any other aspects of professional conduct can also be subject to this kind of "regulation." If the board decides to "reprimand" a licensee, which coincidentally is a casual-sounding penalty that would effectively eliminate practitioners from membership on any managed-care panels or any institutional affiliations, so they could not effectively make a living. The board, after destroying the practitioner's career, may also fine the individual $10,000! It is hard to imagine a more draconian provision, particularly one that violates the constitutional requirement of a specific offense before one's property (money or license) is removed by an agency of the state.

There is an additional provision that permits the board to enjoin summarily and arbitrarily any professional behavior of which it does not approve, with no need to demonstrate public harm before issuing an injunction. Thus, the board can preempt any practice, by any psychologist with which its majority does not agree, by a simple majority vote of the board. Any disapproved behavior, undefined, may subject them to professional discipline. The board is therefore free to use the unlimited police power and financial resources of the state to exhaust individual psychologists who refuse to do what the board (upon an incantation of "professionalism") tells them to do.

WHERE DO WE GO FROM HERE?

Regardless of the interpretation ultimately placed on Maryland House Bill 989 and whether or not it is eventually declared unconstitutional, or is an unwarranted instrument of the executive branch of government, as it stands now this legislation is a problem only to Maryland psychologists. In legal terms, however, bad precedents have a way of working their way around the country, rather like the economic Gresham's axiom that bad money tends to drive out the good. By analogy, bad legal precedents tend to drive out the good as well. *In that sense, there is always the risk that what has taken place in Maryland may "go national."* Nevertheless, like the cognitive intervention for catastrophic thinking, which asks the patient, "how bad can it get?" if a given event takes place, psychologists wondering how bad things can become in the professional-legal sense need only look to this legislation as the answer to this limit-setting question.

As a former president of my state psychological association, I have had occasion to see the dark underbelly of professional practice and regulation. There is no question that any professional self-regulation by APA and by competent ethical and constitutional statutory bodies are needed. I want to emphasize that I continue to support the self-regulation of the field of psychology, regardless of how poor the present regulatory authority and its associated legal apparatus has become. In fact, I continue to believe that boards of examiners can do and are doing much that is worthwhile for the public and for the profession of psychology. Much of this beneficial work, I fear, is regrettably taken for granted (Simon, 1993).

Nevertheless, I am also a firm believer in the rule of law, and in particular the Bill of Rights in the U.S. Constitution. Certainly, I am no constitutional legal scholar, but it seems to me that boards of examiners, despite their "multiple" functions, must operate within the framework of law and that psychologists are entitled to all their constitutional rights when defending themselves against legal charges of wrongdoing. These criteria are obviously violated, as I have attempted to show above, whenever the profession does itself the disservice of adopting vague, behaviorally meaningless verbiage as professional "standards." The same can be said for mindless legislation like H.B. 989, which attempts to subsume "group think" and vacuous authoritarianism for reasonable professional standards and reasonable appeal rights.

It does not matter particularly whether professional tenets are referred to as standards, or "best practices," or "risk management" procedures. To me, all these terms are simply various components of the claptrap of modern postindustrial sloganeering, a sort of managed care for professional regulation, which flies completely in the face of the constitutional requirement for "notice"—the legal term that means a person must be able to interpret a law and apply it before it can be enforced. Psychologists nationally can assist in stemming this trend by supporting changes to the Ethical Principles of Psychologists and Code of Conduct that require an explicit presumption of innocence, freedom of speech, and specific professional standards, as well as accessible, practical appeal rights. An explicit Ethics Code that guarantees due process protections, does away with exhortation and impractical idealization, and emphasizes clear, simple behaviors that truly represent a consensus of the field (e.g., Pope & Vetter, 1992) will be an ideal tool with which to combat the kind of professional fascism represented by H.B. 989.

In my view, it is crucial that psychology as a profession recognize its accountability to the field as a whole, and the legal authority of boards of examiners be accountable, if we intend to make the world safe for the legitimate practice of the profession.

REFERENCES

American Bar Association. (1997). *Model rules of professional conduct* (1998 Edition). Chicago: Author.

American Psychological Association. (1981). Ethical principles of psychologists. *American Psychologist, 36* (6), 633–638.

American Psychological Association. (1992). *Ethical principles of psychologists and code of conduct.* Washington, DC: Author.

American Psychological Association. (2001). Ethics code draft published for comment. *Monitor on Psychology, February,* 76–89.

Bersoff, D. (1994). Explicit ambiguity: The 1992 ethics code as an oxymoron. *Professional Psychology: Research and Practice, 25,* 382–387.

Billet-Ziskin, M. L. (1995). Task force on licensing board disciplinary procedures. *APA Division 31 Newsletter, Spring,* 5.

Fleer, J. (2000). Ambiguities in the ethics code. *The Independent Practitioner, 20,* 259–260.

Hjelt, S. (2000, January). Professional psychology: A view from the bench. *Register Report, 26* (1), 8–13.

House Bill 989. State Board of Examiners of Psychologists—Disciplinary and Regulatory Authority, 1999. 18 Maryland Annotated Code, Section 18-206.1, 18-313.1, and 18-317.1, et seq.

Jones, T. (1995, February 4). The witness's startling stand. *The Washington Post,* D-1, D-8.

Lazarus, A. A. (1998). How do you like these boundaries? *The Clinical Psychologist, 51* (1), 22–25.

Malone, D. (1997). An explanation of "The Investigatory Process" of the Maryland Board of Examiners of Psychologists. *The Maryland Psychologist, 42* (5), 9–10.

Newton, C. (2000, December 8). Psychologist paying price of reporting a claim of abuse. *The Washington Post,* A-53.

Petersen, M. B. (1999). What role does your Association play with regard to regulatory action against your members? *Bulletin of Division 31, Fall,* 4.

Pope, K. S., & Vetter, V. A. (1992). Ethical dilemmas encountered by members of the American Psychological Association: A national survey. *American Psychologist, 47,* 397–411.

Rodgers, D. A. (2000, January/February). The psychology story: 1950–1999. *The National Psychologist, 9* (1), 16, 17.

Saeman, H. (1997, November/December). Cal dispute has cost psychologist $400,000. *The National Psychologist, 3,* 24.

Sall, G. S. (1994). The evil empire II. *The Independent Practitioner, 14,* 275–277.

Saunders, T. R. (2001). After all, this is Baltimore: Distinguished Psychologist of the Year address. *The Independent Practitioner, 21,* 15–18.

Sherven, J. (1994). Guilty until proven innocent. *The Independent Practitioner, 14,* 48–50.

Simon, N. (1993) Licensure issues for the nineties. *The Independent Practitioner, 13,* 27–29.

Striano, J. (1998, July). Lenore Walker "battered" by Colorado licensing board. *NYSPA Notebook, 10* (4), 19.

Thomas, J. (2000, January/February). Rehabilitation or punishment: Newspaper series ponders. *The National Psychologist, 9* (1), 1, 3.

Welch, B. L. (1998, July/August). Why you better pay attention to the 'licensing board' issue. *The National Psychologist, 7* (4), p. 17.

Williams, M. H. (2001). The question of psychologists' maltreatment by state licensing boards: Overcoming denial and seeking remedies. *Professional Psychology: Research and Practice, 32,* 341–344.

Woody, R. H. (2000). Reclaiming mental health services. *The Clinical Psychologist, 53,* 20–23.

Younggren, J. N. (2000, January). Review of Steve Hjelt's view of psychology. *Register Report, 26* (1), 9.

CHAPTER 14

Multiple Relationships

A Malpractice Plaintiff's Litigation Strategy

Martin H. Williams, PhD

The claim that a psychotherapist and a patient had entered into a "multiple relationship" can, unfortunately, serve as an effective centerpiece for a malpractice action against that psychotherapist. Because of a long, evolving history of ethics enforcement against psychotherapists, certain "ethical problems" can appear to be gross deviations from the standard of care, or to represent gross negligence, when, in fact, they are not. The slur, "multiple relationship," is a perfect example. Because of a confusion between that which is risk management and that which constitutes the standard of care—and because some believe that multiple relationships are reliable precursors of therapist-patient sex—some psychotherapists, plaintiff's attorneys, judges, and civil juries will find the mere presence of a multiple relationship to be unethical. That this is a conceptual error provides little comfort to the accused psychotherapist. Today, many psychotherapists blanche at the term "multiple relationship" without giving themselves a chance to carefully consider whether or not such a relationship is either unethical or a treatment problem. This chapter describes the misuse of "multiple relationships" as a slur against treating psychotherapists and explains why this slur has proven so effective in civil court, before licensing boards, and at administrative law hearings as a way to win plaintiff and prosecution cases against psychologists.

The ethics of multiple relationships cannot be understood without an understanding of concerns about therapist-patient sex. These concerns began to be raised systematically in the 1970s and reached a zenith in the mid-1980s (see Pope & Bouhoutsos, 1986). Research indicated that as many as 10% of male psychotherapists had, at some point in their careers, become sexually involved with at least one client. Around the same time period, several very highly publicized lawsuits against egregiously sexually abusive psychotherapists were filed, and large damage awards were made. Some damage awards may have been at least partially predicated on questionable interpretations of published research, which some believed had indicated that therapist-patient sex causes harm universally and that such harm is always devastating and lasting. This issue has been discussed in detail elsewhere (e.g., Williams, 1992). Regardless of the research, however, the psychotherapeutic professions took clear positions that therapist-patient sex is not only unethical; it is repugnant.

Unfortunately, nonsexual multiple relationships also became tainted, in large part because of their potential association with therapist-patient sex. Obviously, a therapist cannot become sexually involved with a patient unless the relationship first evolves from a therapeutic one to a personal one. Thus, the logic goes, there will be a series of steps that gradually transform the relationship from professional, then to personal, and finally to sexual. To prevent therapist-patient sex from occurring, therapists are advised to be very wary of entering into any semblance of a personal relationship with a patient. Hence, we have the current concerns about so-called multiple relationships. As some would have it, a person's psychotherapist ought to have no other relationship or contact with any other aspect of that person's life.

This is a far cry from the logic that initially put dual relationships, as they were then called, into the American Psychological Association (APA, 1953) Ethics Code in the 1950s (e.g., Canter, Bennett, Jones, & Nagy, 1994). Dual relationships were considered to be a problem only when a psychotherapist offered treatment to a member of his or her own family or to another close relative. The profession recognized that one could probably not be objective and offer the best possible treatment to individuals with whom one already had a close relationship. Over the years, though, this concern has evolved to an almost paranoid reaction against offering psychotherapy to nearly anyone with whom one already has, or might in the future have, any other involvement.

Those who endorse such a far-reaching and needless prohibition may assume that most psychotherapists practice in an anonymous, urban setting. In such a setting it may be reasonable to envision a life in which one sees one's patients exclusively in the office. Obviously, this is not the reality of psychotherapists who practice in small towns, on military bases, or in culturally diverse and distinct communities within large urban settings, for example, minority or gay and lesbian communities. Such psychotherapists might find it impossible to avoid benign, multiple relationships with their clients. This notwithstanding, psychotherapists have become concerned about all multiple relationships, despite the fact that not all are necessarily unethical.

THE MINDS OF ATTORNEYS VERSUS THE MINDS OF PSYCHOTHERAPISTS

The existence of a multiple relationship between therapist and patient can and will be used against a psychotherapist before a licensing board, at an administrative law hearing, or in civil court. To understand how this happens, it helps to understand the minds of attorneys. Attorneys are trained in our adversarial system of justice, and they tend to approach problems of right and wrong in a manner that is quite distinct from that taken by psychologists. A psychologist, for example, immediately might try to understand *why* a peer has been accused of wrongdoing. A psychologist might immediately be concerned that "splitting" may have led to a false accusation and may presume that many deteriorating relationships go bad due to the mistakes of *both* parties. Attorneys, by contrast, are trained to think about winning their cases. The focus is not on what caused things to go bad but on how to package the available evidence into a winnable case. Of course there is a spectrum here, with some psychologists being more adversarial themselves and some attorneys very compassionate and understanding people. Nevertheless, if we consider training alone, psychologists are trained to understand and resolve conflicts without becoming adversarial, while attorneys are trained to win while functioning within our adversarial system of justice.

Attorneys, for example, make a study of the art of cross-examination and learn ways to make an opposing witness appear to lack credibility; they study how to make a person look and feel invalidated. Nothing in a psychotherapist's training even remotely resembles such an approach to another human being. This difference in training and disposition must be kept in mind in order to understand why psychologists have such problems once an issue of theirs goes to a licensing board or civil court.

RISK MANAGEMENT

It should also be noted that although multiple relationships can be associated with unethical activities, no psychotherapy profession holds multiple relationships to be unethical per se. Generally, multiple relationships are considered to be unethical only if they involve the risk of harm to the patient, exploitation, or a loss of objectivity by the therapist. Unfortunately, though, some risk-management experts will advise psychotherapists to steer clear of all multiple relationships—not because they are actually unethical, but only because they might increase one's likelihood of being sued. Bear in mind, though, that risk management is neither the ethics standard nor the treatment standard. Risk management is merely a set of cautionary procedures to minimize the chances of being sued. Good treatment and good risk management may sometimes call for mutually exclusive decisions regarding a given patient.

For example, it would probably be good risk management never to treat a potentially suicidal patient. After all, the families of those who commit suicide have been known to sue the psychotherapists who had tried to help the deceased. Most of us would agree that such risk management advice is utter nonsense, because helping those in need is a primary aspiration of the psychotherapy professions. This example illustrates the logic and drawbacks of risk management—its single-minded devotion to avoiding lawsuits and its equally single-minded lack of regard for the primary goals of our work.

As another example, one might recommend that no male therapist should ever treat a female patient. This recommendation, if followed, would probably eliminate most malpractice lawsuits concerning therapist-patient sex, because a variety of researchers have found that the dyad of male therapist and female patient typifies the known cases of this ethics breach. As a result, male psychotherapists would probably go out of business while female patients would be deprived of needed care were this extreme risk management strategy to be followed. With risk management as one's only guide to practice, the baby is very likely to be thrown out with the bath water.

BOUNDARY VIOLATIONS

As part of a licensing board or civil complaint about a multiple relationship, the accuser (plaintiff's attorney or licensing board) will probably attempt to show that there have been "boundary violations." Boundary violations are behaviors that cross the imaginary boundary between a professional relationship and a personal one. Enough of these boundary violations add up to the appearance of a multiple relationship (and, of course, the appearance of a multiple relationship may be confused with an *unethical* multiple relationship). Following is a list of possible boundary violations that might be used to establish in court the appearance of a multiple relationship along with the taint of an ethics problem:

- Self-disclosing information about your life, your family, your experiences, or your feelings—including your positive or negative reactions to the patient you are treating;
- Accompanying your patient to any destination outside your office, such as taking a walk together during a session, having a meal together, accepting a ride should your car be broken, or offering the patient a ride;
- Accepting a small gift from a patient or giving a gift to a patient;
- Hugging a patient or engaging in any other form of nonsexual touching;
- Incorporating forms of therapy that involve physical manipulation of any kind;
- Lending a book or cassette tape to a patient;
- Seeing a patient for one or more treatment sessions without charging a fee;
- Sending a patient a birthday card;
- Giving a "birthday party" during a session for a patient who may never have had his or her birthday celebrated;
- Accepting an invitation from a patient to attend a special event, such as a wedding, bar mitzvah, funeral, or retirement party.

Regardless of one's views on the appropriateness and ethicality of these various behaviors, two things can be said about the items in this list:

1. They have been used in civil and licensing board litigation to document the existence of multiple relationships, for example, unethical, harmful, exploitative, and actionable psychotherapeutic conduct; and
2. They have been used in civil and licensing board litigation as evidence of the existence of an inappropriate sexual relationship between therapist and patient.

Remember, even though there may not even be an allegation of therapist-patient sex, nonsexual multiple relationships can be made to appear to be unethical in court.

A HISTORICAL NOTE

This concept of "boundary violations" has only been around for about 10 years or so. It has replaced "transference abuse" in the plaintiff's lexicon because it is less susceptible to courtroom attack. Transference abuse was the original legal concept that was used by courts to explain what had been wrong with therapist-patient sexual involvement—why it was not simply a form of consenting sex between adults. Courts found that therapists owed a duty to patients to protect them from sexual acting out, because patients are purportedly in the throes of transference and cannot, consequently, make adult decisions regarding sex. The psychoanalytic doctrine of transference posits that the patient regresses in reaction to the analyst providing her with a "blank screen" and other aspects of the psychoanalytic method. The patient projects onto the analyst all unresolved parental issues. Ultimately, longing for sex with the analyst is really a reliving of oedipal longings for sex with her father. Thus, under the circumstances as psychoanalysts viewed them, to take advantage of the patient's longings of this type was more like the statutory rape of a minor than like consenting sex.

There was a significant conceptual problem, though, when "transference abuse" was used to build the plaintiff's case against a defendant accused of therapist-patient sex: Transference is a psychoanalytic concept, and it would only be a matter of time before defense experts figured out that therapists have no obligation to think psychoanalytically or to guide their practice-styles by Freudian notions. As Gutheil (1989) has pointed out: "It seems that professionals who belong to a school of thought that rejects the idea of transference, behaviorists, or psychiatrists who provide only drug treatment, are being held to a standard of care they do not acknowledge" (p. 31).

The concept of "boundary violations" came along to replace "transference abuse." It has been put forward in numerous malpractice cases as something that applies across all theories and all approaches. Juries would hear opinionated expert testimony to the effect that good therapists believe in maintaining certain boundaries and that this holds true across all theories of therapy.

WHY DO PLAINTIFFS NEED "BOUNDARY VIOLATIONS" AND NONSEXUAL MULTIPLE RELATIONSHIPS?

If you pay attention to the newspapers, the cases we hear about often involve obvious and extreme examples of sexual exploitation of patients, and often not of just one but of many patients. I once naïvely wondered why plaintiffs' attorneys might spend a lot of courtroom time discussing minor boundary violations, such as excessive self-disclosure, when it was obvious the case was all about the major boundary violation of a therapist-patient sexual relationship—something that is clearly proscribed by all psychotherapy ethics codes as well as by state law in all 50 states. Why would these attorneys bother to establish that relatively minor boundary violations or a nonsexual multiple relationship had occurred when they clearly have enough evidence to support the more significant claim of therapist-patient sex?

The answer is insurance coverage: nearly all malpractice policies exclude or significantly limit payment of claims for damages resulting from therapist-patient sex. They will pay for a psychotherapist's defense if the allegations are denied, but if sexual wrongdoing is conceded or if the defense loses, there will be no insurance payment. Clearly, in view of this, the plaintiff has every reason to focus on the minor boundary violations or the nonsexual multiple relationship and to try to convince the jury that the psychotherapy that had been carried out was so negligent and so far beneath the standard of care as to have been harmful regardless of whether or not sex had ever taken place.

Some may say that this is fine. After all, if a patient had been harmed by a sexual relationship with a therapist, why shouldn't that patient find a way to get that claim covered? The answer is that this strategy to help compensate victims of therapist-patient sex has a significant cost to the profession: the same multiple relationships that are precursors of therapist-patient sex are sometimes also found in good, ethical psychotherapy. In the past few years, there have been lawsuits filed for boundary violations and multiple relationships alone—where there have been no contentions or intimations that the relationship had become sexualized, and where any harm that befell the patient is very much in the eye of the beholder. *Debatable multiple relationships have been elevated to the status of "negligent acts" by plaintiffs' attorneys seeking their share of damage awards.*

This is a relatively new development, and we'll have to see how winnable these kinds of suits turn out to be over time. Many times the insurance companies and the defendants are willing to settle for a relatively small sum of money, maybe less than $50,000, to make the suit go away. It may take some time before some of these nonsexual multiple relationship cases get to juries and we learn how receptive juries turn out to be.

As an example of a *nonsexual multiple relationship* case, consider this one that I consulted on. A female therapist treated a young borderline woman through her teenage years and nursed her through numerous suicide attempts and a chronic depression. In my mind, what really saved this patient from suicide was the degree of closeness that developed between her and her therapist. There were numerous phone calls, meals together, walks together, and even a special celebration on her 21st birthday, because the patient had for years fantasized about killing herself by that point. There was no doubt in my mind that this therapeutic relationship had been beneficial for the patient, but when the therapist tried to separate from the patient and decrease the intensity of the therapy, the patient felt abandoned and ultimately filed a lawsuit. The lawsuit claimed that the therapist-patient relationship had been overly close, had involved boundary violations, and had therefore been negligent. One of the precipitators of the lawsuit was input to the patient from a relative who was a psychotherapist but who had strong objections to the boundary crossings that were part of the defendant-therapist's customary practice. The case was settled, but had it gone to court, the key issue would have been the motivation of the therapist. The jury would have had to decide whether the inordinate degree of caring and giving the therapist had shown the patient was the result of the therapist's commitment to her profession and to this patient, or was it, as alleged, the result of the therapist's own pathology which caused her to have a uncontrollable need to establish an overly close relationship with the patient.

Consider that any juror can grasp, on a commonsense level, that sexual exploitation is inappropriate. Will jurors also accept the idea that psychotherapy is such an unusual form of social interaction such that even ordinary forms of socializing, with which we are all familiar, become inappropriate and harmful in that context?

QUOTATIONS FROM AUTHORITIES ON BOUNDARIES

The following authors, who put forth a viewpoint that favors strict boundary maintenance, are, I believe, overly focused on the benefits of strict boundaries and not concerned enough about the need for practicing psychotherapists to feel free to practice in innovative ways, to "think outside the box," and to avoid being stifled by a set of needless restrictions on their practice styles.

Pope (1994), for example, states the following: "Establishing safe, reliable, and useful boundaries is one of *the most fundamental responsibilities of the therapist.* The boundaries must create a context in which therapist and patient can do the work of therapy" (p. 70).

Simon (1994) provides the following list of "treatment boundary guidelines," which appears in several of his publications, and which I have seen introduced in court numerous times:

> Maintain therapist neutrality. Foster psychological separateness of patient. Obtain informed consent for treatment and procedures. Interact verbally with clients. Ensure no previous, current, or future personal relationships with patients. Minimize physical contact. Preserve relative anonymity of the therapist. Establish a stable fee policy. Provide a consistent, private, and professional setting. Define length and time of sessions. (p. 514)

And Simon (1994) also offers the following opinion, which has been convincing to jurors around the country: "The boundary violation precursors of therapist-patient sex *can be as psychologically damaging as the actual sexual involvement itself.* Unfortunately, professional ethics codes are usually silent concerning the specific boundary violations that often precede therapist sexual misconduct" (p. 514).

Authors like Simon who are so concerned about avoiding boundary violations may themselves practice in a style of psychotherapy that does not require the crossing of any boundaries—classical psychoanalytic psychotherapy, for example. Perhaps because of the style of practice of the authors who promulgated these boundary guidelines, they may have seen no drawbacks to the profession should the guidelines become widely accepted and enforced as standards of care. They may believe, in other words, that all ethical therapists would automatically find themselves in compliance with the need to maintain boundaries. In the words of Simon (1995), one of the strongest advocates for boundary maintenance, "The boundary guidelines . . . , with appropriate clinical modifications, are a unifying element in the over 450 different forms of psychotherapy currently in existence" (p. 90).

Perhaps Simon is right; that depends on what he meant by the words "appropriate clinical modifications." Simon may have intended to allow for the commonplace ways that humanistic and behavioral practitioners, for example, routinely cross what others perceive as boundaries. Simon may not have anticipated the rigid and unforgiving ways that boundary guidelines would be presented to jurors to make the practices of mainstream humanistic psychotherapists (discussed next), for example, appear to be sleazy.

THE SLIPPERY SLOPE

In addition to this viewpoint that boundary violations are harmful, there is the popular "slippery slope" argument, which suggests that boundary violations often, or inevitably, lead to therapist-patient sex. For example, Strasburger, Jorgenson, and Sutherland (1992) write:

> The slippery slope of boundary violations may be ventured upon first in the form of small, relatively inconsequential actions by the therapist such as scheduling a "favored" patient for the last appointment of the day, extending sessions with the patient beyond the scheduled time, having excessive telephone conversations with the patient, and becoming lax with fees. Violations can involve excessive self-disclosure by the therapist to the patient. . . . Gifts may be exchanged. The therapist may begin to direct the patient's work and personal life choices. . . . Meetings may be arranged outside the office for lunch or dinner. . . . Notice that in this scenario, the therapist has not touched the patient, nor has the therapist said or done anything that is overtly sexual. *The treatment, however, has already become compromised, and the therapist may be found liable civilly. The therapist is also vulnerable to action by a licensing board, should the patient wish to make a complaint.* (p. 547)

HUMANISTS AND BEHAVIORISTS AND OTHER LEGITIMATE BOUNDARY CROSSERS

Unlike therapists who show great concern about maintaining strict boundaries, there are therapists who legitimately cross boundaries, not because it is part of a seduction, but because that is how they do therapy, that is how they get results. These therapists are often humanistic. Here is a quotation from Sid Jourard (1971) on his work:

> In the context of dialogue I don't hesitate to share any of my experience with existential binds roughly comparable to those in which the seeker finds himself (this is now called "modeling"); nor do I hesitate to disclose my experience of him, myself, and our relationship as it unfolds from moment to moment. . . . I might give Freudian or other types of interpretations. I might teach him such Yoga know-how or tricks for expanding body-awareness as I have mastered or engage in arm wrestling or hold hands or hug him, if that is the response that emerges in the dialogue.

> I do not hesitate to play a game of handball with a seeker or visit him in his home—if this unfolds in the dialogue. (p. 159)

Along similar lines, Arnold Lazarus (1994a, 1994b) wrote that he finds in his practice of behavior therapy the need to do ordinary social things with patients, such as asking them to join him for a meal. He strongly believes that to do otherwise would ruin the kind of therapist-patient relationship that he wants to create. Keep in mind that behavior therapy does not come from a tradition in which transference is an issue—in fact, many behavior therapists might laugh at the concept of transference. Lazarus himself has called it a myth. What is important is for behavior therapists to develop a warm and positive relationship with the patient, a relationship that creates the context for the application of the behavioral techniques. Perhaps not everyone would agree with Dr. Lazarus's views regarding how to do therapy, but should anyone have a right to dictate how Dr. Lazarus may practice so long as he does not violate relevant ethics codes?

Here is a cautionary tale cited by Goisman and Gutheil (1992), who provide a poignant example of what might occur when commonplace behavior therapy procedures are held up to psychoanalytic scrutiny regarding boundary maintenance:

> We are aware of a case currently in litigation where a number of the charges against an experienced behavior therapist flowed from the testimony of a psychoanalytically trained expert witness, who faulted the behavior therapist for assigning homework tasks to patients, hiring present and former patients for jobs in psychoeducational programs and other benign interventions, and performing a sexological examination and sensate focus instructions in a case of sexual dysfunction. From a psychoanalytic viewpoint all of these would likely constitute boundary violations of a potentially harmful sort, but from a behavioral viewpoint this is not the case. The legal system in this lawsuit had some difficulty, as is commonly the case, in grasping the distinctions between therapies and the variations of boundary norms appropriate to each type of treatment. (p. 538)

GUTHEIL AND GABBARD'S EXAMPLES

Gutheil and Gabbard (1998) have recently published an article indicating that they believe that the pendulum of boundary violations has swung too far. They have observed instances of boundary violations being used inappropriately and without attention to context. They offer the following examples:

During a visit with her internist, a patient reported having had a number of recent losses through deaths of close family members. Discussion of these losses led her to burst into intense sobbing. Later that evening, the internist called the patent at home to see if she was all right. She reassured him that she was, but she later reported him to her state licensing board for the alleged boundary violation of calling her at home. (p. 412)

A female case manager (a community mental health center staff member given the responsibility of coordinating care and rendering practical assistance to patients) took many trips with a female patient to necessary appointments, accompanied the patient's family to the beach with her own family to encourage socialization and to model parenting, and performed many other out-of-office activities. The patient, a paranoid young woman, formed a strong attachment to the case manager and became furious when the relationship had to end because of the latter's pregnancy. At that point she persuaded her parents to bring an ethics violation complaint against her former helper. In subsequent litigation, no evidence emerged that the patient had been exploited or harmed in any way. But the regulating board hearing the case held the case manager to the standard of a psychoanalyst as to what constituted professional boundaries. (p. 411)

Here is a similar example from my own experience as a defense expert. I'll simplify some of the facts: The plaintiff had been in psychotherapy with the defendant for 11 years. She was a very disturbed individual who had been very resistant to treatment and had fired numerous therapists. She was alleging that her psychiatrist of 11 years had had a sexual relationship with her.

Her psychiatrist had died, and was not involved in the litigation. In fact, as is often the case in such lawsuits, it was the perceived abandonment by the therapist that precipitated the filing of the complaint.

The question that needed to be decided in court was whether there had, in fact, been a sexual relationship. There was no smoking gun— nothing that clearly indicated that a sexual relationship had existed. Lacking this, the plaintiff introduced the following facts as evidence that a sexual relationship *must have existed*:

- The therapist had lent a book to the patient.
- The therapist had accepted small gifts from the patient.
- The therapist had met with the patient at her home when she had been disabled and bedridden with a back injury.
- The therapist had self-disclosed personal information about his family.
- The therapist had called the patient at home when he was dying of a terminal illness.

Basically, the plaintiff tried to link these boundary crossings to sex. The logic of this argument, as already put forth by Strasburger et al. (1992), is that any therapist who has deviated to this extent from the rules (at least the rules that some people accept) for psychotherapy must be a sexual exploiter. It is important to note, by the way, that if a psychotherapist were sexually involved with a patient, one would expect all the same boundary violations to occur: self-disclosure, home visits, gift giving, phone calls. The question we all must face is whether, just because these behaviors often occur in conjunction with illicit therapist-patient sex, we should condemn these behaviors in and of themselves. The question, remember, is only important to those therapists who have an interest in a more humanistic practice style or who practice in some aspect of the health care system that requires them to cross what some consider inviolable boundaries.

A GENERATION GAP

One observation I have made is that most of the defendants I have come across have been middle aged. While it is true that newly trained therapists might intentionally cross boundaries, the fact is that most of them have been inculcated with the viewpoint that stresses the importance of boundaries in graduate or professional schools (see Borys & Pope, 1989). In contrast, many therapists trained in the 1970s or earlier may never have taken an ethics course as part of their training, and they may have been systematically trained in a method or theory that advocates a very loose approach to boundaries. The upshot of this has been the courtroom fighting I have seen between younger expert witnesses honestly testifying that in their view the older defendant should have known that, for example, dining and taking walks together with the patient was inappropriate.

Often, the younger ethics expert has enhanced credibility because of specific responsibilities regarding ethics, such as service on a state or national ethics committee. Or the ethics expert may be someone who has simply taken an interest in ethics and who has attained a certain stature in that area. The defendant may never have thought that boundary issues needed addressing—after all, there is no ethics code prohibition on self-disclosure, taking walks together, and so on. In many cases the outcome of a civil suit is a function of how much the jury seems to like the defendant, the respective experts, and the plaintiff. Unfortunately, what is right and wrong may not play a large role.

CONCLUSION

This chapter has attempted to expose the following fallacious logic: *Multiple relationships are unethical. They are characterized by boundary violations, which are themselves unethical. They are likely to lead to therapist-patient sex, and are signs of negligence whether sex occurs or not.*

I have also tried to show that this viewpoint is an overreaction to two different concerns: the wish to rid our field of therapist-patient sex, and the wish to protect practitioners, through risk management, from lawsuits. Because multiple relationships can be positive, healing aspects of psychotherapy, demonizing them, and demonizing the therapists who make good use of them, has constrained the effective practice of psychotherapy and has led to needless harm to decent, honest psychotherapists who have faced unfair legal actions for engaging in benign multiple relationships. Hopefully, the psychotherapy professions will recognize that the pendulum has swung too far and will take steps to become more supportive of benign multiple relations—relationships that do not lead to harm, do not lead to a loss of objectivity, and are not exploitative.

REFERENCES

American Psychological Association. (1953). *Ethical standards of psychologists.* Washington, DC: Author.

Borys, D. S., & Pope, K. S. (1989). Dual relationships between therapist and client: A national study of psychologists, psychiatrists, and social workers. *Professional Psychology: Research and Practice, 20,* 283–293.

Canter, M., Bennett, B., Jones, S., & Nagy, T. (1994). *Ethics for psychologists: A commentary on the APA ethics code.* Washington, DC: American Psychological Association.

Goisman, R. M., & Gutheil, T. G. (1992). Risk management in the practice of behavior therapy: Boundaries and behavior. *American Journal of Psychotherapy, 46,* 533–543.

Gutheil, T. G. (1989). Patient-therapist sexual relations. *The California Therapist, November/December,* 29–39.

Gutheil, T. G., & Gabbard, G. (1998). Misuses and misunderstandings of boundary theory in clinical and regulatory settings. *American Journal of Psychiatry, 155* (3), 409–414.

Jourard, S. M. (1971). *The transparent self.* New York: D. Van Nostrand.

Lazarus, A. A. (1994a). How certain boundaries and ethics diminish therapeutic effectiveness. *Ethics and Behavior, 4,* 255–261.

Lazarus, A. A. (1994b). The illusion of the therapist's power and the patient's fragility: My rejoinder. *Ethics and Behavior, 4,* 299–306.

Pope, K. S. (1994). *Sexual involvement with therapists.* Washington, DC: American Psychological Association.

Pope, K. S., & Bouhoutsos, J. C. (1986). *Sexual intimacy between therapists and patients.* New York: Praeger.

Simon, R. I. (1994). Transference in therapist-patient sex: The illusion of patient improvement and consent, part 1. *Psychiatric Annals, 24,* 509–515.

Simon, R. I. (1995). The natural history of therapist sexual misconduct: Identification and prevention. *Psychiatric Annals, 25,* 90–94.

Strasburger, L. H., Jorgenson, L., & Sutherland, P. (1992). The prevention of psychotherapy sexual misconduct: Avoiding the slippery slope. *American Journal of Psychotherapy, 46,* 544–555.

Williams, M. H. (1992). Exploitation and inference: Mapping the damage from therapist-patient sexual involvement. *American Psychologist, 47* (3), 412–421.

CHAPTER 15

Psychologists, Licensing Boards, Ethics Committees, and Dehumanizing Attitudes

With Special Reference to Dual Relationships

Arnold A. Lazarus, PhD, ABPP

He looked down at us from the podium, adjusted the microphone (again), and stated flatly, "Any time you cross a professional boundary you place your entire career in jeopardy." He waited for that to sink in. I looked around me. Everyone in the audience seemed to be paying very close attention. This was one of those risk-management seminars in which carefully chosen speakers told us how to hang onto our licenses. I have attended two of those seminars and found them extremely scary. On both occasions, when 4:30 or 5:00 P.M. rolled round and we disbanded, I felt anxious and paranoid. I was not alone. As I

Parts of this chapter are taken from Lazarus, A. A. (2002). Something must be done about the totalitarian mentality of ethics committees and licensing boards. In J. K. Zeig (Ed.). (2002). *The evolution of psychotherapy: The fourth conference.* Phoenix, AZ: Zeig & Tucker.

learned later, most of the seminar attendees felt similarly. It was drilled into us that seeing clients was hazardous. Make one false move and our careers could be plundered. Uncompromising licensing boards and ethics committees would condemn us and strip us of our licenses and livelihoods. The next day (and for 2 or 3 days thereafter) I viewed my clients as dangerous adversaries, as potential litigants, and I was on guard. Fortunately, this soon wore off, and I once again reverted to being the flexible and humane clinician I see myself as.

In both the seminars I attended, we learned the myriad ways in which one can fall foul of a licensing board, and considerable time was spent discussing the perils of dual (or multiple) relationships. One of the lecturers was adamant that any time a therapist entered into a dual relationship, the treatment was likely to be undermined. Unless there was an explicit therapeutic reason to spend time with a client outside the office (as when doing in vivo desensitization for instance), a therapist was well advised to have no dealings with a client in any other setting. Somewhat facetiously, I raised my hand and inquired if it was permissible for a therapist to send out for sandwiches and share them with his or her client in the office. The answer was an emphatic "NO"—unless there happened to be a clear-cut and defensible treatment rationale (such as promoting eating behaviors in an anorexic client). The thinking behind this totalitarian line of reasoning seems to be that seemingly innocent acts can all too readily lead to unethical behaviors. Some "experts" contend that even the most well-intentioned therapist may discover that boundary crossings are likely to foster sexual liaisons. The utter absurdity of this view as a widespread and general probability has been addressed in several places throughout this book so I will not rebut it here.

THE DEFENSELESS PSYCHOLOGIST

The foregoing is not intended to minimize the ubiquitous dangers that mental health practitioners face from their ethics committees and licensing boards. Just how vulnerable are psychologists in front of a state licensing board? In four words—they are *extremely* vulnerable. Bryant Welch, an attorney and psychologist explains exactly why in edition I, 2001, of the document *Insight: Safeguarding Psychologists Against Liability Risks*, published by American Professional Agency, Inc., of the Chubb Group of Insurance Companies. He points out that in our judicial system, the five decision-making functions—investigator, prosecutor, juror, judge, and appellate hearing—are kept separate. Why? So that no single entity can establish domination. This dispersal of authority allows each one to check on the rulings and authority of the others. But as Welch explains, in most states the law permits licensing boards to serve as investigator, prosecutor, judge, jury, and appeals court. "In many cases, the board also serves as the complainant, filing charges against psychologists themselves" (p. 2). He adds, "The biggest problem is that nothing protects a psychologist from an arbitrary or irrational decision by the licensing board" (p. 2).

Welch (2001) also stated that "the cost of a defense before a licensing board is potentially staggering" (p. 5), and he added that some clients had paid $60,000 in attorney fees having "hardly begun their defense" (p. 5). But there is more. In many instances, if you are a professional clinical psychologist or licensed psychotherapist, and are summoned to appear before a licensing board or ethics committee, it may be formidable if not impossible to prove your innocence.

TOTALITARIANISM

Under our system of jurisprudence, if you are accused of committing a crime, you are entitled to a fair trial. You are presumed innocent until proven guilty. But unlike civil and criminal court proceedings, many licensing boards provide no right of discovery. Williams (2000b) makes clear that you may be summoned to a board hearing without having any idea of what the testimony against you will be. In most U.S. states, psychologists cannot take depositions of opposing witnesses to prepare his or her defense. In fact, the defendant may not be permitted to discover who the witnesses will be. Moreover, with many licensing boards there is no statute of limitations. Thus, you may be faced with the impossible task of preparing a defense based on events that occurred years ago and for which exculpatory records and witnesses may be unavailable.

It cannot be overstated that psychologists have lost their licenses without fair hearings, due process of law, or clear standards. A psychologist may pay many thousands of dollars for attorneys and expert witnesses, appear before an administrative law judge, win the case, and be allowed to remain in practice, only to receive a letter from the board revoking his or her license. Yet, as Martin H. Williams (2000a) has underscored, "We must realize that sometimes a defendant who is charged with loathsome ethical violations has, in fact, done nothing wrong" (p. 81). His article, "Victimized by 'Victims' " incisively explains the antecedents, dynamics, and consequences of groundless and false complaints against psychotherapists. The biggest myth of all is that only those who have done something wrong are accused and only those who deserve sanctions get sanctions.

Peterson (2001) documents how blameless psychologists lost "their livelihood, savings, and health because of the practices of their licensing boards" (p. 339). Williams (2001) provides examples of the unfair manner in which state licensing board practices bypass due-process protection. Saunders (2001), in a powerful message against oppression, refers to "a disguised form of professional fascism, embedded in part in the professional regulatory atmosphere of APA, and in particular in the disciplinary process for psychologists operated by State licensing boards" (p. 15).

Consequently, many psychotherapists who are cognizant of the persecutory climate tend to embrace prohibitions and construct rigid boundaries that often undermine their clinical effectiveness, and ironically, render them more susceptible to litigation (C. N. Lazarus, 2001). Terrified providers are apt to permit risk-management principles to take precedence over humane interventions. This is not to gainsay the desirability of constructing a sensitive, intelligent, and pragmatic code of ethics—prescriptions and proscriptions to guide intercollegial conduct, as well as patient and therapist rights and obligations. I stress in my chapter "Something must be done about the totalitarian mentality of many ethics committees and licensing boards" (A. A. Lazarus, 2002), that the enforcement of ethical regulations should follow democratic not autocratic principles.

DUAL RELATIONSHIPS

It is my view that dual relationships may have been so strongly prohibited because many of the people who compiled the ethical rules were psychodynamic thinkers. Psychoanalysis with its clinical-transferential rationale prohibits all forms of dual relationships (despite the fact that Freud and many of his contemporaries and successors crossed boundaries and entered into significant dual relationships). What is viewed as a dual relationship or another boundary crossing in psychoanalytic therapy may be an integral part of behavior therapy. Williams (1997) points out that what cognitive-behavior therapists, existentialists, or humanists may view as salubrious interventions, psychoanalysts would regard as "transference abuse." Must all approaches to therapy work within the confines imposed on us by one theoretical orientation?

Gary Schoener, the executive director of the Walk-In Counseling Center, in Minneapolis, Minnesota, sent me an e-mail on April 4, 2000 in which he discussed "overlapping relationships." He stated, "You run into clients in a church parking lot—that's an 'encounter.' They turn out to go to your church—that's an overlapping relationship. You and they attend a Sunday school class that predominantly involves listening to lectures. That's overlapping with some potential to become dual. The pastor offers a parent support group in which people are to spill their guts about their child-rearing problems. To participate in that group with a current client is riskier and may be a dual relationship with a potential conflict of interest." Personally, I would avoid this degree of overlap or duality.

I receive a similar response from many quarters when mentioning that with some clients, a sense of camaraderie develops when one steps outside the bounds of a sanctioned healer, and this tends to enhance treatment outcomes. "I'm sure this is so," many colleagues have said, "but we trust your judgment in these matters and fully believe that you know when and when not to extend a boundary." They then go on to say that when it comes to many of the other people in practice, their level-headedness and sagacity may be extremely faulty. Thus, they contend that it is in the best interests of their clients, our profession, and society at large, to forbid them to stray beyond strictly prescribed boundaries. My counterargument is that instead of imposing a universal ban, it is better to educate health providers to assess risks and contraindications and for boards and committees to hear complaints and make individualistic case determinations. But the Code of Ethics adopted by the American Psychological Association (1992), the National Association of Social Workers (1999), and the various boards of certified counselors (i.e., American Counseling Association, 1996), and marriage and family therapists (i.e., American Association for Marriage and Family Therapy, 2001; California Association of Marriage and Family Therapists, 1997), are all wary of dual relationships. They all warn against treating friends or family members.

I argued against this prohibition during a talk I gave to the Division of Clinical Psychology at the 1997 American Psychological Association Convention (Lazarus, 1998). I emphasized that my own formative experiences belie the putative dangers that supposedly lurk behind those who provide clinical services to family members, friends, or associates. I mentioned that I have helped many a friend and family member with issues ranging from marital spats to intense phobias. It made no difference if a caring aunt or a total stranger was being treated for claustrophobia via systematic desensitization and in vivo exposure. However, I studiously avoided treating any relative who was unstable or deeply troubled. For example, when one of my relatives requested therapy from me, I referred him to a colleague because, given his bizarre perceptions, had I become professionally involved, the most likely outcome would have been alienation from that wing of the family. This matter goes to the heart of my argument. Let us modify the edict, "Never treat family members or friends," to *"It is advisable to be cautious about treating close associates, and it is inadvisable to treat family or friends who suffer from severe personality disorders or other major psychopathology."*

Ethics committees have expelled psychologists from membership, and state licensing boards have revoked their licenses for having engaged in dual relationships. Ebert (1997) alluded to "unfair and inconsistent decisions . . . used by state licensing authorities" (p. 145) often with catastrophic results. He also stressed that "dual-relationship rules must not impede a psychologist's ability to perform optimum work," and he stressed that "some policies surrounding dual relationships could be considered as gender discrimination" (p. 143). In chapter 29, Miriam Greenspan incisively underscores that whereas an ethic of nonabuse for professional relationships is clearly necessary, she is doubtful if the language of boundaries and the admonition to eschew all dual relationships achieves this objective. In fact she argues that it conceals the political dimension of violence against women. She deplores what she terms "the distance model" and offers instead "a connection model of therapy," and she argues that the rigidification of boundaries may produce more, not less, power abuse in therapy. Similarly, Zur (2000) has shown that the prohibition of nonsexual dual relationships can prove deleterious to the treatment process.

POSTTREATMENT FRIENDSHIPS AND INTIMACIES

Let's segue into a discussion of posttreatment sexual relationships. Though there are some who contend that sex between client and therapist may be salubrious in some instances, I am squarely in the camp that denounces sex with a client. It is fraught with far too many potentially powerful and unpredictable emotions—it is apt to corrode trust, undermine objectivity, and introduce the elements of unfair advantage taking and exploitation (to mention only a few hazards and objections). But what about posttreatment relations? Is friendship or sex permissible when therapy is over and the formal doctor-patient relationship no longer pertains? Two-year and 5-year mandatory waiting periods are on the books in some quarters, whereas others forbid sex with former clients in perpetuity. Blanket rules of this sort strike me as absurd. Surely it is person- and -situation-specific?

For example, say a young, single, heterosexual female client consults a young, unmarried, heterosexual male therapist. She is basically stable and well functioning but is having difficulties at work with an unsympathetic employer. After two role-playing and assertiveness training sessions, she is able to bring matters to a head, and at her third and final session, she reports that she quit her job and found another that augurs well for the future. The therapist recommends a couple of books on assertive behavior to reinforce her newfound skills. Several months later they meet at a party where they have a long and interesting chat and would like to start dating each other. "You have to wait for an additional 16 to 18 months," would be the edict of some, whereas others would decree, "Impermissible! Once a patient, always a patient." The same rules would apply had the client been in therapy for 5 years of intensive treatment for sexual identity problems coupled with a personality disorder, bipolar proclivities, and obsessive-compulsive tendencies. A therapist who worked in a locale that upheld the 2-year posttreatment ban would presumably be permitted to engage in sexual relations with this former client. I submit that in matters of this kind, the "forbidden in perpetuity" rule should pertain. Thus, I am arguing for a case-by-case determination of such matters.

As an extremely wise and perspicacious colleague pointed out to me, the APA Code of Ethics (1992) is a litigator's dream, exposing any psychologist practitioner to being blindsided even though he or she is doing the right thing for the client. Part of the intent behind this book is to disseminate information that may enable matters to be placed on a far more equitable plane.

ACTING DISRESPECTFULLY TOWARD CLIENTS

I have noticed that psychotherapists who are strongly opposed to boundary extensions and adhere to a "strict professionalism" often have what strikes me as an offensive way of relating to their clients. Here is a typical example. I was at a meeting (rather pretentiously called a "Ward Round") where several psychiatric residents took turns presenting cases to about 2 dozen mental health professionals. A young woman was being interviewed by one of the psychiatric residents. The dialogue continued more or less as follows:

Patient: May I ask how old you are?
Resident: Why is that important?
Patient: It's no big deal. I was just curious.
Resident: Why would you be curious about my age?
Patient: Well, you look around 30 and I was just wondering if I am correct.
Resident: What impact would it have if you were not correct?
Patient: None that I can think of. It was just idle curiosity.
Resident: Just idle curiosity?

As I watched these exchanges, I grew uncomfortable. It seemed to me that the patient wished she had never raised the issue in the first place and that she was feeling more and more uneasy. It did not seem that the dialogue was fostering warmth, trust, or rapport. On the contrary, it resembled a cross-examination in a courtroom and appeared adversarial

In psychoanalysis it is deemed important for the analyst to remain neutral and nondisclosing so the patient can project his or her needs, wishes, and fantasies onto this "blank screen." It makes no sense for this to become a rule for *all* therapists to follow. It has always struck me as ill mannered and discourteous to treat people this way.

I recommend the following type of exchange in place of the aforementioned example:

Patient: How old are you?
Resident: I just turned 29. Why do you ask?
Patient: I was just curious. It's no big deal.
Resident: Might you be more comfortable with or have greater confidence in someone older?
Patient: No, not at all.

At this juncture, I would suggest that the topic be dropped. Notice the recommended format. First answer the question and then proceed with an inquiry if necessary. In this way, the patient is validated and not demeaned. Why am I dwelling on such a seemingly trivial issue? Because it is not a minor or frivolous point, and I have observed this type of interaction far too often—usually to the detriment of the therapeutic process. I see it as part and parcel of a dehumanizing penchant among the many rigid thinkers in our field, those who legislate against all dual relationships and deplore all boundary extensions. These are the members of our profession (and they are not a minority) who regard themselves as superior to patients and tend to infantilize and demean them in the process. It is significant that younger and more recently trained psychotherapists endorse more conservative views on ethics and boundaries than those who are older and less recently trained (see Lamb & Catanzaro, 1998).

Regrettably, far too many therapists embrace the widespread belief in the "power differential," which holds that the patient is in a one-down position and is unable to refuse requests and directives from the therapist. It seems to me that some practitioners need to see themselves as omnipotent, thereby rendering all patients readily susceptible to coercion. Thus, their clients are bizarrely overprotected, which, like exploitation, is not beneficial for them and tends to undermine the therapy. It is particularly unfortunate to regard patients as "untouchables" instead of simply treating them as fellow human beings.

REFERENCES

American Association for Marriage and Family Therapists. (2001). *AAMFT code of ethics.* Washington, DC: Author. Retrieved July 8, 2001, from http://www.aamft.org/about/revisedcodeethics.htm

American Counseling Association. (1996). *Code of ethics and standards of practice.* Alexandria, VA: American Counseling Association.

American Psychological Association. (1992). *Ethical principles of psychologists and code of conduct.* Washington, DC: Author.

California Association of Marriage and Family Therapists. (1997). *Ethical standards for marriage and family therapists.* San Diego, CA: Author.

Ebert, B. W. (1997). Dual-relationship prohibitions: A concept whose time never should have come. *Applied & Preventive Psychology, 6,* 137–156.

Lamb, D. H., & Catanzaro, S. J. (1998). Sexual and nonsexual boundary violations involving psychologists, clients, supervisees, and students: Implications for professional practice. *Professional Psychology: Research and Practice, 29,* 498–503.

Lazarus, A. A. (1998). How do you like these boundaries? *The Clinical Psychologist, 51,* 22–25.

Lazarus, A. A. (2002). Something must be done about the totalitarian mentality of many ethics committees and licensing boards. In J. Zeig (Ed.), *The evolution of psychotherapy: The fourth conference.* Phoenix, AZ: Zeig, Tucker.

Lazarus, C. N. (2001). Foundations of pharmacopsychology. In S. Cullari (Ed.), *Counseling and psychotherapy: A practical guidebook for trainees and new professionals* (pp. 246–288). Boston: Allyn and Bacon.

National Association of Social Workers. (1999). *Code of ethics.* Retrieved July 27, 2001, from http://www.naswdc.org/Code/ethics.htm

Peterson, M. B. (2001). Recognizing concerns about how some licensing boards are treating psychologists. *Professional Psychology: Research and Practice, 32,* 339–340.

Saunders, T. T. (2001). After all, this is Baltimore—Distinguished psychologist of the year address. *The Independent Practitioner, Winter,* 15–18.

Welch, B. (2001). *Insight: Safeguarding psychologists against liability risks* (1st ed.). *Caution: State licensing board ahead.* Amityville, NY: American Professional Agency, Inc., Chubb Group of Insurance Companies.

Williams, M. H. (1997). Boundary violations: Do some contended standards of care fail to encompass commonplace procedures of humanistic, behavioral and eclectic psychotherapies? *Psychotherapy, 34,* 239–249.

Williams, M. H. (2000a). Victimized by "victims": A taxonomy of antecedents of false complaints against psychotherapists. *Professional Psychology: Research and Practice, 31,* 75–81.

Williams, M. H. (2000b, winter). APA ethics committee considered prohibiting solo practice. *The Independent Practitioner, 20* (1), 46–49.

Williams, M. H. (2001). The question of psychologists' maltreatment by state licensing boards: Overcoming denial and seeking remedies. *Professional Psychology: Research and Practice, 32,* 341–344.

Zur, O. (2000). In celebration of dual relationships: How prohibition of nonsexual dual relationships increases the chance of exploitation and harm. *The Independent Practitioner, 20,* 97–100.

CHAPTER 16

Dueling Over Dual Relationships

John Fleer, PhD, JD

While writing this chapter, I am awaiting the decision from an administrative law judge who presided over a month-long hearing in which my client, a psychotherapist, was accused by her licensing board of unethical dual relationships. My client, whom I will call Dr. A, practices outpatient psychotherapy with adult clients who have been the victims of extreme trauma in childhood and/or adult life. Many of the clients carry diagnoses of post-traumatic stress disorder and/or dissociative disorders. Some meet DSM–IV (1994) AXIS II criteria for personality disorders as well.

A formal accusation was filed against Dr. A by her licensing board. The accusation was based upon the complaints of two former clients, X and Y. X was in psychotherapy with Dr. A for 4 years. X was, to say the least, a highly demanding and difficult client who was very specific regarding her needs in psychotherapy and the manner in which she wanted to be served. She received outpatient therapy twice a week and made frequent phone calls to Dr. A between office visits. During the 4 years of therapy, Dr. A, on several occasions, conducted sessions at X's home. These were always at the request of X and in response to a crisis situation, or X's inability to leave the home. Dr. A also went on occasional walks with X during the course of sessions, attended four social events (two birthday parties, a graduation party, and New Year's party) at X's invitation (and insistence) and exchanged gifts and cards over the period of treatment. X was often critical regarding the quality and nature of Dr. A's interactions. She provided written grades for Dr. A's performance as a psychotherapist, demanded refunds for therapy, and expressed rage at Dr. A's attempts to place limitations on between-session phone calls.

Ultimately, Dr. A sought impasse consultation for the therapy relationship. The consultant recommended a transition of X to another therapist. The transition period was prolonged and X refused to give up her weekly contacts with Dr. A. Finally, Dr. A formally terminated therapy. X's response was to charge Dr. A with abandonment. Her formal board complaint alleged negligent misdiagnosis, memory implantation, violation of sexual boundaries, breach of confidentiality, and practicing medicine without a license. None of these allegations were factually supported. Ultimately, however, X and the licensing board settled on the claim that Dr. A had engaged in a dual relationship with X, which had caused her harm by virtue of confusing her as to whether Dr. A was her therapist or her friend.

Y was a seriously disordered client who had a long history of inpatient psychiatric hospitalizations for multiple personality disorder (currently, dissociative identity disturbance, per DSM–IV, 1994). Dr. A commenced outpatient treatment with Y with the express intent of limiting hospitalizations. To this end, Dr. A at times had sessions of several hours' duration, due to the unstable and unsafe condition of Y, and also met with Y at her home when physical problems prevented Y from traveling to and from Dr. A's office. With minor exceptions, Dr. A's treatment was successful in keeping Y out of psychiatric hospitals for the year and a half in which she provided treatment. When Y stopped coming to therapy sessions, Dr. A wrote a letter indicating that she would keep session appointments open for 1 month but would formally terminate if she did not hear from Y during that time. When the month passed without contact, Dr. A sent a formal letter of termination. Y's response was to allege abandonment and to file a civil lawsuit (which was ultimately dismissed without any payment on behalf of Dr. A). Y ultimately joined in the licensing board's complaint process and also came to allege that she had been damaged by an unethical dual relationship with Dr. A. She claimed that the lengthy sessions and the meetings at her home had harmed her by their confusing nature. At the administrative hearing, the board presented testimony from both X and Y, in which they claimed to have been damaged by Dr. A. They attributed all subsequent psychotherapy treatment to the harm caused by her dual relationships. The board further presented testimony from an expert who opined that, while none of the alleged boundary violations of Dr. A were in and of themselves unethical (i.e., walks, home visits, gifts, social event attendance), the sum of her acts amounted to gross deviations from the standard of care and violated the ethical standards. This expert further stated that Dr. A's actions were malevolent and had caused pernicious harm.

A month-long battle ensued over the definition of dual relationship, and the question as to whether such a relationship was harmful, exploitive, or impaired the objectivity of the psychotherapist. This dispute was particularly noteworthy because it did not involve any patient-therapist sex and did not involve any financial exploitation of the clients. As noted by the board's own expert, there was no act of Dr. A that could clearly be characterized as unethical. Rather, a Gestalt interpretation was proffered by which the unethical conduct of Dr. A was greater than the sum of its ethical parts.

Dr. A's treatment notes were detailed and comprehensive. Every telephone call, session, and out-of-office contact was meticulously noted. The notes further reflected careful thought prior to the attendance of social events and the giving of any gift. The conscientious nature of Dr. A and her commitment to patient welfare was attested to by a variety of colleagues and consultants. Dr. A expressed her regret that these two clients had not benefited from her treatment, even though there was objective evidence that they both functioned better than they had prior to being treated by her.

In defense of Dr. A, two experts gave testimony. One similarly worked with dissociative clients and trauma victims. This expert has outstanding credentials in these areas and holds positions in professional societies, as well as teaching positions. He is well published in the areas under review. He endorsed Dr. A's treatment approach and her willingness to extend boundaries for the benefit and welfare of her clients. He did not believe that there was any evidence of a dual relationship in either of the two cases under review and further found no exploitation or harm of either of the clients, nor any impaired objectivity on the part of Dr. A.

A well-known ethics expert also testified as to the lack of any ethical violation by Dr. A. He further offered the opinion that, while a knowledgeable psychotherapist might have disagreements regarding the advantages and disadvantages of the treatments provided by Dr. A, these were not matters of ethics, nor did they pertain to matters of standard of care, but reflected differences of opinion regarding theoretical positions and practice styles. He further expressed amazement that a licensing board was pursuing discipline against a therapist, who at worst, had been overly nice, attentive, and responsive to client needs. There was no underlying bad act, such as sexual or financial exploitation, upon which to base testimony that a walk or gift was a conduit to unethical behavior.

We have reached the point where psychotherapists can be charged with misconduct and have their licenses threatened on the basis of therapist conduct that deviates, if only slightly, from rigid models of more or less impersonal conduct. The unhappy or vengeful ex-client can allege confusion or harm without any objective corroboration, and self-styled ethics experts are only too willing to criticize and condemn the overly friendly perpetrator or the clinician whose boundaries are considered too loose. This would almost be humorous, were it not for the sobering fact that licenses and livelihoods are threatened, and therapists often have insufficient funds to cover the significant expenses of defending against these claims. The emotional costs of doing so are also great. Reputations are, of course, damaged by virtue of a complaint or accusation alone.

Courtroom battles concerning psychotherapist dual relationships are likely to increase as ex-patients and their attorneys become more aware of the concept. A vindictive former client can easily allege that the relationship with a former psychotherapist was, in some respects, personal and was pursued by the psychotherapist for his or her own gratification. In the aftermath of long-term treatment, patients are likely to know some personal details of their therapists' lives. These can be recited in court as evidence of unethical self-disclosures. Any contact outside of the therapy office, whether in person or by telephone or letter, can be characterized as a boundary violation. Extended sessions or reduction in fees for services can be characterized as part of the slippery slope that leads to exploitation of the client.

It is ultimately up to mental health professionals to speak out against the overinterpretation of prohibitions against exploitive multiple relationships. Meanwhile, the individual psychotherapist should be aware of the manner in which civil lawsuits and licensing board complaints are adjudicated and the standards that will be applied to make judgments concerning allegations of psychotherapists' unethical dual relationships.

CIVIL LAWSUITS

Civil lawsuits predicated on an alleged unethical dual relationship are usually filed in the form of a professional negligence claim. These are also referred to as malpractice complaints. If the defendant psychotherapist carries professional liability insurance, she or he will usually be provided an attorney to defend the case and will be indemnified for settlements or judgments up to the limits of the insurance policy. If the dual relationship is alleged to have included sexual contact between psychotherapist and client, a civil lawsuit will also typically be brought in the form of a battery claim, in which the psychotherapist will be accused of violating a civil and/or criminal statute prohibiting such sexual contact. These claims are typically not indemnified by liability insurance carriers, although a defense may still be provided by the carrier.

Regardless of the legal theories upon which the civil lawsuit is based, the defendant psychotherapist should contact his or her insurance company or a personal attorney as soon as a notice of the complaint is received. Pertinent treatment records should be secured. No alterations or clarifications should be made to these records. Psychotherapists should prepare no written summaries or descriptions of treatment unless instructed to do so by the insurance carrier or defense counsel. Psychotherapists should also be aware that discussions regarding the specifics of the allegations in the lawsuit are usually not covered by any privilege and could be discoverable by the plaintiff's attorney during the course of the lawsuit. On the other hand, discussions about the case with the insurance carrier representative and defense counsel are confidential.

Each state has its own rules regarding how a lawsuit proceeds from the filing of the complaint through trial and appeal. There is a time limit within which a response must be filed in court once the complaint has been served. Therefore, the insurance carrier and/or attorney should be notified as soon as possible once a complaint has been served.

Before a case goes to trial, both sides have an opportunity to conduct discovery. The testimony of potential witnesses, including the plaintiff and defendant, can be taken by way of deposition. Relevant records can be subpoenaed, and the expert witnesses retained by both sides are usually identified and made available for deposition as well. Thus, in most civil actions, the parties are afforded an opportunity to marshal the relevant evidence and to learn how opposition witnesses will testify prior to trial. Along the way, cases may be dismissed by agreement between the parties or by order from the court. The majority of civil lawsuits are settled prior to trial.

When cases do proceed to trial, either the plaintiff or defendant can assert the right to have the matter heard by a jury. The plaintiff has the burden of proof. This means that the plaintiff bears the obligation of presenting documents and testimony to establish the essential elements of the claim being made. As a practical matter, in the dual relationship-based civil lawsuit, a plaintiff can do so by his or her own testimony, supported by an expert witness who testifies that the defendant psychotherapist has engaged in ethical violations and/or substandard treatment of the plaintiff. The plaintiff in these cases typically asserts as many boundary violations as possible. The expert witness typically refers to Ethics Code statements concerning dual or multiple relationships and expounds upon the way in which such relationships negatively impact, and even exploit, the client.

The defense case similarly rests upon testimony of the psychotherapist defendant, who either denies or explains the nature of alleged boundary violations. Expert witnesses called by the defense need to explain to the judge or jury that the professional society Ethics Codes do not contain specific prohibitions against the therapist's self-disclosures or so-called boundary violations upon which the plaintiff's case is based. Such an expert might also be in a position to offer a professional opinion regarding the plaintiff's underlying psychopathology as it relates to motivations to file a false or distorted claim.

Both sides present testimony on damages. The plaintiff will usually allege that the defendant has caused intense and enduring emotional distress that will itself require extended psychotherapeutic treatment. Plaintiffs are often supported in this regard by psychotherapists they are currently seeing. The defense will argue that damages are nonexistent or less extensive than those being claimed.

In regard to the negligence claim, a jury or judge deciding the civil lawsuit will need to determine whether it is more likely than not that the defendant breached the standard of care and thereby caused damage to the plaintiff. The standard of care is determined by reference to the practices of other reputable psychotherapists with similar education, training, and practice to that of the defendant. This is the topic upon which the expert witnesses called by either side most commonly express disagreement. The plaintiff's expert or experts will testify that the conduct of the defendant psychotherapist was outside the standard of care and would not be engaged in during similar circumstances by reputable practitioners. The defense expert or experts may well testify that the acts of the defendant would similarly have been engaged in by other reputable practitioners under the same or similar circumstances. They will explain that the standard of care consists of a broad range of therapeutic choices.

Because the standard of care is not something with which a layperson (juror) would be familiar, the quality of expert witness testimony is probably the most important factor in determining the outcome of a judge's or jury's deliberations. Expert witnesses retained by the defense should be well-familiar with pertinent Ethics Code provisions regarding dual or multiple relationships, and should be able to communicate with the judge or jury in easy to understand language. They must have a good grasp of the standard of care concept and should be comfortable defending opinions under rigorous cross-examination.

Participation in a civil trial is an unpleasant and even traumatic experience for defendants. Nevertheless, professional negligence claims for health care providers in general are more often decided in favor of the defendants than the plaintiffs, if they proceed through trial. Even if a verdict is in favor of the plaintiff, the defendant is usually sufficiently covered by insurance for the judgment amount and is provided further defense on appeal on those cases in which an appeal is warranted. For the psychotherapist against whom a judgment has been rendered, the most negative consequence may well be that the judgment is reported to the state board that licenses the psychotherapist. This report may lead to a further investigation and disciplinary proceedings.

LICENSING BOARD COMPLAINTS

State licensing boards can, in most states, initiate an investigation of a licensee in response to a report of a settlement or a judgment against the psychotherapist. State boards also commonly investigate complaints made by ex-clients who may or may not also have filed civil lawsuits. Licensing boards conduct investigations and hearings in accordance with administrative law statutes, which differ from civil proceedings. The adjudicatory process again differs state by state, but, in general, the psychotherapist who is faced with disciplinary charges from her or his licensing board is afforded fewer due process protections than a defendant in either civil or criminal proceedings. Details of the board's investigation are usually not disclosed to the licensee until after they have been completed. The licensee usually has no or extremely limited discovery rights and does not have the opportunity to take depositions of the complaining party or expert witnesses who will be called to testify in the case.

If a psychotherapist is formally charged with intentional misconduct, gross negligence, or repeated acts of negligence, the hearing is usually held before an administrative law judge or the licensing agency itself (that is, the same party that is bringing the charges!). There is no right to a jury. Even if the administrative law judge finds in favor of the psychotherapist, the licensing board may refuse to adopt the administrative law judge's decision.

Currently, most professional liability insurance policies provide for some payment of a psychotherapist's licensing board defense costs. The amount of such coverage has traditionally been inadequate to pay attorney and expert witness fees should the matter proceed to hearing. However, some insurance companies now offer significantly higher levels of defense costs coverage in exchange for a relatively small premium surcharge. There is, in any event, no insurance against the negative consequences of an adverse finding against the psychotherapist. There is no insurance for suspension or revocation of the psychotherapist's license.

Despite the differences between the administrative and civil law systems, the trial-hearing still revolves around the concept of standard of care. Expert witness testimony supporting the accused psychotherapist remains the single most important element in a successful defense. Administrative law judges and members of licensing board agencies require education on the nature of professional Ethics Codes and the inclusiveness of standard of care as applied to the case at hand.

CONCLUSION

The battle over dual relationships is increasingly being played out in civil litigation and licensing board disciplinary proceedings. The psychotherapist who is targeted in either a civil lawsuit or a disciplinary complaint should seek prompt assistance from legal counsel and his or her professional liability insurance carrier. In matters that proceed to trial or hearing, the retention of competent expert witnesses on behalf of the psychotherapist is of paramount importance.

REFERENCE

American Psychological Association. (1994). *Diagnostic and statistical manual of mental disorders.* Washington, DC: Author.

CHAPTER 17

Are Dual Relationships Antitherapeutic?

Alan W. Scheflin, BA, JD, LLM, MA

What causes people to heal? This is the central question guiding physical medicine and mental therapy, and it is the standard by which all treatments and procedures must be measured. Techniques that do not facilitate cure must be discarded; methods that make people well must be endorsed. It is by this yardstick that dual relationships should be evaluated.

Prohibitions against dual relationships have been a recognized part of the ethics of therapy since the creation of psychoanalysis more than a century ago. Indeed, if we include sexual relationships as part of the class of dual relationships, the ethical prohibition goes back at least as far as Hippocrates, who warned, in the still viable Hippocratic Oath: "Whatever houses I may visit, I will come for the benefit of the sick, remaining free of all intentional injustice, of all mischief and, in particular, of sexual relations with both female and male persons, be they free or slave." In this chapter, I will not address sexual dual relationships, so that no part of the following discussion should be applied to that topic.

SOCIAL DUAL RELATIONSHIPS AND THE LAW

The first appearance of the dual relationship issue in courts of law is *Landau v. Werner* (1961) where the English Court of Appeal held a

257

psychiatrist responsible for the consequences of mishandling the transference phenomenon. The patient was an intelligent, middle-aged woman in an anxiety state. The psychiatrist gave her psychoanalytic treatment in his office. After 4 or 5 months the plaintiff was much better but felt she had fallen in love with the doctor, even though he explained this to her as being part of the process of transference. Feeling that a sudden withdrawal on his part might cause a relapse, over the next 7 or 8 months the doctor took her out to tea and dinner in restaurants on a number of occasions. He visited her once in her bed–sitting room, and he had some conversations about their spending a holiday together. Unfortunately, the plaintiff's condition deteriorated so the doctor resumed formal treatment, but to no avail. The plaintiff became incapable of work. After bringing a suit against the doctor, she recovered a judgment of six thousand pounds. The appellate court upheld the verdict and noted that the medical evidence was all one way in condemning social contacts. Furthermore, the doctor had failed to convince the judge that his departure from standard practice was justified and was a reasonable development in this young science. The judge concluded that this treatment was unwise and that it led to the grave deterioration in the plaintiff's health. In essence, the court refused to tolerate any deviation from the current standard of care, thus stifling innovation (Scheflin, 1997).

In the frequently cited legal case of *Zipkin v. Freeman* (1968), the Supreme Court of Missouri addressed the issue of whether a defendant-psychiatrist's patient could recover money and property from the psychiatrist's insurance carrier after a sexual relationship ended. This is a rather complex and convoluted case, which I will not dwell on because it is not a pure example of a *nonsexual* dual relationship. Nevertheless, it is worth reporting the verbatim comments of an expert, a Dr. Flynn, who testified that apart from the sexual aspect of the case, to take the relationship outside the office into social relationships "would allow the patient to develop all sorts of unusual ideas just around the feelings that she has about the doctor" (p. 761), and that a psychiatrist should no more take an overnight trip with a patient than shoot her. Flynn further stated that "patients have enough trouble with their feelings that they develop about the doctor without adding to them by actual events" (p. 761). He concluded by saying that transference should be handled in the office situation exclusively. The appellate court found the psychiatrist at fault noting that "It is pretty clear from the medical evidence that the damage would have been done to Mrs. Zipkin even if the trips outside the state were carefully chaperoned, the swimming done with suits on, and if there had been ballroom dancing instead of sexual relations" (p. 761).

The Zipkin case (1968) points out that the ethical issue of social dual relationships had not become a serious *legal* problem. As of 1968, when Zipkin was decided, only one English case (*Landau v. Werner*, 1961) had discussed social dual relationships. After Zipkin, the subject of social dual relationships has received virtually no judicial attention. Only three other cases have touched upon the subject.

The legal literature cites several instances in which therapists went beyond constructive boundary crossings—which is probably why the profession as a whole is apt to censure and denounce dual relationships. For example, in *Poliak v. Board of Psychology* (1997), a 50-year-old female psychologist became overly concerned with her 34-year-old patient. Gradually, the relationship moved from professional to personal when the psychologist visited the patient's place of business. Soon afterward, the psychologist sent her daughters to the patient's business for facials and then massages. The psychologist drove the patient to various appointments, treated her to lunches and dinners, and let the patient take care of her dog for a week. In therapy, when the patient made overtures, the psychologist tried to discuss transference issues but the patient withdrew on these occasions. At a particular point, both patient and psychologist realized that their relationship had become personal and so the therapy was terminated, but no referral to another therapist was made. After termination, the patient and the psychologist spent time together and went to Europe together. They started a sexual relationship 7 months after the termination, though the psychologist was heterosexual. The patient was invited to move into the psychologist's home. Eventually, the patient was asked to leave and the relationship ended. The board revoked her license, but the court of appeals reversed. The court's opinion only dealt with the posttermination sexual relationship. It is perhaps cases like this one that have mistakenly led many to believe in the inevitability of a so-called slippery slope that leads to sexual liaisons.

In *Harris v. Leader* (1998), a borderline patient sued her psychiatrist alleging that he allowed her to hold and kiss his hand during certain therapy sessions, sit at his feet and wrap her arms around his legs, and hug at the end of the sessions. The psychiatrist claimed that the patient was insistent for this contact and that it lasted a very short time. He felt that the contact would be good for the patient on creating a bond that would facilitate treatment. The patient claimed that the treatment made her totally dependent on the psychiatrist, believing she could not live without him and that he was God. The court rejected the patient's claims noting that the dependence was part of the borderline condition and the patient had initiated the physical contact. The court also rejected the claim that the psychiatrist acted inappropriately by engaging in self-disclosure to the patient, including telling her that he had sexual fantasies about her. According to the court, some schools of therapy believed that self-disclosure was valuable in facilitating cure.

SOCIAL DUAL RELATIONSHIPS AND ETHICS

It was not until the late 1980s that ethics committees of professional mental health organizations paid serious attention to nonsexual involvement in the lives of patients. The few authors who wrote on the topic were in agreement that defining the term was virtually impossible. They did not agree, however, on the ethical implications of dual relationships. Some authors argued that all dual relationships were unethical; other authors took a more pragmatic viewpoint and argued that under some circumstances because dual relationships were almost unavoidable, only some of them, those which exploit or harm the patient, were unethical (Younggren & Skorka, 1992).

Initially, the American Psychological Association's (APA) *Ethical Principles of Psychologists* simply stated that "psychologists make every effort to avoid dual relationships with clients and/or relationships which might impair their professional judgment or increase the risk of client exploitation" (APA, 1981, p. 636). It should be noted that this definition did not forbid dual relationships. It condemned only those dual relationships that (a) impaired professional judgment, or (b) increased the risk of exploiting the patient. As so stated, the ethics for mental health professionals paralleled the ethics for attorneys. Both groups of professionals are considered in law to be in a "fiduciary" relationship with the client-patient. This relationship requires the highest duty of loyalty known to the law (Frankel, 1983). Loyalty requires that the revelations and secrets of the client-patient be kept confidential and that the professional avoid all adverse conflicts of interest where the loyalty owed to the client-patient could be diluted by self-interest or concern for others. Thus, the proper source of a rule against dual relationships is the fiduciary nature of the work done by mental health professionals. Accordingly, dual relationships that impair the psychologists' judgment, or that harm the patient, are by definition unethical and legally actionable.

Unlike the more stringent rules that exist for psychotherapists, lawyers then, and still, have enjoyed greater latitude and a wide range of dual relationships with clients, including sexual relationships, which are permitted except in very rare circumstances (where they impair judgment or prejudice the client's legal interests). It is not unusual for lawyers to enter into a wide variety of business relationships with their clients, as well as many other types of social contact (American Bar Association, 1983).

What are social (nonsexual) dual relationships? They are relationships or contacts between a therapist and patient that are concurrent with, or a consequence of, the therapeutic relationship. Herlihy and Corey (1992) note that "dual relationships include personal, social, business, and secondary financial relationships" (p. 6).

There are some commentators who even regard boundary crossings, such as accepting a Christmas present from a client, or disclosure of personal information by the therapist to the client, as a dual relationship.

Should all of these social dual relationships be deemed unethical? The most recent version of the American Psychological Association *Ethical Principles of Psychologists and Code of Conduct* (1992) contains three expanded sections:

1.17 Multiple Relationships does not prohibit dual relationships unless "it appears likely that such a relationship reasonably might impair the psychologist's objectivity or otherwise interfere with the psychologist's effectively performing his or her functions as a psychologist, or might harm or exploit the other party" (p. 5). If harm to the patient was not foreseen, and a relationship is created which might be detrimental to healing, the therapist should resolve the situation with the best interests of the patient in mind.

1.18 Barter (With Patients or Clients) suggests that bartering goods, services, or other nonmonetary payment generally has an "inherent potential for conflicts, exploitation, and distortion of the professional relationship" (p. 6). However, bartering is permitted "*only* if (a) it is not clinically contraindicated, *and* (b) the relationship is not exploitative" (p. 6).

1.19 Exploitative Relationships are forbidden with patients, students, supervisees, employees, and research participants.

The earlier literature on dual relationships tended to focus on identifying and defining these relationships, similar to the way an archaeologist categorizes relics. Once labeled, they were declared to be unethical. This early view began to change in the late 1980s when the focus shifted away from definitions and toward consequences. Dual relationships were now seen to be unethical not because they were dual relationships, but rather because such relationships tended to result in exploitation of the patient or a breach of trust, loyalty, and independence. The evil was thus not the existence of the relationship, but rather the exploitation, impairment, or harm that could be caused by them. As a result of this shift in view, state disciplinary boards now look more closely to see whether a patient's interests have been abused. If so, then the dual relationship is held to be unethical.

Dual relationships by their very nature involve an additional element of bonding with the patient. This bonding, in turn, opens up new channels of communication that might not be available in the strict therapy room setting. For example, social contact might permit the therapist to see how the patient actually functions in the world, rather than simply hearing the patient's description of how he or she functions. Thus, dual relationships generally involve real world contact, and they place the patient in an action oriented, rather than purely verbal, mode.

Should social dual relationships be encouraged, prohibited, or regulated? The answer should depend upon whether such relationships enhance therapy.

WHAT MAKES THERAPISTS EFFECTIVE?

Modern medicine, mental or physical, involves healing. Much research has been conducted into why healing occurs. In a survey of a variety of therapies that produced outcome data, Lambert (1992) discovered that only 15% of the variance involving cure was based on therapeutic technique. According to his research, extratherapeutic change (the patient's ego strength, environmental factors including social support, etc.) accounted for 40%; common factors (rapport, warmth, etc.) accounted for 30%; and expectancy (placebo effects) accounted for the final 15%. Thus, *placebo* and *rapport* are an essential part of the healing process. Patients are more likely to improve if they have a good rapport with their healers and if there is a strong placebo effect in operation. Do social dual relationships enhance the personal factors that account for most of the healing process?

There are three components to the personal characteristics that make the healer more likely to succeed. First, the patient must trust the healer's ability to bring about a cure. This aspect of the relationship is defined by expectancy, or the placebo effect. Second, the healer must be a nurturer, expressing warmth, compassion, and understanding. This aspect of the therapeutic alliance is called "rapport." Finally, there must be a dimension of positive thinking, which for religious patients is dealt with by prayer, and for secular patients is handled by optimism. Brief exploration of these three dimensions will disclose that social dual relationships, handled with competence and care, empowers the therapist by enhancing the patient's will to heal.

Placebo and Rapport

In Latin, placebo means "I shall please." The placebo effect as a powerful aspect of healing was first expressly noticed by Beecher (1955). According to Scheflin and Opton, Jr. (1978): "It would be difficult indeed to overestimate the importance of the placebo effect in medicine. The effect is especially strong when fortified by strong devotion to the doctor" (p. 278).

Bishop (1977) quotes the remarkable conclusion of a report published the prior year in the Proceedings of the Mayo Clinic: "From antiquity to this era of medical enlightenment, (the) placebo has been the single most potent and versatile tool for relieving the sufferings that man is heir to. . . . Be it mother's kiss or voodoo drums, leeches, purgatives, poultices or snake oil, the wondrous effect of placebo therapy is undeniably evident" (p. 1). Goleman (1993) reports on recent research in which two-thirds of just under 7,000 patients suffering from asthma, duodenal ulcer, and herpes improved, at least temporarily, despite being given medically useless surgical and chemical treatments. According to Goleman: "New findings show that the placebo effect—in which patients given an inactive treatment believe that it can cure them—is most powerful when a trusted physician enthusiastically offers a patient a new therapy" (p. C-3). Thus, placebo healing is most effective when the patient likes and respects the healer and when both patient and healer are very enthusiastic about the curative aspects of a new treatment (Shapiro & Shapiro, 1997). Two Danish researchers have claimed that the placebo effect is a myth. Asbjorn Hrobjartsson and Peter C. Gotzsche (2001) studied 114 publications that involved about 7,500 patients with 40 different conditions. They concluded that there was no support for the current belief that approximately one-third of these patients would have improved if given an inert pill that they were told was active. The Danish scientists theorized that most diseases wax and wane so that the improvement is a phase of the disease cycle, not of the placebo effect. When they compared studies in which patients had received no treatment, not even a placebo, the rate of recovery was about the same as when placebos were given. The one exception was in studies of pain, or where there was a subjective reporting requirement. In those cases, the placebo patients reported lower pain than did the no treatment patients. The Danish researchers admitted that placebos are still important in clinical research. But they argued that in clinical practice, it is probably no more than a reporting bias whereby the patient seeks to please the doctor (Kolata, 2001).

Because the Danish study did not evaluate the impact of rapport, it fails to address the curative power of personal contact with the patient. It might well be suggested that the placebo effect is itself an aspect of rapport, otherwise known as "the therapeutic alliance." Many contend that the relationship with the therapist is *the* single most important factor in healing. That relationship will enhance the placebo effect, but it will be neutral with regard to the actual therapy techniques used.

This is not to gainsay that there are established empirically supported techniques for several conditions. Nevertheless, the primacy of the therapeutic relationship makes it almost imperative for a clinician or counselor to avoid anything that may dilute or undermine it. Hence, proponents of dual relationships support such therapist-patient interactions because they tend to foster rapport.[1]

Prayer and Optimism

A mirror image of placebo and rapport is prayer and optimism. As noted by Scheflin and Opton, Jr. (1978): "Healing by faith, hope, prayer, and sacrificial submission to higher powers *works*. It is only the explanation that is in doubt. Does the healing power of prayer descend from God or arise from the supplicant's faith?" (p. 279). In *People v. Pierson* (1903), the court made these observations:

---

[1]Placebos are not without their own ethical issues. If placebos are so effective in healing, should they be used without the informed consent of the patient? Does the ethical and legal requirement of informed consent impair the practice of effective therapy? Despite the increasing evidence of the importance and efficacy of the placebo effect, the ethics of the placebo remain murky. After all, as Byerly (spring 1976) has noted, the use of placebos always involves a deception of the patient. Informed consent is impossible. Does the use of the placebo effect constitute an "exploitation" of the patient? If placebos are successful because of the bond between the healer and the patient, then the type of healing practiced does not make any significant difference (White, Tursky, & Schwartz, 1983). If this is true, why license mental health professionals? Some cab drivers, barbers, nail salon employees, and bartenders may have more to teach to therapists than do the creators of new techniques.

We are aware that there are people who believe that the Divine power may be invoked to heal the sick, and that faith is all that is required. There are others who believe that the Creator has supplied the earth, nature's store-house, with everything that man may want for his support and maintenance, including the restoration and preservation of his health, and that he is left to work out his own salvation, under fixed natural laws. There are still others who believe that Christianity and science go hand in hand, both proceeding from the Creator; that science is but the agent of the Almighty through which he accomplishes results, and that both science and Divine power may be invoked together to restore diseased and suffering humanity. But, sitting as a court of law for the purpose of construing and determining the meaning of statutes, we have nothing to do with these variances in religious beliefs and have no power to determine which is correct. We place no limitations upon the power of the mind over the body, the power of faith to dispel disease, or the power of the Supreme Being to heal the sick. We merely declare the law as given us by the legislature. (pp. 211–212)

Prayer is relevant to a discussion of dual relationships because it creates another dimension of interaction with the therapist and leads to increase clients' familiarity of and trust in their therapists. Indeed, some patients seek out therapists mainly because this faith dimension can be shared. Prayer builds rapport, enhances hope, and triggers optimism. On the other hand, a therapist who imposed his or her religious beliefs on a patient would be engaged in an impermissible exploitative relationship. There are therapists who, in concert with the client's wishes, will resort to prayer in the middle of a session. This is, in a sense, a dual relationship, but if the net result is positive, it is foolish to disallow it. The basic rules apply—do not use coercion, exploitation, or deception in counseling and therapy.

Is religious faith itself a form of placebo effect? The crucial issue has yet to be directly addressed: Is it faith that helps heal, or is it something else with faith being one category or subtype of that something else? In other words, it may be that a positive mind-set is what cures—the power of positive thinking. If so, and there is support for the idea that positive thinking is curative, then faith, which is an aspect of positive thinking, may heal in the same way placebo heals and the same way optimism heals. If this latter point is found to be correct, then it is not faith, but rather the positive outlook faith brings, that is the crucial variable.

Recent research raises the interesting prospect that although there is value in positive thinking, the real value may actually be found in the avoidance of negative thinking. A research project conducted at Ohio State University found that optimism and pessimism are actually independent variables, and that pessimism was an effective predictor of future psychological and physical health. While pessimism predicted anxiety, stress, and ill-health, optimism did not predict anything (Robinson-Whelan, Kim, MacCallum, & Kiecolt-Glaser, 1997).

SOME CAUTIONS CONCERNING SOCIAL DUAL RELATIONSHIPS

Some restrictions on social dual relationships make sense. London (1997) has correctly observed that a responsible clinician uses sound professional judgment, establishes a positive therapeutic alliance, obtains necessary positive consultations, and documents what is done on a regular basis. He writes that "We should not become so fearful of our legal vulnerabilities that we cease to use our sound training and professional judgment. Nor should we allow other professions or the uninformed to determine the standard of care" (p. 6). Although this is generally sound advice, mental health professionals have permitted lawyers to set the appropriate standard of care, to the detriment of patients who will now be handled by the practice of defensive medicine (Scheflin, 2000). A substantial number of Milton Erickson's brilliant cures involved dual relationships. Recently, one of Erickson's sons told me that if his father were practicing today, he would be repeatedly sued for boundary violations (Scheflin, 2001).

At least two arguments supporting caution in developing social dual relationships are worth mentioning. The first deals with the fact that therapists, especially beginners, may feel the need for the structure and support provided by strict boundaries. It has been argued that better education about intimacy and boundary issues should form part of all good training curricula. Thus, instead of admonishing young therapists and trainees to avoid dual relationships, they should learn how to manage them—to the ultimate benefit of the client. On the other hand, it is has been stated that very clear boundary lines protect novice therapists from patient contacts they are not ready to handle. This argument, however, may justify the voluntary imposition of clear boundaries on the therapy relationship; it does not justify compelled universal avoidance.

A final argument concerns the fact that some classes of patients may appear the most likely candidates for social dual relationships, but these relationships may actually contribute to patient pathology (Brown & Scheflin, 1999; Scheflin & Brown, 1999). For some patients, maintaining absolute strict boundaries may be essential to their cure. Several of the contributors to this book have explicitly emphasized the importance of *not* pursuing dual relationships with highly dependent, borderline, histrionic, antisocial, and other seriously disturbed individuals.

A MODEST PROPOSAL

A new study in the March 10, 2001 issue of *The Lancet* (Rostler, 2001) found that doctors who showed empathy and acknowledged their patients' fears and concerns were more effective than doctors who maintained a strict professional demeanor keeping their patients at an emotional arm's length. The establishment of a therapeutic *partnership*, emotional and medical, was a powerful inducement to cure. To the extent that therapy is moving toward brief encounters with stricter boundaries, the health of the patients is being put at risk.

Herlihy and Corey (1997) have pointed out that dual relationships are often unavoidable. Indeed, Corey, Corey, and Callahan (1998) suggest that "Dual relationships are inherent in the work of all helping professionals" (p. 228). Lazarus (1994) has persuasively argued that some ethical rules and legal risk management practices actually diminish therapeutic effectiveness. He numbers the restrictions on dual relationships among them, as does Zur (2000) who also makes a strong case for permitting out-of-office contacts (Zur, 2001).

Office visits do not present a full, complete, and necessarily accurate picture of how the patient copes with the real world. Furthermore, while some patients might take advantage of lowered boundaries, other patients would benefit from the additional care and concern.

A prohibition on social dual relationship might better be replaced with a focus on the therapist's fiduciary responsibility. Mental health professionals owe the highest duty of loyalty to their patients. Every act or omission by a healer must be justified as being exclusively for the benefit of the patient. Judge Benjamin Cardozo (*Meinhard v. Salmon*, 1928) provided a much quoted description of fiduciary duty: "Not honesty alone, but the punctilio of an honor the most sensitive, is then the standard of behavior" (p. 546). Thus, a therapist is answerable to the patient and the disciplinary board whenever the treatment given cannot be proven to have been undertaken exclusively for the patient's well-being and cure. After all, does it make therapeutic sense to focus on *technique*, that often accounts for a fraction of the cure, and inhibit *rapport* that accounts for most of it?

REFERENCES

American Bar Association. (1983). *Model rules of professional conduct* (as amended 2001). Chicago: Author.

American Psychological Association. (1981). Ethical principles of psychologists (Approved 1997). *American Psychologist, 36* (6), 633–638.

American Psychological Association. (1992). *Ethical principles of psychologists and code of conduct.* Washington, DC: Author.

Beecher, H. K. (1955). The powerful placebo. *Journal of the American Medical Association, 159,* 1602–1606.

Bishop, J. E. (1977, August 25). Potent nondrugs: Placebos are harmless, but they work, posing problems for medicine. *Wall Street Journal,* p. 1.

Brown, D., & Scheflin, A. W. (1999, fall-winter). Factitious disorders and trauma-related diagnoses. *Journal of Psychiatry & Law, 27,* 373–422.

Byerly, H. (1976, spring). Explaining and exploiting placebo effects. *Perspectives in Biology and Medicine, 19,* 423–436.

Corey, G., Corey, M. S., & Callahan, P. (1998). *Issues and ethics in the helping professions* (5th ed.). Boston: Brooks/Cole.

Frankel, T. (1983). Fiduciary law. *California Law Review, 71,* 795–836.

Goleman, D. (1993, August 17). Placebo effect is shown to be twice as powerful as expected. *New York Times,* p. C-3.

Harris v. Leader. (1998). 1998 W.L. 122411 (Georgia App.).

Herlihy, B., & Corey, G. (1992). *Dual relationships in counseling.* Alexandria, VA: American Counseling Association.

Herlihy, B., & Corey, G. (1997). *Boundary issues in counseling: Multiple roles and responsibilities.* Alexandria, VA: American Counseling Association.

Hrobjartsson, A., & Gotzsche, P. C. (2001, May). Is the placebo powerless? An analysis of clinical trials comparing placebo with no treatment. *New England Journal of Medicine, 344*(21), 1594–1602.

Kolata, G. (2001, May 24). Researchers say placebo effect is fiction, not fact. *The Oregonian,* p. 1.

Lambert, M. J. (1992). Psychotherapy outcome research: Implications for integrative and eclectic therapists. In J. C. Norcross & M. R. Goldfried (Eds.), *Handbook of psychotherapy integration* (pp. 94–129). New York: Basic Books.

Landau v. Werner. (1961). 105 Solicitor's Journal 1008.

Lazarus, A. A. (1994). How certain boundaries and ethics diminish therapeutic effectiveness. *Ethics and Behavior, 4* (3), 255–261.

London, R. L. (1997, January). Forensic and legal implications in clinical practice: A master class commentary. *International Journal of Clinical and Experimental Hypnosis, 45* (1), 6–17.

Meinhard v. Salmon. (1928). 249 N.Y. 458, 164 N.E. 545.

People v. Pierson. (1903). 176 N.Y. 201, 68 N.E. 243.

Poliak v. Board of Psychology. (1997). 55 Cal.App.4th 342, 63 Cal. Rptr.2d 866 (3rd Dist.)

Robinson-Whelan, S., Kim, C., MacCallum, R. C., & Kiecolt-Glaser, J. K. (1997). Distinguishing optimism from pessimism in older adults: Is it more important to be optimistic or not to be pessimistic? *Journal of Personality and Social Psychology, 73*, 1345–1353.

Rostler, S. (2001, March 10). Empathy, warmth can be potent medicine. *Reuters Health*. Retrieved June 10, 2001, from reutershealth.com

Scheflin, A. W. (1997). Ethics and hypnosis: Unorthodox or innovative therapies and the legal standard of care. In W. Matthews & J. Edgette (Eds.), *Current thinking and research in brief therapy: Solutions, strategies, narratives* (Vol. 1, pp. 41–62). New York: Brunner/Mazel.

Scheflin, A. W. (2000, spring). The evolving standard of care in the practice of trauma and Dissociative Disorder Therapy. *Bulletin of the Menninger Clinic 64* (2), 197–234.

Scheflin, A. W. (2001). Caveat therapist: Ethical and legal dangers in the use of Ericksonian techniques. In B. B. Geary & J. K. Zeig (Eds.), *Clinical handbook of Ericksonian hypnosis and psychotherapy* (in press). Phoeniz, AZ: Zeig, Tucker & Theisen.

Scheflin, A. W., & Brown, D. (1999, fall-winter). The false litigant syndrome: "Nobody would say that unless it was the truth." *Journal of Psychiatry & Law, 27*, 649–705.

Scheflin, A. W., & Opton, Jr., E. M. (1978). *The mind manipulators*. New York: Paddington Press.

Shapiro, A. K., & Shapiro, E. (1997). *The powerful placebo: From ancient priest to modern physician*. Baltimore: The Johns Hopkins University Press.

White, L., Tursky, B., & Schwartz, G. E. (Eds.). (1983). *Placebo: Theory, research, and mechanisms*. New York: The Guilford Press.

Younggren, J. N., & Skorka, D. (1992). The nontherapeutic psychotherapy relationship. *Law & Psychology Rev., 16*, 13–28.

Zipkin v. Freeman. (1968). 436 S.W.2d 753 (Mo.), rehearing denied Feb. 10, 1969.

Zur, O. (2000). Going too far in the right direction: Reflections on the mythic ban of dual relationships. *California Psychologist, 23* (4), 14, 16.

Zur, O. (2001). Out-of-office experience: When crossing office boundaries and engaging in dual relationships are clinically beneficial and ethically sound. *The Independent Practitioner, 21* (2), 96–100.

PART 5

Dual Relationships in Special Populations

Part 5 focuses on the inevitability and importance of dual and multiple relationships in small tight-knit societies, such as rural, military, deaf, spiritual, and other small communities. It outlines how dual relationships are part of the rich web of connection that cannot be isolated from the community as encouraged by the urban-analytic and risk-management model. In chapter 18, Barnett and Yutrzenka describe the inevitability of dual relationships in the military and in rural communities and provide 11 suggestions on how to handle them. In chapter 19, Guthmann and Sandberg show how social dual relationships are a vital part of deaf communities, which are inherently highly interdependent and close due to the language barrier. Llewellyn (chapter 20) clarifies how dual relationships, familiarity, and trust in the church community are almost prerequisites to spiritual counseling. In chapter 21, Zur and Gonzalez outline the unique and complex unavoidable multirelationship situations in which military psychologists find themselves. These situations include sharing a tent with a client during training, having a superior as a client, or the understanding that the Department of Defense is your primary client rather than the service member you are treating. Kertész adds a cultural dimension in chapter 22 to the discussion of dual relationships with his elaboration on important and expected boundary crossings and multirelationships between therapists and clients in the Latino culture.

CHAPTER 18

Nonsexual Dual Relationships in Professional Practice, With Special Applications to Rural and Military Communities

Jeffrey E. Barnett, PhD
and Barbara A. Yutrzenka, PhD

Numerous articles as well as changes in law, licensing regulations, and ethical standards have sensitized psychologists to the nature of their professional relationships as psychotherapists, supervisors, teachers, employers, and researchers. Inherent in these professional relationships is an obligation to ensure that professional boundaries are not violated and that psychologists should avoid exploitation of the consumer's trust and confidence.

Reproduced by permission of the Division of Psychologists in Independent Practice of the American Psychological Association. Barnett, J. E., and Yutrzenka, B. A. (1994). Nonsexual dual relationships in professional practice, with special applications to rural and military communities. *The Independent Practitioner, 14* (5), 243–248.

Dual relationships—relationships with consumers outside the context of an established professional relationship—can pose a serious threat to professional boundaries and open the door for consumer exploitation and harm. However, does harm *always* follow dual relationships? The answer is a resounding, "That depends." While most authors agree that all dual relationships have the *potential* for harm and certainly create ethical dilemmas, only those involving sexual intimacies with current or recently terminated clients have been studied extensively and have received clear legal, ethical, and/or regulatory prohibitions. The research base for understanding nonsexual dual relationships is limited; and legal and regulatory guidelines are either nonexistent or vaguely written.

The purpose of this chapter is to address some of the ethical issues surrounding nonsexual dual relationships in professional practice and to examine these issues as they specifically apply to rural and military communities. A brief review of the literature relevant to dual relationships and their inclusion in ethical principles follows.

DUAL RELATIONSHIPS INVOLVING SEXUAL INTIMACY

The majority of the literature examining the scope and implications of dual relationships has focused on those involving sexually intimate behavior occurring in the context of psychotherapy. For reviews of this literature, refer to Gabbard (1989), Keith-Spiegel and Koocher (1985), and Pope (1990). Writers have commented on issues such as potential dilemmas experienced when engaging in nonerotic physical contact in the therapy relationship (Holub & Lee, 1990; Pope & Vasquez, 1991), the potential connection between nonerotic physical contact and sexual intimacy in the therapy relationship (Holroyd & Brodsky, 1977, 1980; Stake & Oliver, 1991), sexual intimacies with current patients and clients (Folman, 1991; Pope & Bouhoutsos, 1986; Pope & Vetter, 1991), and sexual involvement with former patients and clients (Bouhoutsos, Holroyd, Lerman, Forer, & Greenberg, 1983; Gabbard & Pope, 1989).

With few exceptions, research has consistently revealed that sexual intimacies between therapist and client are damaging to the client (Holroyd & Brodsky, 1977; Pope, 1988, 1990). Parallel studies examining sexualized dual relationships within academic or supervisory relationships (Glaser & Thorpe, 1986; Pope, 1989) have indicated that exploitation and harm also occur in these relationships. In addition, an increasing number of psychologists have experienced the damaging effects of these relationships as they become defendants in litigation and/or actions taken by licensing boards or state and national psychological associations based on consumer complaints (Gottlieb, Sell, & Schoenfeld, 1988; Pope & Vetter, 1992).

NONSEXUAL DUAL RELATIONSHIPS

The scope and implications of nonsexual dual relationships have not received extensive attention in the literature. For reviews of the nonsexual dual relationship literature, please refer to Borys and Pope (1989), Pope (1991), and Younggren and Skorka (1992). Why the limited attention to nonsexual dual relationship when, as with sexualized dual relationships, they involve a broad and diverse range of potentially harmful behaviors? Keith-Spiegel and Koocher (1985) speculated that perhaps one of the reasons for this limited attention is because "the role superimpositions are often not inherently controversial or riddled with moral overtones" (p. 267). Other possible reasons may be related to the complexity of the phenomenon itself and the inadequacy of existing definitions. Kitchner (1988) suggested that inadequate definitions have led to limited understanding of the ethical problems that dual relationships create. Utilizing role theory, she proposed that dual role relationships consist of individuals in competing and inequitable roles. Potential for exploitation in these relationships increases as the roles diverge. That is, there is a greater risk for exploitation within the psychotherapy relationship (high divergence in roles) than between friends (low divergence in roles):

> When the conflict of interests is great, the power differential large, and the role expectations incompatible, the potential for harm is so great that the relationships should be considered *a priori* unethical. At the other extreme, when the conflict of interests is small or nonexistent, the power differential small, and the role expectations compatible, there is little danger of harm. (Kitchner, 1988, p. 220)

Thus, she recognized that while all dual relationships are "ethically problematic" (Kitchner, 1988, p. 217), not all result in exploitation or harm. However, according to Kitchner all professionals need to be cognizant of potential role conflicts and work toward minimizing their impact.

Borys and Pope (1989), in what is currently the most comprehensive study on the topic of nonsexual dual relationships, reported that beliefs and behaviors regarding dual relationships vary as a function of therapist gender, profession (psychologist, psychiatrist, social worker), region of residence, practice locale (size of community), and theoretical orientation. For example, male therapists tended to rate dual professional roles, including those involving social and/or financial relationships, as more ethical and reported engaging in these behaviors with more clients than did the female therapists. Respondents who live and work in a small town tended to rate dual professional roles as more ethical than respondents who live and work in suburban or urban settings, but only differed from these latter groups in actual behavior in the domain of financial involvements (i.e., small town respondents were more likely to engage in these behaviors). Finally, while there were no significant differences between the three mental health professions regarding engaging in sexual and nonsexual dual relationships, psychiatrists tended to view nonsexual dual relationships as less ethical than either social workers or psychologists. Not only does this study identify several variables involved in beliefs about and participation in dual relationships, its results point to the complexities involved.

Definitional concerns have also been recently addressed in a project designed to mirror the original methodology underlying the establishment of the original American Psychological Association (APA) Ethical Standards for Psychology (1953). Utilizing a single item, critical-incident survey format, Pope and Vetter (1992) invited a representative sample of APA members to "describe, in a few words or more detail, an incident that you or a colleague have faced in the past year or two that was ethically challenging or troubling to you" (p. 398). As in the 1953 study, the authors intended to utilize these comments in APA's 1992 revision of the Ethical Principles.

A 51% response rate resulted in 703 separate ethical incidents in 23 different categories. Of the categories receiving the highest percentage of the total number of responses, incidents involving the maintenance of "clear, reasonable, and therapeutic boundaries around the professional relationships with a client" (Pope & Vetter, 1992, p. 400) received 17% of the responses, second only to incidents pertaining to confidentiality (18%).

Numerous examples highlighted the need for clear and explicit definitions of nonsexual dual relationships. In response to these data, Pope and Vetter offered three specific recommendations for consideration in revisions of the ethical principles. First, they recommend that dual relationships need to be more carefully defined and that ethical principles need to state clearly "if and when (dual relationships) are ever therapeutically indicated or acceptable" (p. 400). Second, they suggested that dual relationships need to be distinguished from *accidental* or *incidental* extratherapeutic contacts (e.g., unexpectedly sitting next to your client at a concert; encountering a client at a health club). Finally, with over one-third of the incidents in this category involving practice dilemmas in rural communities, small towns, or other remote locales, Pope and Vetter emphatically stated that the ethical principles must "clearly and realistically" (p. 400) address geographic contexts.

ETHICAL STANDARDS AND DUAL RELATIONSHIPS

Results of research have supported and perhaps even propelled changes in ethical standards, state licensing board regulations, and state laws involving criminalization of sexual involvement with current, and in some cases, prior therapy clients. The initial version of the Ethical Principles of Psychologists (APA, 1953) addressed the issue of dual relationships in Section B: Safeguarding Welfare of Clients. It advised psychologists not to enter into clinical relationships with members of one's own family, with intimate friends " . . . or with persons so close that their welfare might be jeopardized by the dual relationship" (p. 4).

Concern for the welfare of clients is paramount in professional relationships, and, of particular concern when dual relationships exist, has consistently appeared as one of the primary tenets of ethical behavior throughout the various revisions of the Ethical Principles. The most recent revision of the Principles reflects an increased attention, both in amount and specifically of information, to this concern for consumer welfare. For example, in comparison with its 1981 predecessor, in which a single paragraph addressed guidelines for consideration regarding dual relationships (Principle 6a), the current *Ethical Principles of Psychologists and Code of Conduct* (APA, 1992; hereafter referred to as the Ethics Code) dedicates several sections to the topic. The Preamble, Principle B, and Principle E reiterate the commitment of the profession to the welfare and protection of consumers (individuals/groups with whom psychologists work). Principle B: Integrity, specifically directs psychologists to "avoid improper and potentially harmful dual relationships" (p. 1599). In addition, Principle E addresses concern for the welfare of others, implicit in which are directives not to "exploit or mislead other people during or after professional relationships" (p. 1600). By design, these statements are intentionally broad goals for ethical practice. Specific prohibitions and rules of conduct regarding dual relationships are relegated to the Ethical Standards within the Ethics Code.

It is not surprising that some of the clearest statements about dual relationships in the Ethics code are directed toward those involving sexual intimacies. For example, Standard 1.19: Exploitative Relationships, explicitly prohibits sexual relationships with students or supervisees "over whom the psychologist has evaluative or direct authority" (p. 1602). Standard 4.05: Sexual Intimacies with Current Patients or Clients, definitively states that "Psychologists do not engage in sexual intimacies with current patients or clients" (p. 1605). Psychologists are also instructed not to "accept as therapy patients persons with whom they have previously engaged in sexual intimacies" (Standard 4.06, p. 1605), again because of the clearly harmful dual relationship which is likely to ensue in such a circumstance. Furthermore, Standard 4.07: Sexual Intimacies with Former Therapy Patients, provides specific instructions that psychologists do not become sexually intimate with a former client until a minimum of 2 years has passed since termination of therapy services. However, due to the controversial nature of this directive, a caveat is added that advises against this "except in the most unusual circumstances" (p. 1605) because of the potential for harm to or exploitation of the former client due to the previous therapy relationship.

The inclusion of specific standards in the Ethics Code that address nonsexual dual relationships is a notable improvement over previous documents. Individual sections on misuse of psychologists' influence (1.15), multiple relationships (1.17), bartering (1.18), and exploitative relationships (1.19) address some of the issues raised in recent research (Borys & Pope, 1989; Pope & Vetter, 1992) and draw attention to these ethical issues. For example, Standard 1.17: Multiple Relationships, recognizes that a work setting (rural, urban) is relevant when considering ethical solutions to potentially unavoidable multiple (dual) relationships. Younggren and Skorka (1992) noted that the inclusion of a specific section on multiple relationships reflects a movement "away from the implication that all dual relationships are harmful and towards a position that is tied to patient exploitation and harm" (p. 23). They support that this shift to outcome variables (patient harm, exploitation, impact on treatment) rather than attempts to define all potential variables involved in dual relationships will, in the long run, assist regulatory efforts.

In addition to the APA Ethics code, a number of state licensing boards have adopted the American Association of State and Provincial

Psychology Boards' (AASPPB) Code of Conduct (1991) as the standards by which they will judge ethical violations. Consistent with the parallel discussions in the APA Ethics Code, Section B, Impaired Objectivity and Dual Relationships in the AASPPB's Code, specifically prohibits the establishment or continuation of a professional relationship with a client when current or previous nonclinical relationships with that same client affect the psychologist's objectivity or competency. The Code clearly prohibits any sexual behaviors or sexual intimacies with a current or previous client with whom services have been rendered in the past 24 months. The same time line is applied to a prohibition from entering a financial or other potentially exploitative relationship with a current or former client.

NONSEXUAL DUAL RELATIONSHIPS IN RURAL AND MILITARY COMMUNITIES

As described above, researchers have attempted to define the scope and impact of nonsexual dual relationships. Similarly, ethical standards and codes of conduct have attempted to provide guidelines for ethical solutions when faced with dual relationship dilemmas. It would seem to follow that psychologists committed to ethical practice are familiar with this information, apply it to their practices, and, as a result, are able to minimize or even eliminate the risk of becoming involved in dual relationships with consumers of their professional services. However, in communities in which choice of service provider is limited either because of setting (e.g., rural communities) or because of setting and employer (e.g., military communities), nonsexual dual relationships are not a matter of "if" as much as "when." Psychologists working in these settings routinely face ethical dilemmas involving dual or multiple relationships. Hargrove (1986b) proposed that "Ethical behavior in mental health practice is forged from the interplay between practice and the environment in which it occurs" (p. 20). Focusing on rural communities in particular, Hargrove (1982a, 1982b, 1986a, 1986b, 1993) and others (Keller & Murray, 1982; Murray & Keller, 1986; Sobel, 1992; Templeman, 1989) have identified general characteristics of rural communities that create a context from which dual relationship dilemmas emerge: sparse population, geographic distance/isolation, limited health/mental health service choices, limited personal privacy, and overlapping or multiple levels of personal and professional relationships.

These factors contribute to greater interdependence among individuals within communities. Thus, for psychologists living and working in rural communities, some variation of a nonsexual dual relationship with consumers of their services is inevitable. Furthermore, the longer a practitioner stays in a rural area, the greater the likelihood of community leadership and increased community development. Thus, as Hargrove (1986b) noted "the longer the person is in the role of the clinician in the community, the more likely dual relationships will occur" (p. 22). Consider the following examples:

Case A: Dr. Givvme Openland moved to a small farming community in the midwest where she works as the only mental health clinician in a community mental health center satellite clinic. The nearest community with other mental health providers is an hour away and the nearest urban center is 2 hours away. She frequently sees her clients or their family members in the grocery store or other local businesses, and at church and community gatherings. She is often acquainted with her clients prior to initiating therapy. In many cases, individuals seek her out specifically because they know her or because they cannot travel the distance to receive alternative services.

Case B: Dr. Itsa Smallworld is one of six mental health professionals (and the only psychologist) in a rural community mental health center. His wife owns a clothing store in town and his children attend the local schools. He and his family participate in church, school, and civic activities. After years of involvement in the local PTA, he decides to run for one of two vacant positions on the school board. He is surprised to learn that one of his current clients is also a candidate for the positions.

Both of these examples typify the experiences of rural psychologists. Unlike their urban counterparts, overlapping professional-personal boundaries are often unavoidable. If rural psychologists refrain from treating individuals with whom they have had any contact outside of therapy, the availability of appropriate mental health treatment for many in the community will be severely limited.

Similar ethical dilemmas are frequently encountered by psychologists serving in the military.

Consider the following examples:

Case C: Major Bee Allucanby is one of three mental health professionals stationed at a small isolated military post. Like the others stationed at this post, she and her husband live in post housing and do the bulk of their shopping and socializing at post facilities. Limited mental health services are available to service men and women and their dependents off-post, but are rarely used.

Case D: *After his internship, Captain Ric Ranger is assigned to a special military unit. He is the sole mental health provider for unit members, the unit commander and his immediate supervisors, as well as for their spouses and families. He trains with the unit's members, consults organizationally to its command structure, and serves in administrative capacities within the unit. He also socializes with unit members and their families.*

As in rural communities, it is neither appropriate nor possible to refrain from multiple relationships with current or former clients in military settings, if one wants to function effectively both personally and professionally as a member of the community/unit. According to Barnett (1987), referrals to other practitioners are not always feasible "due to such factors as professional isolation, security considerations, or the fact that units frequently expect 'their' psychologist to treat 'their' soldiers" (p. 4).

How do rural or military psychologists deal with the continual personal and professional challenges that nonsexual multiple relationships create for them? The APA Ethics Code (1992) offers the clear dictum that at all times "The welfare and protection of the individuals and groups with whom psychologists work" (p. 1599) should form the basis for all ethical decisions. Standard 1.17 applies this specifically to the unavoidable multiple relationships that occur in rural and military communities by mandating that "Psychologists must always be sensitive to the potential harmful effects of other contacts on their work and on the persons with whom they deal" (p. 1602). These and other relevant sections of the Ethics Code provide basic guidelines for rural or military psychologists to consider when faced with the dilemma of dual relationships. However, they are not designed to anticipate or address every possible permutation of this (or any other) ethically troubling situation. According to Pope and Vasquez (1991):

> Ethics codes, standards, or rules can never legitimately serve as a substitute for a thoughtful, creative, and conscientious approach to our work. They can never relieve us of the responsibility to struggle with competing demands, multiple perspectives, evolving situations, and the prospect of uncertain consequences . . . (they) serve best to awaken us to the potential pitfalls, but also to opportunities, to guide and inform our attempts to help without hurting. They cannot do our work for us. (pp. 49–50)

Thus, ethics codes on standards are *necessary but not sufficient* when rural and military psychologists are faced with difficult ethical decisions regarding professional-personal boundaries. These decisions also rely on experience and the context within which they work, as well as the professional training they receive. Standards for practice in rural or military settings are needed. Here are other suggestions:

1. **Acknowledge the facts.** Dual relationships are a reality in rural and military communities. Unless you choose to live the life of an isolate in your community, multiple levels of interaction with clients or former clients are inevitable. Face this head on and be prepared!

2. **Be sensitive to community expectations.** Another reality is that you share "life in a fish bowl" with other members in the community. As highlighted by Hargrove (1982a, 1986b) and Keller (1982), certain personal or professional behaviors, especially those that differ from the norms of the community, may go unnoticed or unquestioned in large communities. However, in rural settings, these behaviors may reduce your credibility and effectiveness within the community. For military psychologists, community expectations are expanded to include the standards and protocol of military life.

3. **Compartmentalize roles, not relationships.** Dunbar (1982) states that psychologists in rural settings cannot afford to be warm and caring in therapy and aloof and distant outside of therapy. To avoid this, you must establish a clear demarcation between the different roles you have ascribed to you, but try to maintain a constant interpersonal style. Discuss the issue of outside-therapy contacts openly at the beginning of therapy, and reintroduce this discussion as needed throughout the course of therapy. This will sensitize both professional and consumer to the issues involved.

4. **Know thyself.** When treading in gray ethical areas, such as non-sexual dual relationships, it is crucial that you have a solid understanding of who you are, that you monitor your personal and professional needs, and that you remain cognizant of your possible influence in the lives of others. *You* should be the first to know when dual relationships are negatively affecting your professional responsibility to clients or former clients. Do not wait for a client (or lawyer) to inform you there is a problem.

5. **Know others.** It is important to identify psychologists in your community or state with whom to consult when questions of ethical practice surface. Have them help you become aware of any attempts to

rationalize, deny, or trivialize potential harm or exploitation that might occur from dual relationships (Borys & Pope, 1989).

6. **Nurture networks and resources.** Familiarize yourself with the other service providers in your community or surrounding area. Know what is available and know the service providers. Nurture these networks. Battles over "turf" may limit your ability to work effectively in the community and with your clients.

7. **Make referrals.** If referral options exist within your community or if consumers have the resources to utilize referrals to service providers in proximate communities, dual relationship dilemmas can be minimized if not eliminated. In fact, Keith-Spiegel and Koocher (1985) stated that psychologists who know in advance of treatment that a dual relationship conflict exists, and who also know that alternatives exist (e.g., referral to another practitioner) *will* be held culpable if they choose to undertake the professional relationship.

8. **Remain cognizant of confidentiality.** The APA Ethics Code (1992) provides guidelines for maintaining the confidentiality of and within professional relationships. Unique challenges to these guidelines exist in rural and military settings. For example, because it is likely that you will interact with your clients outside therapy, you must be careful not to diminish your clients' right to privacy. You indirectly receive unsolicited information about your clients simply by observing them in the community. Others who know your clients may unwittingly or knowingly share information with you. In some cases, you may be expected to share information about your clients without their consent. This latter example is particularly true in "need to know" situations in the military (Jeffrey, Rankin, & Jeffrey, 1992). A thorough discussion about confidentiality, including limitations, should occur at the outset of treatment.

9. **Document, document, document.** Carefully and meticulously document all deliberations with consultants and with clients regarding dual relationship dilemmas. Include a statement of rationale behind all decisions. While you cannot foresee all possible circumstances in every relationship, recording this process may serve to document your efforts to meet a reasonable standard of care and your efforts to protect your clients' best interests.

10. **Remain current on professional issues.** To minimize the risk of "ingrown thinking" (Swihart, as cited in Hargrove, 1982a, p. 178) or ethics "drift" (Murray, 1990, p. 17), participate in continuing education activities in your community, state, or region. For information about professional training opportunities in your state, contact your local

mental health, state psychological association, state division of mental health, and/or the closest clinical psychology training program. At a minimum, be a consumer of the professional literature.

11. **Enter the professional dialogue and be a part of needed changes.** Share your experiences with others so they can listen, learn, react, and respond. Write or make presentations about the dilemmas you have faced, the solutions you have chosen, and the outcome of those solutions. Join in the dialogue with state and national ethics committees as they strive to make ethics standards and codes "contemporary and realistic" (Pope & Vetter, 1992, p. 438) and applicable for *all* psychologists. Conduct or collaborate in research projects that will guide ethical decision making in the future.

REFERENCES

American Association of State Psychology Boards. (1991). *AASPB Code of Conduct.* Author.

American Psychological Association. (1953). *Ethical standards of psychologists.* Washington, DC: Author.

American Psychological Association. (1992). Ethical principles of psychologists and code of conduct. *American Psychologist, 47,* 1597–1611.

Barnett, J. E. (1987). Ethical dilemmas for military psychologists. *The Army Psychologist, 1,* 4–6.

Borys, D. S., & Pope, K. S. (1989). Dual relationships between therapist and client: A national study of psychologists, psychiatrists, and social workers. *Professional Psychology: Research and Practice, 20,* 283–293.

Bouhoutsos, J., Holroyd, J., Lerman, H., Forer, B., & Greenberg, M. (1983). Sexual intimacy between psychotherapists and patients. *Professional Psychology: Research and Practice, 14,* 185–196.

Dunbar, E. (1982). Educating social workers for rural mental health settings. In H. A. Dengerink & H. J. Cross (Eds.), *Training professionals for rural mental health* (pp. 54–69). Lincoln, NE: University of Nebraska Press.

Folman, R. Z. (1991). Therapist-patient sex: Attraction and boundary problems. *Psychotherapy, 28,* 168–173.

Gabbard, G. (Ed.). (1989). *Sexual exploitation in professional relationships.* Washington, DC: American Psychiatric Press.

Gabbard, G., & Pope, K. (1989). Sexual intimacies after termination: Clinical, ethical, and legal aspects. In G. Gabbard (Ed.), *Sexual exploitation in professional relationships* (pp. 115–127). Washington, DC: American Psychiatric Press.

Glaser, R. D., & Thorpe, J. S. (1986). Unethical intimacy: A survey of sexual contact and advances between psychology educators and female graduate students. *American Psychologist, 41,* 43–51.

Gottlieb, M. C., Sell, J. M., & Schoenfeld, L. S. (1988). Social/romantic relationships with present and former clients: State licensing board actions. *Professional Psychology: Research and Practice, 19,* 459–462.

Hargrove, D. S. (1982a). An overview of professional considerations in the rural community. In P. Keller & J. D. Murray (Eds.), *Handbook of rural community mental health.* New York: Human Sciences Press.

Hargrove, D. S. (1982b). The rural psychologist as generalist: A challenge for professional identity. *Professional Psychology, 13,* 302–308.

Hargrove, D. S. (1986a). A commentary on rural mental health training. In J. D. Murray & P. A. Keller (Ed.), *Innovations in rural community mental health* (pp. 239–249). Mansfield, PA: Rural Services Institute.

Hargrove, D. S. (1986b). Ethical issues in rural mental health practice. *Professional Psychology: Research and Practice, 17,* 20–23.

Hargrove, D. S. (1993). Psychologists and rural services: Addressing a new agenda. *Professional Psychology: Research and Practice, 24,* 319–324.

Holroyd, J. C., & Brodsky, A. M. (1977). Psychologists' attitudes and practices regarding erotic and nonerotic physical contact with clients. *American Psychologist, 32,* 843–849.

Holroyd, J. C., & Brodsky, A. M. (1980). Does touching patients lead to sexual intercourse? *Professional Psychology, 11,* 807–811.

Holub, E. A., & Lee, S. S. (1990). Therapists' use of nonerotic physical contact: Ethical concerns. *Professional Psychology: Research and Practice, 21,* 115–117.

Jeffrey, T. B., Rankin, R. J., & Jeffrey, L. K. (1992). In service of two masters: The ethical-legal dilemma faced by military psychologists. *Professional Psychology: Research and Practice, 23,* 91–95.

Keith-Spiegel, P., & Koocher, G. (1985). *Ethics in psychology.* New York: Random House.

Keller, P. A. (1982). Training models for master's level community psychologists. In H. A. Dengerink & H. J. Cross (Eds.), *Training professionals for rural mental health* (pp. 40–53). Lincoln, NE: University of Nebraska Press.

Keller, P. A., & Murray, J. D. (Eds.). (1982). *Handbook of rural community mental health.* New York: Human Sciences Press.

Kitchner, K. S. (1988). Dual role relationships: What makes them so problematic? *Journal of Counseling and Development, 67,* 217–221.

Murray, J. D. (1990). Professional survival and success in the rural community. *The Clinical Psychologist, 10,* 16–21.

Murray, J. D., & Keller, P. A. (Eds.). (1986). *Innovations in rural community mental health.* Mansfield, PA: Mansfield University Rural Services Institute.

Pope, K. S. (1988). How clients are harmed by sexual contact with mental health professionals: The syndrome and its prevalence. *Journal of Counseling and Development, 67,* 222–226.

Pope, K. S. (1989). Sexual intimacies between psychologists and their students and supervisees: Research, standards and professional liability. *The Independent Practitioner, 9,* 33–41.

Pope, K. S. (1990). Therapist-patient sexual involvement: A review of the research. *Clinical Psychology Review, 10,* 447–490.

Pope, K. S. (1991). Dual relationships in psychotherapy. *Ethics and Behavior, 1,* 21–34.

Pope, K. S., & Bouhoutsos, J. (1986). *Sexual intimacy between therapists and patients.* New York: Praeger.

Pope, K. S., & Vasquez, M. J. T. (1991). *Ethics in psychotherapy and counseling: A practical guide for psychologists.* San Francisco: Jossey-Bass.

Pope, K. S., & Vetter, V. A. (1991). Prior therapist-patient sexual involvement among patients seen by psychologists. *Psychotherapy, 28,* 429–438.

Pope, K. S., & Vetter, V. A. (1992). Ethical dilemmas encountered by members of the American Psychological Association. *American Psychologist, 47,* 397–411.

Sobel, S. B. (1992). Small town practice of psychotherapy: Ethical and personal dilemmas. *Psychotherapy and Private Practice, 10,* 61–69.

Stake, J. E., & Oliver, J. (1991). Sexual contact and touching between therapist and client: A survey of psychologist's attitudes and behavior. *Professional Psychology: Research and Practice, 22,* 297–307.

Templeman, T. L. (1989). Dual relationships in rural practices. *Journal of the Oregon Psychological Association, 35,* 12–14.

Younggren, J., & Skorka, D. (1992). The nontherapeutic psychotherapy relationship. *Law and Psychology Review, 16,* 13–28.

CHAPTER 19

Dual Relationships in the Deaf Community

When Dual Relationships Are Unavoidable and Essential

Debra Guthmann, EdD
and Katherine A. Sandberg, LADC

Deaf communities present a unique environment for mental health professionals who work in them. Professionals who work with deaf individuals frequently encounter their clients outside of the work environment, serve in more than one professional capacity, or share common history. Such dual or multiple relationships are often unavoidable in the deaf community. Owing to these special circumstances, the deaf community is a distinctive category when it comes to dual relationships in therapy.

This chapter will explore the complexities of dual relationships in the deaf community, using the following questions: Should professionals who work with deaf clients in vocational rehabilitation, social work, mental health, educational settings, or other human service agencies socialize with their clients? Should they work with people with whom they have dual or multiple relationships? How should professionals deal with potential or unavoidable dual-relationship issues? Is the significance of dual relationships different for hearing and deaf professionals?

It is the purpose of this chapter to shed light on the special, intimate nature of the deaf community and the practicality, mechanics, and benefits of dual relationships in such communities. Though the potential for dual relationships exists in a variety of human service settings, the framework for clinical considerations about dual relationships in counseling settings with deaf clients is a separate matter because of aspects specific to the deaf community. It is similar to issues of dual relationships that are raised in rural and small communities, such as ethnic minority, military, spiritual, and recovery. It is hoped that the explanation of this framework will enable clinicians to enter into dual relationships, when appropriate, with a greater understanding of how to make them contribute favorably to the welfare of clients and the community.

Professionals who work with deaf clients have grown from being a relatively small group of service providers to a full complement of specialists in a wide range of human services. Simply being able to communicate with consumers is no longer sufficient. In order to provide effective services, it is essential that counselors, social workers, psychologists, psychiatrists, and other professionals accept and understand the social and cultural considerations that consumers who are deaf bring into the therapeutic setting.

COMMUNICATION AND CULTURE
IN THE DEAF COMMUNITY

Deafness is often referred to as a hidden disability because it does not become evident until the person begins to communicate or experiences problems with communication. Relational difficulties are common in families with a deaf member because 90% of deaf children have hearing parents (Schein & Delk, 1974) who often do not communicate effectively with their children. Many deaf people grow up in families and attend schools where their language isolates them from the normal information flow. For the 90% of deaf children born to hearing parents, American Sign Language (ASL) is not their first language. Like adults, deaf children in a non-ASL environment are left out of the everyday conversation in their homes and schools. When deaf children ask about what has been said or what is being talked about, they are often given an abbreviated version of the conversation or told that it is not important. This leads them to feel left out or less important than others.

Due to language problems, deaf children begin to spend more time with deaf peers and less time with their parents. The child's acquisition of ASL naturally grows with repeated exposure, whereas parents often have limited exposure to the language (Guthmann, 1999; Guthmann, Heines, & Kolvitz, 2000). These factors increase fear among parents of losing their children to the deaf community and intensify feelings of guilt and discord within the family. Growing up with feelings of alienation, inadequacy, and defectiveness naturally augments a desire to belong and be understood.

Among deaf people, voices are rarely used, even by people who have intelligible speech. Instead, deaf people tend to conduct all human interactions using ASL, a language of nonverbal communication with an emphasis on facial expressions and body language. Used daily by more than half a million Americans, ASL enables deaf people to communicate with one another and function in society. Getting someone's attention can include flashing lights, waving, tapping on the floor or table (which produces vibrations that can be felt), or even throwing things. These are aspects of the deaf community in America, a population whose culture is characterized by a strong affinity derived from the collective bond of being deaf. Many deaf people consider themselves members of a "language minority" rather than persons with a pathological condition or disability. The deaf community is comprised of deaf individuals who share a common language, common experiences, and common values (Padden & Humphries, 1988).

Although lipreading is commonly thought to be an effective way of communicating with deaf people, the use of lipreading alone is not adequate. Research shows that only 20% of spoken language is visible on the lips (Jeffers & Barley, 1971). The daily experience of a deaf person using lipreading or speech reading might be simulated by attempting to understand a television program without sound. Lipreading is not a dependable means of communication for the majority of deaf individuals. A more effective way for a deaf person to communicate with a hearing person is to make use of interpreters. However, the impersonal and potentially intrusive nature of this form of communication makes it difficult, limiting, and at times inappropriate for personal and intimate conversations.

Members of deaf communities socialize together, go to the same educational institutions, social clubs, and restaurants, and spend time in the company of other signing people. There is a strong sense of community primarily because of the opportunities to freely communicate. For many children, going to a deaf residential school is their first opportunity to be fully included in all conversations. For some deaf adults who didn't attend school with deaf peers, discovering the rich social opportunities in the deaf community and realizing that they are fully included is a life-changing experience.

There are very few culturally affirming postsecondary programs available to deaf students. Workplaces for deaf people tend to also be few in number. Many communities have very limited social service resources that are culturally capable of providing services to deaf people. Establishing, fostering, and maintaining social ties with other deaf people is of the utmost value. These ties are necessary for the formation of intimate relationships and general survivability. It is common to have friendships with deaf people in other towns, states, and throughout the country. Deaf social events attract deaf people from hundreds or even thousands of miles away. Residential schools for the deaf, found in most states, have historically been the core of deaf education and the center of the deaf community. A close-knit group of people, the deaf community has a strong network through which information is shared on a national basis. It is clear how the deaf community has a small town feel despite its geographic size.

In summary, the bond that exists between fellow members of the deaf community is inimitable. The level of understanding and trust that comes from having experienced the same feelings of isolation, incompetence, discrimination, and inferiority is at the heart of this bond among deaf people. As described before, the deaf community is an interconnected and interdependent close-knit society whose members rely on each other for survival and growth.

DUAL RELATIONSHIPS WITHIN THE DEAF COMMUNITY

Dual relationships are an important ethical consideration for psychotherapists. Herlihy and Corey (1992) have addressed many issues relating to dual relationships that occur "when professionals assume two roles simultaneously or sequentially with a person seeking help" (p. 3). Defined as such, dual relationships include situations, such as a therapist-client relationship taking place concurrently with a friendship or business relationship, and when a therapist's former schoolmates, colleagues, or friends enter into a therapeutic relationship with him or her.

In small communities, such as deaf communities, some form of dual relationship is more likely to be the rule than the exception. And although often perceived in negative terms, dual relationships are not inherently problematic or unethical. The tight-knit nature of deaf communities is such that therapist-patient relationships within these communities often involve dual relationships. Dual relationships in deaf communities are often realistic and unavoidable. Due to the nature of the deaf community, as articulated previously, therapists in deaf communities are very likely to have known their patients in a nontherapeutic context beforehand, as a teacher, peer, colleague, acquaintance, teammate, friend, coach, or in many other roles.

In preparing this chapter, a survey (Guthmann et al., 2000) was mailed to more than 200 hearing members of the American Deafness and Rehabilitation Association, an organization for professionals who work with deaf and hard-of-hearing individuals. The survey asked a number of questions related to ethical challenges faced by hearing professionals in their work with deaf patients. Individuals who responded to the survey felt that refusing to provide counseling to individuals with whom one has another relationship would prevent people from receiving assistance. To deny therapeutic services in order to avoid dual relationships on principle is unethical.

The survey (Guthmann et al., 2000) highlighted the issue of professionals serving in a sequence of different roles with a deaf person. Many respondents work in positions that may constitute a combination of roles: administrator, counselor-therapist, interpreter, friend, or colleague. In one example, an individual worked with a deaf person first as his counselor, later as his supervisor, and finally as a colleague. In another instance, the professional was originally the deaf person's teacher, then counselor, and finally supervisor. Again, with the small-town feel of the deaf community, these situations occur frequently.

Professionals in service to the deaf community are often called upon to function in dual and multiple roles, since it may not be feasible or desirable for them to avoid professional, social, or other contact outside the therapeutic setting. The limited amount of available options means that sometimes socializing with clients in the deaf community is unavoidable. It is also acceptable and likely to be beneficial. Respondents to the survey (Guthmann et al., 2000) felt that professionals should be allowed to choose their own social contacts regardless of hearing status. For hearing professionals, involvement in the deaf community is a way to learn the culture and build trust with community members. For deaf professionals, the deaf community is their home!

While it may be complex, it can be ethical to counsel an acquaintance, peer, colleague, friend of a friend, relative of a friend, or a friend directly. In the context of the deaf community, it is unrealistic for counselors to expect to have no other relationship with their clients, prior to or simultaneously with treatment. Often clients seek out professionals *because* they are known and are not complete strangers. In fact, maintaining a more traditional therapeutic detached role when working with deaf clients has a different impact than in the general population. Hearing professionals may establish boundaries that are misinterpreted by the deaf community as aloofness, superiority, coldness, and disinterest. The deaf community may think hearing professionals, including interpreters, use the deaf community for financial or professional gains. Some hearing professionals make a special effort to build trust in the deaf community by their personal involvement.

A common dual relationship issue involves confidentiality. Because of the intimate nature of the deaf community, professionals may learn something about a client outside of the counseling setting. For example, a clinician sees a client at a deaf event where the client appears to be drinking alcohol. In the office, the individual reports continued sobriety. Another example might be a social worker who realizes that a new client is in a relationship with an individual who is rumored to be HIV positive. These situations raise difficult questions about the limits of confidentiality. Counselors may encounter situations where members of the deaf community make statements about their client's therapy. It can be tempting to "set the record straight" about the content of counseling. Maintaining confidentiality can be challenging when one's professional reputation is threatened. Despite the difficulty, the professional still has an obligation to serve the client and maintain confidentiality.

The ability to communicate well is vital, and working with a nonsigning therapist requires an interpreter. Because the nature of therapy is personal and confidential, the use of an interpreter is obviously not the best choice for a therapeutic setting. Writing notes back and forth is also a poor substitute for direct dialogue. A better solution is to seek therapy from professionals who are fluent in ASL and familiar with deaf culture. Whether deaf or hearing, such signing therapists are likely to understand, through personal experience or extensive second-hand experience, the patient's point of reference as a deaf person in a hearing world.

The interconnected nature of deaf communities, as inspired by the intense need for a strong communal structure and collective support and companionship, dictates that very often, therapeutic relationships in deaf communities are preceded or accompanied by some other type of relationship. The values of personal connection, knowledge, understanding, and shared history that characterize the deaf community account for the usefulness of dual relationships in therapy. The implementation of dual relationships in the deaf community, while at times complex, is often the reason that therapy in these situations is appealing and helpful to the client.

RECOMMENDATIONS

For deaf professionals, common social, educational, background, and cultural experiences with deaf clients often enhance the relationship, but sometimes bring about conflicts. The challenge of dual relationships is determining which relationships will be helpful and which will be harmful. Of utmost importance is whether or not the dual relationship interferes with the professional's ability to ethically and appropriately provide counseling. It is important for counselors and other professionals to have a process for making these determinations. The following recommendations may be helpful in the development of such a process:

1. There is a need to be flexible in balancing the delicate issues of providing effective services while maintaining clinically appropriate boundaries. The boundaries established in the deaf community may appear to be more fluid and flexible than those established when working with other groups due to the nature of the deaf culture.

2. Informed consent needs to occur at the beginning and throughout the therapeutic relationship. It is important to have disclosure statements or informed consent documents that include a description of the agency or therapist's policy pertaining to professional versus personal, social, or business relationships. This written statement can serve as a springboard for discussion and clarification. Written materials can be supplemented by explanations provided in ASL, either in person or on videotape.

3. If dual relationships arise during counseling, they should be discussed in a frank and open manner. Clients should be encouraged to raise any concerns they might have. Professionals who are open to these discussions help clients to be honest about dual relationship issues. Discussion and clarification is an ongoing process.

4. Set healthy and appropriate boundaries from the beginning of the professional relationship. If your agency does not have a specific policy regarding dual relationships, it is suggested that

supervisors and supervisees develop a clear and shared under-standing of the kind of professional boundaries expected from employees of the agency. Professionals may decide to establish firm boundaries around their private lives. The function of boundaries is to accommodate the needs of clients while still attending to the therapists' desires for privacy. Some clients are likely to benefit from casual boundaries, others from more clear and consistent ones. Educate the client about boundaries and involve the client in setting the boundaries of the professional relationship. Although the ultimate responsibility for main-taining appropriate boundaries rests with the professional, cli-ents can be active partners in discussing and clarifying the nature of the relationship as well as expectations. Because of the cultural expectations in the deaf community, deaf clients may be especially in need of this kind of education.

5. Develop a treatment plan that is based on the client's situation, presenting problem, personality, and subculture. When applica-ble, include dual relationships as part of the treatment plan.

6. Documentation is an especially important ethical precaution when it comes to dual relationships. Good therapy records should include accurate accounts of all interactions with clients, risk benefit analysis, documentation of consultations, informed consents, treatment plans, and so on.

7. Before becoming involved in a dual relationship, professionals should analyze their own motivations. Deaf professionals also enjoy membership in deaf clubs, teams, and other organizations. It would be very easy to rationalize by thinking "It's okay with the client" or "I can keep my roles separate." Make sure it is discussed and clarified with the client.

8. Make a risk benefit analysis. The onus is on the professional to decrease the likelihood of problems with dual relationships and increase their possible benefits. Most important, the therapist must be conscious and aware of the complexities associated with multiple roles.

9. Practitioners are advised to use consultation around dual-rela-tionship issues. Routine consultation with other professionals can be useful in gaining an objective perspective and identifying potential difficulties in dual relationships. A consultant or super-visor can help construct a well-articulated treatment plan to promote safe and productive dual relationships. For profession-als serving deaf clients, it may be difficult to find a consultant

or supervisor with expertise in the area of deafness. In these situations, counselors may seek outside expert consultation.

10. Be aware that the roles of friend and clinician in the deaf community may be beneficial but can also be complex and at times incompatible. The counselor may hesitate to confront the client in therapy for fear of damaging the friendship. Mandatory reporting requirements of the counselor can strain the friendship. Clients may hesitate to talk about deeper struggles for fear that their counselor-friend will lose respect for them. It is imperative that the clinician be aware of these and other examples of conflict of interest.

11. Knowledge of the ethical codes and relevant laws is important. All codes of ethics of major professional associations ban sexual dual relationships and consider unethical only the dual relationships that impair therapists' judgment or may harm and exploit clients. None of these codes prohibit nonsexual dual relationships across the board.

12. Do not hesitate to refer the client to another professional if you are unqualified to conduct therapy with a member of the deaf community, if the dual relationship has a high likelihood of interfering with treatment, or if the dual relationship makes you significantly uncomfortable for any reason.

13. Practitioners who are involved in dual relationships need to keep in mind that, despite informed consent and the frank discussion of potential risks at the outset, unforeseen problems and conflicts can arise. Reassess the dual relationship, consult with an expert, discuss it with the client, and choose a course of treatment that will most benefit the client. This can include changing the nature of the dual relationship, terminating the dual relationship, or terminating treatment and providing the appropriate referrals.

CONCLUSION

Deaf communities are special because of the overlapping relationships of its members. The concept of community and support can be no better demonstrated than in a collection of people in which a therapist can treat a former or current student, colleague, or friend. Knowledge of each other in a variety of contexts is an excellent base from which therapeutic progress can ensue.

A glaring reason for clients to seek treatment from within their own deaf communities is to avoid the necessity for interpreters. If the priority was to avoid all dual relationships, deaf consumers would be forced to seek therapy from professionals outside the deaf community and make use of interpreters for therapy sessions. The dynamics of therapy would change drastically for the worse, and privacy would be absent by the simple fact that a third party is present to serve as a translator.

The many benefits of dual relationships in the deaf community, as described in this chapter, warrant attention by practitioners and consumers within and outside the deaf community. Treatment of fellow members of the deaf community enhances the welfare and progress of clients by providing a therapeutic environment in which both parties speak the same language (literally) and the client starts from a place of trust and has a sense of being understood and feeling comfortable.

Counselors and other professionals who work with deaf people face challenges as well as rewards in their work. Dilemmas with regard to ethical behavior will surface, whether the issue is one of role, relationships, boundaries, personal motivations, confidentiality, conflict of interest, or referral. Some behavior, such as sexual relationships and failure to perform mandatory reporting, are clearly unethical and unacceptable. Other actions lie in gray areas, which must be explored independently for different cases in order to best fit the client's needs.

The trials of role delineation, establishing boundaries, and working in a unique cultural environment are likely to remain a part of the profession, but there are measures practitioners can take to be better prepared for the complexities of being many things to a client. Self-awareness and acknowledgment of inner conflicts, strengths, limitations, values, beliefs, and needs on the part of the therapist are essential for an ethical practice. Also, by developing systems of support, providing training opportunities in ethics, and raising intricate ethical dilemmas for discussion, professionals can continue to build upon services that are respectful of and helpful to deaf people. The joy of seeing a client overcome communication barriers and other obstacles makes the effort worthwhile.

Deaf communities are a prime example of the practicality and functionality of dual relationships in therapy. The structure of the social scene of deaf communities provides for the likelihood that members of the community, professionals and consumers alike, know or have known each other in a nontherapeutic capacity. Educational institutions and workplaces for the deaf are other settings in which deaf people have contact and spend time with other members of the deaf community. There are clients in the deaf community who recognize that a foundation for therapy is already in place, and they choose their therapists because of the already existing knowledge, understanding, and trust.

Dual relationships may comprise a fundamental part of therapy in deaf communities, because they relieve deaf consumers of the burdens of communicating with nonsigning therapists outside the deaf community. Clients are freed from having to participate in therapy with an outside practitioner who does not understand deafness and thus adds to the feelings of being misunderstood and the sense of isolation that typify the lives of so many deaf persons. To deny deaf persons therapy with members of their own communities with whom they have other relationships is to stifle the values of deaf communities and evoke the distrust associated with the severance of deaf persons from each other in a hearing world.

REFERENCES

Guthmann, D. (1999). *The gray area: Ethics in providing clinical services to deaf and hard of hearing individuals.* Retrieved July 16, 2001, from http://www.mncddeaf.org/articles/ethics_ad.htm

Guthmann, D., Heines, W., & Kolvitz, M. (2000). One client: Many provider roles—dual relationships in human service settings. *Journal of American Deafness and Rehabilitation Association, 33,* 1–13.

Herlihy, B., & Corey, G. (1992). *Dual relationships in counseling.* Alexandria, VA: American Association for Counseling and Development.

Jeffers, J., & Barley, M. (1971). *Speechreading (lipreading).* Springfield, IL: Charles C Thomas.

Padden, C. A., & Humphries, T. (1988). *Deaf in America: Voices from a culture.* Cambridge, MA: Harvard University Press.

Schein, J., & Delk, M. (1974). *The deaf population of the United States.* Silver Springs, MD: National Association of the Deaf.

CHAPTER 20

Sanity and Sanctity

The Counselor and Multiple Relationships in the Church

Russ Llewellyn, ThM, PhD

Pastoral counseling and psychotherapy in church settings provide a unique environment in which dual relationships often play an essential role in the pastor-therapist-client relationship. One of the reasons that dual relationships are especially important for pastors is that they are very often the first person to whom people turn during times of mental or spiritual anguish. Dual relationships in this context are relationships in which the pastoral counselor or psychotherapist has more than one role or relationship with clients. Common examples of dual relationships in pastoral counseling are when therapists work with clients who are also fellow members of the congregation, fellow committee members, or associates in church business (Geyer, 1994; Montgomery & DeBell, 1997).

Most counseling by Christian counselors has an inherent duality in its practice due to clients' conscious intent to integrate faith into the psychotherapy experience. In such settings, clients hire clinicians to provide dual skills: clinical expertise and specialization of Christian spiritual integration. This duality commonly manifests itself in a single therapy setting when working with clients who view spirituality as part of their mental health. In addition, there is also the very common dual role that occurs in the relatively small church community, where therapists, not only the pastors, work with people with whom they have other relationships in the church community.

I am a seminary-trained Christian psychologist with degrees both in theology and in clinical psychology. There are many Christians who have been trained as psychologists, psychiatrists, counselors, marriage and family counselors, social workers and pastoral counselors. Many, myself included, have specific training in the integration of Christian spirituality into psychotherapy. Some of us have offices or counseling centers on church grounds. Before my training as a clinical psychologist, I was a pastor and started a church, providing pastoral counseling in that role. My clinical psychology training included a significant component of Christian spirituality. I specialize in working with personality disorders, self-esteem, dissociative identity disorder, and application of Christian spirituality and the use of prayer in psychotherapy.

Since I've been involved in the church leadership over a period of decades, I have served in many capacities, including counselor on the church property, board member, adult education teacher, and seminar leader. I was also involved in starting what became a psychological center, which is part of the church ministry. In these roles I have experienced many multiple relationships in the church setting. Besides being a clinical psychologist, I am now also the church prayer coordinator and leader of the Healing Prayer services both at church and in our home. Our children grew up in the church, and my wife is one of the teaching leaders in a lay counseling work as well as a member of the ruling council of the church. As a couple we have been in small "care groups" designed for a 1-year Christian community experience of support. We participate in worship services, and I have in the past been part of the planning and preparation for them.

Some church ministries offer additional services, such as outreach programs for the homeless and others in need, crisis hotlines, and help and support for unwed or expectant mothers. Our church has a 1,000-member community center where about 3,500 people from the church and general community do fitness training, swim, play tennis, and participate in other programs.

Obviously, members of the church interact with one another in many different spiritual and secular ways, and pastoral counselors are no exception. Fellow members of the congregation show support for one another and the church by helping each other in a variety of contexts. The church setting has a similar dynamic to rural settings, where dual relationships are unavoidable and in fact essential for establishing trust (Montgomery & DeBell, 1997; Schank & Skovholt, 1997). There are many creative ways churches reach out to care for the community and extend the love God has for others. Accordingly, pastoral counselors' personal involvement in these activities or programs offers numerous potentials for multiple relationships.

Most of the dual relationships of which I've been a part of developed in the context of my memberships, activities, and duties in the church. People got to know me in a variety of roles, such as fellow committee member, former pastor, fellow worshiper, leader of prayer groups, father of children attending Sunday school, or husband of the woman who trains people for lay counseling services and is a member of the church ruling board. Observing me in these roles and becoming accustomed to and informed about my spiritual beliefs and convictions, as well as my style, personality, attributes, and behaviors, has led many people to seek my services as a psychotherapist. Unlike what many therapists believe, these people choose me as their therapist precisely *because* they are familiar with me and especially because they know me as a devoted and practicing Christian.

The familiarity is of course a two-way street. Not only do many of my clients choose me because they know me in the church, but also my familiarity with them has a positive affect on the therapeutic process. As Zur (2001) describes, familiarity with clients outside the office is likely to speed up the clinical process by facilitating faster development of trust and making clinical interventions more relevant and effective.

MULTIPLE RELATIONSHIPS IN THE CHURCH SETTING

Following are a few examples of beneficial dual relationships in the church community.

- In my clinical practice I saw the husband of one staff member of our church with whom subsequently I had an almost 3-decades-long relationship through the church. Both he and his wife were glad that I knew him, his background, and shared history in the church because it facilitated faster resolution of the presenting problem. There were probably some critical times when feedback from me as a friend who knew him kept clinical intervention from being necessary. The three of us agreed that the clinical experience added a richness, meaning, and depth to our long-term friendship.

- When my practice was first getting started and I was the only Christian-trained clinical psychologist in the county, I saw a number of Christian women in counseling. They were women whom my wife and I also knew through the church. We liked and respected these women. After they finished their work with me, five of them, along with one whom I had not seen, but had done some business consulting with her husband, formed a Christian women's support group with my wife. This leaderless group of women developed a rich history of relationship, meeting once monthly for discussion and support for almost 25 years.
- Many years ago, in my early days of establishing myself as a counselor, I began developing a friendship with a man from church who soon after became a client. We also played racquetball together. He sought my clinical services because he knew me as a person, sports partner, and as a Christian. We continued our church activities and friendship, including playing racquetball, after he became a client. As he had a compulsive personality, playing racquetball with him gave me very important data about how he was managing his compulsions, anger, and drivenness. I could observe changes in his coping style due to therapy on the racquetball court. There was never any good reason not to continue this mutually enhancing and beneficial multiple role.
- I had an occasion in which I was in one of the prayer stations after a worship service and a previous client chose to sit down with me to pray for her. She especially benefited from the exchange because I was already spiritually attuned to her and her struggles due to our clinical experience.
- A father I knew from church asked me to visit his son who lay dying of cancer in the hospital. This young man struggled because he perceived himself as not at peace with God. I had seen him in therapy nearly 2 decades ago as a young teenager, in which his thoughts about God were one of our main topics of discussion. I talked with his father about what my role would be and whether it would be a role of psychologist and/or pastor. The father insisted that it was only as a single role as Christian psychologist, even though prayer would be a part of the experience. I told him I was willing to do it only if his son wanted to see me. It was also a multiple role in that my wife and I prayed for him and the family apart from the time I spent seeing him. Our prayers joined those of 200 other people praying for him. Not doing this service would have been against my religious beliefs. Because of the significant

roles I had played in his life, the family asked me to give his memorial service address.

- One couple I got to know as fellow participants in a small "care group," though we had friendly relations with them, never became personal friends. More than 2 decades later they, and especially she, sought my help for them and their family. After termination, there has developed a greater bond of interest and caring. Our therapeutic contact enhanced the bond of affection in our ongoing church association. When they learned of our adult daughter's brain tumor, they made it a point to let us know they were praying for her and our family on a regular basis.

- The multiple role of therapist and minister who performs a marriage ceremony was presented to me once by a couple who were former clients. While I did not perform this particular ceremony, before declining the offer I thought it out carefully. I followed the cue of a friend of mine who is both a therapist and a minister, to whom this situation has also been presented. He has performed two such ceremonies with a client or former client. In each instance he underwent thorough deliberation before making his decision. This process included talking about it with colleagues and obtaining outside "arm's length" professional ethical and legal counsel to ensure that he would act in a manner beneficial to the client and the therapeutic work.

- One young woman I watched grew up in the church around the same age as my daughter. She would talk with my wife on occasion as a teenager and my wife and I would talk about concern for her apparent depression and distress. She had completed work with a couple of therapists before she sought me out as an adult. Our prior relationship and the familiarity with my family enabled her to begin with a high level of trust in and respect for me. That has been invaluable to our difficult work uncovering and working with traumas in her life. Also the fact that I had known both her parents helped me understand her and helped her feel seen and known.

Because I am involved in the community through the church, I have the opportunity to meet a variety of people within and outside the church. In many cases, people gain trust in me through church activities and then decide to seek me out as a counselor because they know me and my spiritual values. Some other clients know me first as a therapist and later make use of other services I offer in the church. My appeal as a prayer leader or as a fellow church member is increased by the knowledge and understanding I have of clients' needs, character, values, and interests from experience with them in therapy.

THE ETHICS OF PASTORAL COUNSELING

Pastoral counseling often involves several sets of codes of ethics. To me, the first and foremost is the Christian Association for Psychological Studies (CAPS International). I have been a member of this 45-year-old, 2,000-member Christian psychological organization for almost half of its existence. Its *Statement of Ethical Guidelines* (1992) does not use the term "dual relationships." Rather, Section 2 addresses "Loving Concern for Clients," which emphasizes accepting people without discrimination, appreciating the value of the individual person, maintaining a commitment to not act based on the interest of self, taking appropriate action to help or protect others, avoiding having sexual contact with or otherwise exploiting clients, making financial arrangements that are clear, and protecting the best interests of clients.

The most extensive and detailed code is the Christian Counseling Code of Ethics (1998) of the American Association of Christian Counselors (AACC), an organization that represents over 35,000 members worldwide. This Code presents a confusing and conflicting message. Section 1-140 states:

> Some dual relationships are not unethical—it is client exploitation that is wrong, not the dual relationship itself. Based on an absolute application that harms membership bonds in the body of Christ, we oppose the ethical-legal view that all dual relationships are per se harmful and therefore invalid on their face. Many dual relationships are wrong and indefensible, but some dual relationships are worthwhile and defensible. (Dual and Multiple Relationships section, para. 2)

In the same section, the Code states: "Dual relationships involve the breakdown of proper professional or ministerial boundaries" (AACC, 1998, Dual and Multiple Relationships section, para. 1). And Section 1-141 states: "Christian Counselors do not engage in dual relationships with counselees" (The Rule of Dual Relationships section, para. 1). Paradoxically, this AACC Code of Ethics states that it opposes an absolutizing of the ethical-legal prohibition and makes an absolute statement of prohibition.

Besides the AACC Code of Ethics (1998), therapists are also mandated to follow the Code of Ethics of their specific professional organizations, such as the American Psychological Association (APA) *Ethical Principles of Psychologists and Code of Conduct* (1992; also see chapter 5).

Another code that may be relevant is the American Counseling Association (ACA) Code of Ethics (1996). Section A.1.d., Family Involvement, states: "Counselors recognize that families are usually important in clients' lives and *strive to enlist family* understanding and involvement as a positive resource, when appropriate" (Client Welfare section, para. 4 [emphasis added]). Section A.6.a, Dual Relationships, states:

> *Avoid when possible.* Counselors are aware of their influential positions with respect to clients, and they avoid exploiting the trust and dependency of clients. Counselors make every effort to avoid dual relationships with clients *that could impair professional judgment or increase the risk of harm* to clients. (Examples of such relationships include, but are not limited to, familial, social, financial, business, or close personal relationships with clients.) When a dual relationship *cannot be avoided,* counselors take appropriate professional precautions such as informed consent, consultation, supervision, and documentation *to ensure that judgment is not impaired and no exploitation occurs.* (The Counseling Relationship section, para. 6 [emphasis added])

The National Association of Social Workers (NASW) Ethical Standards (1999), Standard 1.06.c, states:

> Social workers should not engage in dual or multiple relationships with clients or former clients in which there is a risk of exploitation or potential harm to the client. In instances when dual or multiple relationships are unavoidable, social workers should take steps to protect clients and are responsible for setting clear, appropriate, and culturally sensitive boundaries. (Dual or multiple relationships occur when social workers relate to clients in more than one relationship, whether professional, social, or business. Dual or multiple relationships can occur simultaneously or consecutively.) (Conflict of Interest section, para. 3)

All major professional organizations, while condemning exploitation and sexual dual relationships, do not have clear mandate to avoid all nonsexual dual relationships. Indeed, as documented in the previous section, there may be some circumstances in which knowing the client in another setting is therapeutically beneficial to the client and ethically appropriate. It has been articulated before that in some settings and situations it is impossible to avoid all dual relationships and that, in fact, not all dual relationships are necessarily harmful (Huber, 1994; Kitchener, 1988; Koocher & Keith-Spiegel, 1998; Schank & Skovholt, 1997; Zur, 2000).

Another aspect of the ethics of spiritually oriented counseling is the volume of discrepancy, if any, between therapist and client about religious values. In such cases, the therapist needs to examine compatibility in offering help, and possibly make referrals. APA, *Ethical Principles of Psychologists and Code of Conduct* (1992), Principle D. states, "Psychologists are aware of culture, individual, and role differences, including those due to age, gender, race, ethnicity, national origin, *religion*, sexual orientation, disability, language, and socioeconomic status" (APA, 1992, p. 1599 [emphasis added]). These guidelines for therapists to be sensitive, aware, and considerate of cultural and spiritual differences is the common theme among professional codes of ethics.

While in many cases, as documented above, dual relationships are ethical and beneficial, in other cases they may serve otherwise. Such was the case of a former client who wanted to be a part of the leadership in my healing prayer team, of which my wife is a part. My clinical assessment was that these two roles were incompatible for this client and not likely to benefit him. Due to his personality and the type of problem he was encountering at the time, I was concerned that participating in the leadership team and working closely with my wife would interfere with future clinical work. He had terminated therapy with important unresolved issues years earlier. I knew that it was likely he would want to seek therapy from me again. We discussed at length and agreed that he would not pursue future therapy with me so he could assume a role in the healing prayer team. We also agreed that I would provide a professional referral to another Christian therapist. I later gave the referral, which he made use of. The man continues to value the connection and even now, years later, both my wife and I have the opportunity to mentor and guide him on his spiritual path.

Susan came to me as a teenager with great conflicts and was one of the people in whom I invested a lot of energy and care. She left therapy to attend a university in her late teens and transferred to another therapist to continue her work. She appeared in our lives again about 7 years later, interested in exploring a social relationship. I wondered how much healing she had experienced in the abandonment feelings of her previous negative father transference to me, which we worked on during therapy, and whether we would be able to transition into friends. The transition from therapy to friendship was predictably complex, since my relationship with her as a therapist had been essentially a transference relationship. I discussed openly with her my concerns, and she believed at the time that she had resolved these issues in her subsequent therapies. When she had a daughter, some old mixed feelings toward me resurfaced. Because of these difficulties we mutually decided to end the friendship. For me, the importance lies in that we knew how to disengage when the sequential dual relationship was no longer beneficial and enhancing.

The church environment as illustrated above provides a complex and fertile ground for multiple relationships between pastors, therapists, and clients. In situations when conflicts of interests are clear and have the potential to negatively impact the therapeutic environment, dual relationships should certainly be avoided.

A prime example is that a minister should not provide psychotherapy for any of his employees or staff. Accordingly, therapists at our church psychological center will not see a staff person for therapy, although they will see someone from the congregation. Simply being the member of the same congregation and having that multiple-role relationship is not a reason to avoid seeing a potential client. The director of the center has a very complex network of multiple-role relationships: he is employed by the church, licensed by the denomination, and supervised by a pastor. The director manages staff and is a colleague to other independent contractors on staff, including his wife. His family is also part of the church community. The director's participation in this array of roles enables the center to be effective as a part of the larger church community.

The use of a spiritual intervention is within the scope and training and the ethical guidelines of pastors and therapists. It creates an inherent duality where mental health and spirituality overlap, and if fact may not be distinguishable. Similarly, the church setting does not allow for utter avoidance of dual and multiple relationships among pastors, therapists, clients, and members of the church. It's the risk-free commentary of absolute prohibition of dual relationships that injects the unethical poison of fear under the guise of concern for our clients' safety. As documented in this chapter, dual relationships can be ethical—the examples from the previous section show that they can be helpful as well. But examples from this chapter also show that they can be complex. Particularly in pastoral counseling, dual relationships are accepted and embraced; congregants in quest of therapy and spiritual guidance seek out pastoral counselors to help them grow from more than one angle. Parishioners can build a strong foundation of trust by seeing their therapist and pastor active in the church and community and get to know them in these different contexts. If a therapeutic relationship commences from this place of trust, progress and effectiveness increase substantially.

CHRISTIANITY AND DUAL RELATIONSHIPS

Beliefs about the spiritual nature of life can create affinities or distance between a client and counselor. Following are the results of a study done by Eck (2001): Natural scientists' belief in God was 39.3%. Ninety-five percent of Americans say they believe in God. Forty-eight percent of psychologists report religion is important or fairly important while 73% of them have the same beliefs about spirituality. Ninety-three percent of the general population identify with a religious group and 84% try to live according to their religious beliefs. Forty-eight to 53% of psychologists and psychotherapists reported that religion was valuable, and 65% of psychologists and 77% of all therapists reported consistent effort to live their lives in accordance with their religious beliefs.

Another very positive blend of complementary roles, which is unique to the church setting, is my involvement in the healing prayer ministry. I have found that the objectives in the healing of emotional wounds through prayer are often the same as those I would have as a therapist, although the means are different. In a few cases, people receiving help from this ministry have wanted to seek more psychological help because the issues were complex, and they believed I could be of assistance. In those cases in which I have been willing to see the person professionally, I explained the ramifications of our dual-role relationship to get their informed consent for psychotherapy. Some therapists pray for clients in areas not related to their psychotherapy, but still in the clinical setting. This dual role in a single setting is also done by informed consent. When not related to psychotherapy, this prayer is done without charge.

Different cultural perspectives affect the perception of dual relationships. Rather than an individualistic Western standpoint, the church has a community-oriented Eastern view. The individual is defined as a member of a wider community, the "body of Christ." Colleague Willene Pursell reflects, "Whenever a person who is a Christian comes to me for therapy, whether I know them or not, I automatically enter into a dual relationship with them because they are members of the body of Christ" (W. V. Pursell, personal communication, August, 17, 2001).

Oordt (1997) concurs that like psychotherapy, Christianity is also based on relationships. This is supported by passages such as: "The Christian church is a community of individuals called into relationship with each other as a unified body" (Acts 4:32–35; 1 Cor. 1:10); "The Christian ethic is rooted in how we relate to one another" (Matt. 5:42–43; Matt. 19:18–19); "The Christian view of relationship has boundaries outlined in Scripture, ranging from how we treat those in need" (Matt. 25:34–40); "to the use of discretion in sexual intimacies" (1 Cor. 6).

Eighty-seven percent of the general population believes that God answers prayers and 53% report they have felt the direct presence of God. Seventy-nine percent of clients who identify themselves as religious prefer the use of prayer and Scripture in counseling as opposed to therapy that does not integrate Christian faith. The same 79% also favor religious counselors with congruent values, and explicitly religious themes in counseling (Worthington, Kurusu, McCullough, & Sanders, 1996). Therapist-client compatibility is one of the reasons many Christian therapists choose to identify themselves as Christian and practice in church settings.

Members of the church tend to have a more accepting view of dual relationships because of the cultural and religious emphasis on spiritual connection and care, as opposed to individualistic boundaries and separation. Dual relationships are part of the church community, as its members join together on a variety of tasks, journeys, and celebrations. Weight is given to relationships between people and with God. Dual relationships in the Christian community are welcomed and encouraged because they build a strong bond between therapist and client.

DEMONIZATION OF DUAL RELATIONSHIPS

Professionals in the field of psychology often lock themselves into clinical settings for reasons of therapist convenience, theoretical perspective, confidentiality, and insurance economics. This halts the personal growth fueled by multiple roles in multiple settings. Paul Clement reflected, "If you want learning to generalize the least, then see a person the same hour of the week in the same place" (P. W. Clement, personal communication, May 2, 1970). One of the benefits of sharing a community, such as the church setting, with clients is enhanced learning in multiple settings.

There are clinicians who get nervous about the topic "dual relationships" because it is a term often used as equivalent to "unethical" or "exploitative." The majority of this stigma originated from APA's *Ethical Principles of Psychologists* of 1990, which essentially advocated that all dual relationships were unethical. There are many counselors who engage in dual relationships and are not open about what they do because of the stigma surrounding multiple roles in therapy. One of the problems that results from these attitudes is that therapists avoid seeking advice and counsel from colleagues and experts in an attempt to avoid negative stigma and judgment. There is substantial evidence that if an accusation of a dual relationship is made, the Board of Consumer Affairs will investigate the allegation and assume that an unethical dual relationship exists unless proven otherwise. There is, therefore, a great need to document everything regarding therapist judgments and informed consent about entering into multiple relationships with a client. This fear-driven advice advocates the presumption of guilt until innocence is proved and has a punishing impact on the psyche of a counselor trying to assess objectively the potential benefits or detriments of a multiple role relationship.

I had a first-hand experience with such a situation. I was giving testimony about a friend of mine who was also a doctor I saw for another professional nontherapeutic service. In his profession, a dual relationship with me is not unethical. The Board of Consumer Affairs interviewer inquired about the nature of our relationship, beginning with whether or not he had ever seen me in therapy, which he had not. The next question was if I had ever given him psychological advice. To my detriment, I mistakenly used the term "consult" to describe an informal discussion I had with my friend, who was in therapy at the time, about the mode of some therapy options.

The interviewer abruptly ended our dialogue and left the room with the declaration that he would be back shortly. Upon his return, I was informed that he had talked with his supervisor to discuss whether or not they needed to investigate me for having a "dual relationship." Their suspicion arose from my inadvertent use of the technical term "consult" to describe the extended conversation with my friend. It was never our intent to be in a professional psychological relationship, even briefly. Even though no investigation was pursued, this encounter had a chilling effect on me.

Practitioners making decisions about the implementation of dual relationships should consider only the factors relevant to the welfare of the client and their own competence and comfort. When fear of licensing boards contaminates the assessment of dual relationships, the client suffers because his or her best interests are not the first priority.

PRINCIPLES IN NEGOTIATING DUAL RELATIONSHIPS IN PASTORAL COUNSELING

I am assuming the uniform ethical position of all major codes of ethics as a starting place: Do good, do not harm, do not use the therapists' position of trust and power for selfish advantage or exploitation of the client, avoid sexual involvement with the client, and avoid role relationships in which your objectivity or judgment may be impaired. The following are principles that can be helpful in the application of ethical and productive dual relationships in pastoral counseling.

- *Arm's-length consultation.* After you identify the complexity of the case, seek "arm's length" ethical, legal, or clinical consultation with an expert (who is not a colleague or a friend) in dual relations before proceeding. Document your consultation in your case notes, including the issues discussed and advice received. Be open to further consultation if so needed. Consultation is helpful as an objective perspective in anticipating aspects of dual relationships best discovered by an outsider, and facilitating progress through ethical, helpful dual relationships.
- *Informed consent.* Use informed consent at the beginning and throughout the therapeutic relationship. As new issues surrounding dual relationships and informed consent arise during the course of therapy, discuss them fully with the client. Informed consent can also include discussion of how you might approach the issues of the community as well as those of the client. The effect of a client's actions on the community is a relevant issue for people in positions of leadership or who are otherwise high profile.
- *Willingness to address conflict.* Conflict of needs is much more likely to be problematic if it goes unaddressed. Multiple relationships in the church setting can lead to unexpected conflict of interest. Such conflict must be openly acknowledged and discussed. The solution can range from dissolving the conflict of interest situation to termination of therapy. What is important is that full dialogue takes place and the resolution is conducive to the well-being of the client.
- *Flexibility of approach.* Therapy, in the church or elsewhere, should be tailored to the client. Different clients have different needs and work best with approaches that suit them. Rather than assuming that one tactic or setting fits all clients' needs, counselors should explore with the client what works best for him or her and go from there. In doing clinical work both on and off the church campus, I learned that some people are more comfortable in a church counseling center, while others prefer to see someone in a clinical setting off the church campus. While some clients put more emphasis on their spiritual practices, others may emphasize

cognitive or behavioral aspects of their functioning. There are a variety of factors that influence how and where a client is best served therapeutically, one of which is the desired level of privacy. The key is to be aware of clients as individuals and attentive to the kinds of treatment to which they are most receptive.

- *Maturity, boundaries, and maintaining therapists' space.* Clarity of roles, boundaries, and expectations on the part of both therapists and clients makes it easier to maintain multiple roles and avoid confusions and misunderstandings. The ego strength of clients, level of functioning, and personality should be assessed, along with the ability, willingness, and desire of both parties to enter a multiple role or more mutual relationship. Dual relationships are an excellent opportunity for clients to practice problem solving and expressing needs. Therapists need to be clear on what their needs are for individual space. Therapists must take care and keep their space from being taken over by a client. If the situation does arise where a therapist feels that space or privacy is invaded, mature and open handling of competing needs can remedy the situation.
- *Transference issues.* Early developmental issues as a subject for therapy and a long therapeutic relationship can increase the likelihood that either the client or therapist will have difficulty transitioning to a relationship in which mutual needs are the relationship expectation. The more complex shift is often on the part of the client. As demonstrated by the example of Susan, frustration is brought into the new relationship if clients have not resolved their negative transference and internal growth issues. In such cases, a mutual relationship, like a friendship with a previous therapist, is not advisable.

Huber (1994), Kitchener (1988), and Lukens (1997) offer additional considerations that are helpful in thinking through the involvement of clients and counselors in church settings and their consequent engagement in dual relationships.

1. A wide discrepancy of obligations in dual relationships creates a greater possibility for conflict of interest and consequent loss of objectivity on the part of the therapist.
2. Isolated or tight-knit communities are environments in which dual relationships are not avoidable. This is because of location, number of available practitioners, and the general interconnected way of life in small and close communities.

3. Both therapist and client must be willing and able to set and maintain applicable boundaries. Clarity of boundaries lowers the probability of confusion on the part of the client with regard to expectations about the dual relationship (Kitchener, 1988).

4. Dual relationships are more problematic when there is a definite power-prestige differential (Geyer, 1994). The potential for exploitation or harm to the client is proportional to the amount of power the therapist has over the client (Kitchener, 1988).

5. Issues of confidentiality may arise in the course of dual relationships that take place in certain social settings. Concerns about confidentiality should be discussed with the client throughout treatment as needed.

This section gives guidance for practitioners on how to handle dual relationships in a manner that is most beneficial for the client and respectful of the practitioner's need for privacy.

THE INDISPENSABILITY OF DUAL RELATIONSHIPS IN PASTORAL COUNSELING

Through examples, relevant ethics, and helpful principles, this chapter sheds light on how dual relationships in pastoral counseling are normal, important, unavoidable, and helpful. Most clients in the Christian community expect and welcome the participation of their therapists in church services and activities. In fact, many clients are attracted to their therapists in the first place by gaining knowledge and understanding of them as pastors and fellow Christians.

In small towns and close communities, multiple relationships occur regularly and are a part of life (Schank & Skovholt, 1997; Zur 2000). Practitioners interact with former and current clients at grocery stores, their children's' schools, community events, and social gatherings. Nowhere is this more true than in the church community. The same social norms of familiarity and interconnectedness that apply to rural communities, the military, and close-knit groups, such as the deaf, or fellowships of recovering alcoholics, apply also to religious communities, such as the Christian church. In these settings, multiple-role relationships are unavoidable, expected, and embraced.

Social acceptance or rejection of dual relationships depends mainly on cultural outlook. Abi-Hashem, a consultant and teacher of psychology in other nations of the world, especially the Mid-East, states: "Dual roles is not an issue in other nations of the world. It is primarily an issue in the United States" (N. Abi-Hashem, personal communication, July 9, 2001). There are predisposing worldview factors that influence how one sees the individual in relation to the community. The western worldview emphasizes autonomy and individualism over community. The eastern worldview emphasizes interdependence and sees the individual as a member and a part of community.

This chapter illustrates that dual relationships are not only unavoidable in pastoral counseling, but in fact are essential and crucial. They provide an incredible richness and depth to the therapeutic process, benefiting counselees, pastoral counselors, and the spiritual communities in which they take place.

I hope this chapter has brought some sanity and humanity into the discussions about how the people who are clients and the people who serve clients can live in a common community based on commitment to the church. The therapeutic relationship and the community of the church are both designed in part to function as sanctuary. The combined power of sanctuary in the church community and dual relationships in pastoral counseling serve both the church community and the therapeutic relationships contained in them, or it serves neither. We as Christians, counselors and clients alike, live inseparably in the community.

REFERENCES

American Association of Christian Counselors. (1998). *Christian counseling code of ethics.* Retrieved August 20, 2001, from http://www.aacc.net/downloads/ethics.pdf

American Counseling Association. (1996). *Code of ethics and standards of practice.* Alexandria, VA: Author. Retrieved July 8, 2001, from http://www.cacd.org/codeofethics.html

American Psychological Association. (1990). Ethical principles of psychologists. (Amended June 2, 1989) *American Psychologist, 45,* 390–395.

American Psychological Association. (1992). Ethical principles of psychologists and code of conduct. *American Psychologist, 47,* 1597–1611.

Christian Association for Psychological Studies. (1992). *Statement of ethical guidelines.* Retrieved August 20, 2001, from http://www.caps.net/join.htm#ethics

Eck, B. E. (2001). *A review and exploration of the therapeutic use of spiritual disciplines.* Paper presented at the annual meeting of the Christian Association for Psychological Studies, Western Region, San Diego, CA.

Geyer, M. C. (1994). Dual role relationships and christian counseling. *Journal of Psychology and Theology, 22* (3), 187–195.

Huber, C. H. (1994). *Ethical, legal and professional issues in the practice of marriage and family therapy* (2nd ed.). New York: Macmillan.

Kitchener, K. S. (1988). Dual role relationships: What makes them so problematic? *Journal of Counseling and Development, 67,* 217–221.

Koocher, G. P., & Keith-Spiegel, P. (1998). *Ethics in psychology: Professional standards and cases.* New York: Oxford University Press.

Lukens, H. C., Jr. (1997). Essential elements for ethical counseling. In R. K. Sanders (Ed.), *Christian counseling ethics: A handbook for therapists, pastors and counselors* (pp. 43–56). Downers Grove, IL: Inter-Varsity Press.

Montgomery, M. J., & DeBell, C. (1997). Dual relationships and pastoral counseling: Asset or liability? *Counseling and Values, 42* (1), 30–41.

National Association of Social Workers. (1999). *Code of ethics.* Retrieved July 27, 2001, from http://www.naswdc.org/Code/ethics.htm

Oordt, M. S. (1997). The ethical behavior of Christian therapists. In R. K. Sanders (Ed.), *Christian counseling ethics: A handbook for therapists, pastors and counselors* (pp. 326–331). Downers Grove, IL: Inter-Varsity Press.

Schank, J. A., & Skovholt, T. M. (1997). Dual-relationship dilemmas of rural and small-community psychologists. *Professional Psychology: Research and Practice, 28* (1), 44–49.

Worthington, E. L., Kurusu, T. A., McCullough, M. E., & Sanders, S. J. (1996). Empirical research on religion and psychotherapeutic processes and outcomes: A 10-year review and research prospectus. *Psychological Bulletin, 119,* 443–487.

Zur, O. (2000). In celebration of dual relationships: How prohibition of nonsexual dual relationships increases the chance of exploitation and harm. *The Independent Practitioner, 20* (3), 97–100.

Zur, O. (2001). Out-of-office experience: When crossing office boundaries and engaging in dual relationships are clinically beneficial and ethically sound. *The Independent Practitioner, 21* (2), 96–100.

CHAPTER 21

Multiple Relationships in Military Psychology

Ofer Zur, PhD and Steve Gonzalez, PsyD

> At approximately 9:00 A.M. Eastern Standard Time on September 11, 2001, my long-term "therapeutic relationship" with most of my patients unexpectedly changed. When the World Trade Center in New York City and the Pentagon military installation in Washington, DC, were attacked, my relationship with my patients immediately became a clear dual relationship. War had been declared against and by the United States, and at that moment it became perfectly evident that my primary role was no longer as psychologist but as a Naval Officer with a secondary function as staff psychologist. When our unit was mobilized a short time later, my patients and I became shipmates: the office was replaced with a ship and the couch with bunks. We were no longer doctor and patient, but comrades in arms with the common goal of national defense.
>
> —Steve Gonzalez, PsyD Lt. MSC, U.S. Navy

GENERAL BACKGROUND OF MILITARY PSYCHOLOGY

The practice of psychology or psychiatry in the military is a unique situation and is markedly different from private practice and most other

The views expressed in this chapter are maintained by the authors and are not to be attributed to the Department of Defense or the Navy.

nonmilitary settings. Active duty military clinical psychologists or psychiatrists fulfill dual roles as therapists-clinicians and commissioned military officers. In addition to these multiple roles, psychologists also have dual agency as they carry responsibility for and loyalty to their clients as well as the military or the Department of Defense (DOD) (Hines, Adler, Chang, & Rundell, 1998). Johnson (1995) describes military psychologists as "serving two masters."

The opening example of this chapter illustrates such multiple roles. Functioning within the framework of multiple relationships is part and parcel of what military psychologists do on an everyday basis. More often than not, these circumstantial multiple roles are unavoidable. Comparisons have been made between military psychologists and rural, small-town, correctional, or hospital psychologists. However, the unique status of military psychologists stems from the often isolated nature of military bases and even more so from their binding commissioned status, where they are required to place military interests and national security above the interests of their clients.

Concerns about dual relationships in the military are part of the larger concern of the armed forces about fraternization. Fraternization, one form of multiple relationship, is defined by the Air Force Instruction 36-2909 as "a personal relationship between an officer and an enlisted member which violates the customary bounds of acceptable behavior" (Professional and Unprofessional Relationships, 1996, p. 2, cited in Staal and King, 2000). Staal and King then describe how the power imbalance between officers and enlisted members is evident by the stressed importance of rank. They go on to explain the reasons the military gives this much attention to fraternization, which are: the risk of depreciation of the superior's authority; conflict of interest; or fostering concern about favoritism among the surrounding members.

UNAVOIDABILITY OF DUAL RELATIONSHIPS IN THE MILITARY

Following are descriptions of the four types of dual relationships with which military psychologists are faced as part of their daily reality.

1. *When therapist and client are members of a small close-knit military community.* The most apparent aspect of dual relationships in the military consists of the same dynamics as any rural, isolated, or small community. Military psychologists are likely to interact regularly with their clients

in numerous settings, such as at the only general store on the base, in a recreational league, in a band, at parties, at children's school activities, at community gatherings, or in committees. Many military bases are located in remote, isolated, or highly secured areas. Others are overseas where they are isolated not only with fences but also with language and cultural barriers. Invariably, the focus on security leads such communities toward self-containment, self-sufficiency, and often, for security reasons, intentional isolation. Needless to say, in many of these settings psychologists have only one general store at which they can shop, one school to which they can send their children, and one baseball league or band in which they can play. In some situations dual relationships with one's dentist, physician, or supervisee can be avoided by a referral to another military or to an off-base clinician. However, in many other situations of deployments, assignments to remote locations, or the availability of only one psychiatrist or psychologist, there is no option of referral and dual relationships necessarily come into play.

This one aspect of dual relationships in the military bares close resemblance to the prevalent and unavoidable dual relationships in other small close-knit communities, such as *rural* (Barnett & Yutrzenka, 1994; Hargrove, 1986; Jennings, 1992; Schank & Skovholt, 1997); *religious* (Geyer, 1994; Montgomery & DeBell, 1997); *feminist* (Greenspan, 1995; Lerman & Porter, 1990; Stockman, 1990); *gay* (Brown, 1991; Smith, 1990); and *ethnic minorities* (Sears, 1990).

The literature on dual relationships in general has warned practitioners about the dangers of dual relationships and the problem of a "slippery slope," where nonsexual dual relationships end up, through a snowball-type escalation, as exploitive and/or sexual relationships (Bersoff, 1999; Borys, 1992; Kitchener, 1988; Koocher & Keith-Spiegel, 1998; Pope, 1991; Pope & Vasquez, 1998) and Woody (1998). There is no evidence to suggest that psychologists who interact with their patients as shipmates, colleagues, or acquaintances, as is done routinely in the military, in any way hinder the therapy process. Zur's (2001a, 2001b) account of dual relationships and familiarity as beneficial to therapy in small nonmilitary communities also applies to military settings.

2.   *When psychologists are also consultants to the military.* Unlike almost all other clinical settings, in the military, superior officers or an individual's commanders have the authority to assign individuals under their command or supervision to seek mental health services or undergo an evaluation in accordance with various military regulations (Mental Health, 1997; Requirements, 1997; Staal & King, 2000). The result of such assignments is dual or multiple relationships between psychologists and their clients.

An important aspect of these dual relationships is the primacy of the military role over the clinical. This primacy is known throughout the military community as the "need to know" clause, which refers to the right of a commanding officer to view or be privy to specific patient information that would in all other nonmilitary circumstances be considered confidential. Specifically, if the information revealed in a session is deemed by the psychologist to be a threat to national security or a potential safety hazard or concern, the patient's commanding officer must be notified, and he or she could potentially initiate administrative or legal action against the patient. Recent patient impassivity, depression, chemical dependency, and self-mutilative behavior are common examples of a much broader list of possibilities that put this clause into effect. As noted above, supervisors not only have the authority to demand a psychological evaluation but also the right to know significant clinical information if it has any potential bearing on national security.

A related dual relationship that military psychologists face is their dual role as clinician and forensic evaluator. In general, the clinical role comes first and the psychologist is later ordered by the military to perform an evaluation of competency or suitability for service determination. Similar complexities are often experienced by therapists in private practice with regard to child custody and other forensic situations. However, therapists in these nonmilitary settings have the choice of whether or not to step into the forensic role; or if they do not, the option is still available to protest being deposed to a judge. Such choices do not apply to military psychologists.

Johnson (1995) reflects on clinical-forensic dual relationships: "It is quite common for military psychologists to engage in clinical functions only to later serve in a DOD 'gatekeeper' role, recommending discharge from service or, worse, divulging sensitive material in a forensic format. In this case, as in many others, the client was inadequately prepared for this role switch" (p. 11).

3. *When the client is also the therapist's superior.* A dual relationship circumstance that evokes difficult, if not impossible, ethical dilemmas for military psychologists is the issue of treating or assessing a service member of a higher rank. All active duty psychologists are commissioned officers, and the majority of patients seen are from the enlisted community. Nevertheless, there are individuals who present to the clinic of a higher rank than the provider. This situation frequently causes confusion and discomfort, if not anxiety and trepidation in the treating psychologists. These situations are even more difficult if the involved depositions or the evaluation will be used to determine the (superior)

patient's fitness or suitability to perform certain military duties. In these situations, the challenge for psychologists is to remain as objective as they would if the patient was their subordinate and not lose their clinical or military bearings.

When psychologists are ordered to evaluate senior members within their own chain of command, they can protest and argue with their direct supervisors against the assignment. However, ultimately they have no choice but to obey the order. Staal and King (2000) present such a case and discuss what may happen if the evaluation of such a case included the presence of a mental health condition. This evaluation could result in negative consequences, such as the revocation of responsibilities or privileges; restriction of entry to certain areas or access to security information; or demotion of the individual from his or her position of command. Such a recommendation is likely to affect the attitude and behavior of the restricted superior toward the therapist in post or during nonclinical contacts.

4. *When the client becomes a comrade.* Other dual relationships unique to the military are those derived from the fact that the primary role of the psychologist is not that of a clinician but of an enlisted person. The opening vignette of this chapter illustrates how quickly the role of a military psychologist can shift from clinician to comrade. Staal and King (2000) describe a case in which the psychologist was assigned to the same tent as the client during military exercises. One must take into account that the majority of military organizations combine all ranks of enlisted personnel during training and other exercises for the sake of building comaraderie and unity among members. This in turn increases the probability that future professional or social contact will occur. As members become better acquainted with one another and branch out to meet other servicemen, the web of connection in the military unit as a whole thickens. The result is even more dual relationships.

WHO IS THE CLIENT?

In most nonmilitary settings, the question of who the client is remains relatively straightforward. This is not the case in the military. One of the main issues among the many difficult dilemmas encountered by military psychologists on a daily basis is the identification of the client. Who do military psychologists serve? And where do their loyalties lie? Simply put, is the client the service member sitting in the office, or the DOD (or the military or the government)? Or both?

The ultimate client is the military or DOD and *not* the actual person who is sitting in the office. This fact has profound significance for the therapeutic encounter. This is a unique dual-relationship situation in which the military psychologist is faced with dual allegiances and dual loyalties. This is especially true if a service member is directed by his or her commanding officer to appear for a psychiatric evaluation as per specific military instructions (Mental Health Evaluations of Members of the Armed Forces, 1997). In these circumstances, neither the patient nor the psychologist has a choice of whether or not to enter into the clinical relationship (Johnson, 1995; Staal & King, 2000). While psychologists attempt to assess thoroughly and accurately, they are aware that in these situations the client is the referral source, which is the Army, Navy, military, government, or DOD, but is *not* the individual service member who is sitting in the office. Remaining objective is an absolute requirement for military psychologists and must be sought at all costs. Responding to the referral source's specific questions is the undisputed assigned obligation of psychologists even if it may have adverse effects, such as dismissal, for the service member.

The question of who the client is becomes even more acute when, as described above, the original clinical or client focus of therapy switches to an evaluation of military seemliness. The difficulty in these cases lies in the sequential dual relationships where the primary obligation shifts from the service member being treated to the military. Acknowledging and coming to terms with the issue of who the client is continues to be essential in order for military psychologists to perform their duties. Informing clients about the implication of this fact prior to the onset of treatment or evaluation is the ethical, clinical, and moral obligation of the therapist.

POWER AND "UNUSUAL AUTHORITY"

Unlike most clinical settings, psychologists in the military often have an enormous amount of power over their service member clients. Orme and Doerman (2001) describe the notion of "unusual authority" that military psychologists have over their patients by virtue of the psychiatric diagnosis or recommendations that are being made. If during the assessment of a service member for fitness and suitability for a position, severe mental health pathology conditions are evidenced and the member is found unfit or unsuitable during assessment of a service member for fitness or suitability for a military position, a specific recommendation for administrative separation from the service will be made to the member's commanding officer. Such a recommendation by a psychologist may in essence terminate the service member's military career.

The question then becomes, How does the psychologist balance the needs of the individual service member in conjunction with satisfying the obligation to and directive of the "ultimate client," the military? In these "need to know" situations where the fitness of the service member is questioned, the service member's livelihood, identity, or ability to provide for a family can be in direct conflict of with the military's need to retain fit, competent, and reliable soldiers. While obtaining an Informed Consent from clients at the onset of the clinical encounter as the ethical and moral act, the dilemma psychologists face is still extremely difficult. Psychologists must obey the order to conduct and report an objective evaluation and also try to attend to the individual wishes and needs of the service member. These kinds of power relationships are often part of forensic and other evaluations pertaining to fitness for duty or Workers' compensation. However, military evaluations are more complex because often neither the individual patient nor the psychologist has much choice in the matter.

The power of military psychologists over their individual member clients is real and tangible. This form of power must be clearly differentiated from therapists' power as described by Austin (1998), Bersoff (1999), Borys (1992), Brown (1994), Kitchener (1988), Koocher and Keith-Spiegel (1998), Pope (1991), Pope and Vasquez (1998), and Woody (1998). Their argument is that because of the power differential between therapists and clients in regular private practice settings, the latter are vulnerable and incapable of free choice and hence exploitation in the course of dual relationships is likely to occur, therapeutic benefits are significantly compromised, and harm often results. Lazarus (1994) responds to these assertions by articulating the illusion of power that so many therapists believe they have over their clients. Dineen (1996) describes how professional boundaries are in fact self-serving as they increase therapists' power. Zur (2001a) articulates how rigid boundaries, isolation, and the avoidance of dual relationships also increase therapists' power and the chance for exploitation.

In a similar vein a lot has been written about the illusive slippery slope phenomenon (Borys & Pope, 1989; Gabbard, 1994; Pope, 1990; Sonne, 1994; Strasburger, Jorgenson, & Sutherland, 1992). This term, popularized by Strasburger et al. (1992), has been described as follows: " . . . the crossing of one boundary without obvious catastrophic results (making) it easier to cross the next boundary" (Gabbard, 1994, p.

284). This snowball concept has come under intense critique for being irrational and syllogistic (Lazarus, 1994; Zur 2000, 2001a). One would think that if there is one place where the slippery slope phenomenon would manifest itself the most, it would be the military due to the inherent dual role, dual loyalty, and the real and significant power discrepancy that psychologists assume in these settings. However, Hines et al. (1998) who studied dual agency and compared military, HMOs, and other civilian psychiatrists report that " . . . military psychiatrists reported the fewest boundary violations from dual relationships" (p. 831).

Another concern about power in military psychology is the form of a multiple relationship in which psychologists enter into the therapeutic relationship as an advocate for the individual service member-patient but end up in an evaluatory or reporting role. After such a change psychologists are often viewed by the patient no longer as supportive but as an adversary or even worse, advocate for their parent military command. The struggle between maintaining a role of patient advocacy versus adversary is an issue military psychologists face and deal with on a regular basis. This is commonly seen in the military-forensic realm, where the military psychologist may be called in to testify by the patient's attorney as both a fact and expert witness. The clinical testimony provided, although ideally intended to serve the best interest of the patient, may actually strengthen the case against the patient (i.e., a clinical explanation of antisocial personality disorder). This dilemma may also arise if there are questions regarding the competency or sanity of patients.

All military psychologists are officers. That means that most psychologists are in positions of authority and supervision over lower ranking enlisted members. Because 80 to 85% of all military members are not officers, military psychologists are in a position of power over most military members even without a clinical relationship. If one adds the therapeutic connection, the "need to know" principle and the "unusual authority," the power status of the military psychologist becomes enormously clear. Its significance cannot be undermined.

CONFIDENTIALITY

Due to the dual role and multiple relationships that are inherent in the practice of military psychology, confidentiality concerns take a different form in the military than in any civilian setting. The military position in regards to confidentiality has been described as a "strong anti-privilege position." The general rule is that national security and military concerns override the confidentiality of doctor-client relationships. Consistent with this "need to know" clause, court-martial and other military authorities do not recognize any ethical obligation in regard to confidentiality (Johnson, 1995).

In addition to the overriding lack of protection of confidentiality, the military psychologist must follow the standard exceptions to privilege to which most nonmilitary clinicians are bound, such as danger to self or others and child- and elderly-abuse reporting. The military psychologist also has a duty to report spouse or child abuse to the service member's command. In military settings, access to confidential clinical files and other threats to confidentiality pertain to several sources: clients' command, military or DOD investigative or legal services, spousal abuse investigations, drug and alcohol abuse investigations, and military personnel in charge of health records (Johnson, 1995).

Informed Consent is of utmost importance in any clinical setting, especially in the military. While all service members learn some of the information contained in Informed Consent as part of their original employment contract, there must be also an Informed Consent before the onset of treatment. Besides clinical information and clients' rights, the written and the verbal consent must include a thorough explanation of the limits of confidentiality, privacy concerns, the potential for multiple relationships and the concern about who the client is (e.g., Department of Defense vs. the individual patient). More specifically the Informed Consent must outline the fact that if the psychologist is under the impression that the client's mental health problems are likely to affect national security, fitness to duty, or ability to perform, this must be reported to the client's supervisor. Johnson (1995) and others have stated the obvious implication of lack of confidentiality rules, which is the avoidance of utilization of mental health services by military personnel who fear the damage to their military career that can result from a mental health consultation.

CONFLICT BETWEEN THE MILITARY AND PROFESSIONAL ETHICS CODES

The American Psychological Association (APA, 1992) has acknowledged the inevitability of multiple relationships in some settings, primarily the military and rural communities (Barnett & Yutrzenka, 1994; Zur, 2000).

Nevertheless, military psychology presents clinicians with unique and extremely complex and difficult ethical dilemmas. Please refer to the 1992 APA Code of Ethics (see chapter 5) for explicit terms.

Principle D in the Code states, "They respect the rights of individuals to privacy, confidentiality, self-determination, and autonomy, mindful that legal and other obligations may lead to inconsistency and conflict with the exercise of these rights" (APA, 1992, p. 1599). Principle E states, "When conflicts occur among psychologists' obligations or concerns, they attempt to resolve these conflicts and to perform their roles in a responsible fashion that avoids or minimizes harm" (APA, 1992, p. 1599). Last, Ethical Standard 1.02, Relationships, states, "If psychologists' ethical responsibilities conflict with law, psychologists make known their commitment to the Ethics Code and take steps to resolve the conflict in a responsible manner" (APA, 1992, p. 1600).

These guidelines (APA, 1992) are an improvement over former ones, as they acknowledge that some dual relationships are unavoidable. However, these guidelines pose more difficulties than assistance or guidance. Almost all ethical codes emphasize and focus on psychologists' responsibly, loyalty and care for their individual clients. This does not fully apply to the military setting in which the DOD is defined as the client. The complexities of dual relationships and conflicts of loyalties that occur in the military are not addressed in APA's Code of Ethics or that of any other professional psychotherapy association.

Several places in Section 1.17 (APA, 1992) state that psychologists should refrain from entering into professional dual relationships if such a relationship reasonably "might harm" or "create a risk of harm." These guidelines cannot be implemented in military psychology, as dual relationships are inevitable. Psychological reports can cause severe harm to the service-member clients if such reporting causes them to lose their specific position or even their employment and enlistment status.

The main problem with the Code (APA, 1992) is that it does not take into consideration the two rules by which military psychologists must abide. Johnson (1995) states, "Frequently, simultaneous allegiance to professional (ethical guidelines) and military (federal statutes) requirements is not possible, placing the military psychologist in ethical quandaries that lack elegant resolution and create a continuing environment of risk" (p. 281). Johnson describes the effort by military psychologists to satisfy the competing demands of APA and DOD as "damage control." He then calls for collaboration between APA and DOD for the purpose of providing clear, manageable, and unified ethical guidelines. Jeffrey, Rankin, and Jeffrey (1992, cited in Johnson, 1995) describe a couple of cases that delineate the vulnerability of military psychologists to sanction. One case involved a military psychologist who was sanctioned by APA for failing to maintain the confidentiality of a service member. The second case was of a military psychologist who upheld the principle of confidentiality and was sanctioned by his commanding officer for failing to report a violation of the Uniform Code of Military Justice.

Staal and King (2000) confirm the lack of acknowledgment about the impracticality and at times impossibility of applying APA ethical principles to military settings. Although they display a clear comprehension of the complexities of military psychology, Staal and King still attempt to apply Gottlieb's (1993) general ethical decision-making model to the military setting. Gottlieb's model may be of some help in ethical decision-making in private practice and other civilian settings where therapists have choices and options about who they treat and whether or not they engage in dual relationships. However, termination of treatment, referrals to other practitioners, protection of confidentiality, avoidance of dual relationships, or refusal to treat are generally not available options for psychologists in a military setting. Hence the utility of Gottlieb's model in military settings is nullified.

The incompatibility of the dual agency or dual loyalty with APA Code ethics was best expressed by Johnson (1995) who states that while the "mission of the military might most parsimoniously be stated, 'to fight and win any battle as directed by appropriate authority,' the mission of the psychologist's professional code (APA, 1992) is the welfare and protection of the individuals and groups with whom psychologists work" (p. 291).

CONCLUSION

The military setting presents one of the most complex dual-relationship situations for clinicians. These complexities derive from the fact that active duty military clinical psychologists or psychiatrists always engage the dual roles of therapist-clinician and commissioned military officer. Consequently, military psychologists have dual agency as they carry responsibility and loyalty toward their individual clients and toward their ultimate client, the military or the DOD.

This chapter identifies several types of unavoidable nonsexual dual relationships in the military and emphasizes the unique power position that psychologists have over their individual clients. Dual relationships in the military stem from the isolated nature of the location of military bases and the fact that psychologists must report any concern about their individual client's fitness for duty or the possibility of threat to national security. The "need to know" clause and the "unusual authority" described above give military psychologists the power to determine the service person's enlistment status.

The concern with power in the military is not focused on sexual or other types of exploitation but instead on the impact of the dual agency or dual loyalty on the therapeutic process. These dualities place military psychologists in extremely difficult ethical and moral impasses where they must give primacy to the need and demands of the military over those of individual clients. This has far-reaching implications on issues of confidentiality and privilege. While securing an Informed Consent is of high importance, ethically and otherwise, it does not resolve concerns about the protection of the therapeutic process. As previously described, the unfortunate result of the DOD or the military's almost unrestrained access to confidential mental health records and the "need to know" clause is a low utilization of mental health services in the military.

The conflict between military laws and regulations and professional ethics codes, such as those of APA (1992), place an enormous burden on military psychologists due to incompatibility of these two guidelines. Serving the two masters of individual clients and the military and being bound by two conflicting sets of regulations leaves psychologists in convoluted situations. Johnson's (1995) appeal for the intense collaboration of APA with the DOD is of paramount importance in order to help psychologists deal with conflicting pressures and ethical quandaries.

REFERENCES

American Psychological Association. (1992). *Ethical principles of psychologists and code of conduct.* Washington, DC: Author.

Austin, K. M. (1998). *Dangers for therapists.* Redlands, CA: California Selected Books.

Barnett, J. E., & Yutrzenka, B. A. (1994). Nonsexual dual relationships in professional practice, with special applications to rural and military communities. *The Independent Practitioner, 14* (5), 243–248.

Bersoff, D. N. (1999). Ethical conflicts in psychology. In D. N. Bersoff (Ed.), *Ethical conflicts in psychology* (pp. 207–208). Washington, DC: American Psychological Association.

Borys, D. S. (1992). Nonsexual dual relationships. In L. Vandecreek, S. Knapp, & T. L. Jackson (Eds.), *Innovations in clinical practice: A source book* (Vol. 11, pp. 443–454). Sarasota, FL: Professional Resource Exchange.

Borys, D. S., & Pope, K. S. (1989). Dual relationships between therapist and client: A national study of psychologists, psychiatrists, and social workers. *Professional Psychology: Research and Practice, 20,* 283–293.

Brown, L. S. (1991). Ethical issues in feminist therapy. *Psychology of Women Quarterly, 15,* 323–336.

Brown, L. S. (1994). Boundaries in feminist therapy: A conceptual formulation. *Women and Therapy, 15,* 29–38.

Dineen, T. (1996). *Manufacturing victims: What the psychology industry is doing to people.* Toronto: Robert Davies Publishing.

Gabbard, G. O. (1994). Teetering on the precipice: A commentary on Lazarus's "How certain boundaries and ethics diminish therapeutic effectiveness." *Ethics & Behavior, 4* (3), 283–286.

Geyer, M. C. (1994). Dual role relationships and Christian counseling. *Journal of Psychology and Theology, 22* (3), 187–195.

Gottlieb, M. C. (1993). Avoiding exploitative dual relationships: A decision-making model. *Psychotherapy, 30,* 41–48.

Greenspan, M. (1995). Out of bounds. *Common Boundary Magazine, July/August,* 51–56.

Hargrove, D. S. (1986). Ethical issues in rural mental health practice. *Professional Psychology: Research and Practice, 17,* 20–23.

Hines, A. H., Ader, D. N., Chang, A. S., & Rundell, J. R. (1998). Dual agency, dual relationships, boundary crossings, and associated boundary violations: A survey of military and civilian psychiatrists. *Military Medicine, 163,* 826–833.

Jennings, F. L. (1992). Ethics of rural practice. *Psychotherapy in Private Practice (Special Issue: Psychological Practice in Small Towns and Rural Areas), 10* (3), 85–104.

Johnson, W. B. (1995). Perennial ethical quandaries in military psychology: Toward American Psychological Association and Department of Defense collaboration. *Professional Psychology: Research and Practice, 26,* 281–287.

Kitchener, K. S. (1988). Dual relationships: What makes them so problematic? *Journal of Counseling and Development, 67,* 217–221.

Koocher, G. P., & Keith-Spiegel, P. (1998). *Ethics in psychology: Professional standards and cases* (2nd ed.). New York: Oxford University Press.

Lazarus, A. A. (1994). The illusion of the therapist's power and the patient's fragility: My rejoinder. *Ethics and Behavior, 4,* 299–306.

Lerman, H., & Porter, N. (Eds.). (1990). *Feminist ethics in psychotherapy.* New York: Springer.

Mental Health Evaluations of Members of the Armed Forces, Department of Defense Directive 6490.1 (October 1997). Washington, DC: U.S. Government Printing Office.

Montgomery, M. J., & DeBell, C. (1997). Dual relationships and pastoral counseling: Asset or liability? *Counseling and Values, 42* (1), 30–41.

Orme, D. R., & Doerman, A. L. (2001). Ethical dilemmas and U.S. Air Force clinical psychologists: A survey. *Professional Psychology: Research and Practice, 32* (3), 305–311.

Pope, K. S. (1990). Therapist-patient sexual involvement: A review of the research. *Clinical Psychology Review, 10,* 477–490.

Pope, K. S. (1991). Dual roles and sexual intimacy in psychotherapy. *Ethics and Behavior, 1* (1), 21–34.

Pope, K. S., & Vasquez, M. J. T. (1998). *Ethics in psychotherapy and counseling: A practical guide* (2nd ed.). San Francisco: Jossey-Bass.

Requirements for Mental Health Evaluations of Members of the Armed Forces, Department of Defense Instruction 6490.4 (August 1997). Washington, DC: U.S. Government Printing Office.

Schank, J. A., & Skovholt, T. M. (1997). Dual-relationship dilemmas of rural and small-community psychologists. *Professional Psychology: Research and Practice, 28* (1), 44–49.

Sears, V. L. (1990). On being an "only" one. In H. Lerman & N. Porter (Eds.), *Feminist ethics in psychotherapy* (pp. 102–105). New York: Springer.

Smith, A. J. (1990). Working within the lesbian community: The dilemma of overlapping relationships. In H. Lerman & N. Porter (Eds.), *Feminist ethics in psychotherapy* (pp. 92–96). New York: Springer.

Sonne, J. L. (1994). Multiple relationships: Does the new ethics code answer the right questions? *Professional Psychology: Research and Practice, 25* (40), 336–343.

Staal, M. A., & King, R. E. (2000). Managing a multiple relationship environment: The ethics of military psychology. *Professional Psychology: Research and Practice, 31* (6), 698–705.

Stockman, A. F. (1990). Dual relationships in rural mental health practice: An ethical dilemma. *Journal of Rural Community Psychology, 11* (2), 31–45.

Strasburger, L. H., Jorgenson, L., & Sutherland, P. (1992). The prevention of psychotherapist sexual misconduct: Avoiding the slippery slope. *American Journal of Psychotherapy, 46* (4), 544–555.

Woody, R. H. (1998). *Fifty ways to avoid malpractice.* Sarasota, FL: Professional Resource Exchange.

Zur, O. (2000). In celebration of dual relationships: How prohibition of nonsexual dual relationships increases the chance of exploitation and harm. *The Independent Practitioner, 20* (3), 97–100.

Zur, O. (2001a). Out-of-office experience: When crossing office boundaries and engaging in dual relationships are clinically beneficial and ethically sound. *Independent Practitioner, 21* (1), 96–100.

Zur, O. (2001b). On analysis, transference and dual relationships A rejoinder to Dr. Pepper. *The Independent Practitioner, 21* (3), 201–204.

CHAPTER 22

Dual Relationships in Psychotherapy in Latin America

Roberto Kertész, MD, PhD

Dual relationships are the extension of the therapeutic contract between therapist and patient to other kinds of interactions. They most commonly include social events or business ventures. Obviously, the therapeutic contract has precedence over any other link. The needs and welfare of the client are primary. The patient's trust must never be violated. Psychotherapy in Latin America brings additional and unique complexities to the dynamics of dual relationships.

As observed during my experiences in most of the countries of this wide area of Latin America, as lecturer, therapist, and consultant, family bonds tend to be closer than in Anglo-Saxon countries. Family and community alliances are much more predominant than individual bonds. For example, it is comparatively rare for adolescents to leave their homes to attend a college in another state. Religious differences also exert their influence. Catholic value systems enhance sacrifice and compassion more than protestant ones, which place greater emphasis on work success. These "warmer" human relations and communal ethics spill over into our therapeutic work both in individual- and group-therapy settings, and in my experience favor the establishment of more than a single bond between therapists and clients.

Practicing psychotherapy in the Latin culture often presents psycho-therapists with opportunities to develop healthy and productive dual and multiple relationships with their clients. Unlike the Anglo culture, these kinds of relationships are seen as more of the norm rather than a dangerous deviation from a rigid distance model of therapy and a punitive code of ethics.

MULTIRELATIONSHIPS IN THERAPY IN A LATIN CULTURE

Following are a few examples of multiple relationships that I have employed successfully in my psychotherapy in Argentina. These multiple relationships are not unusual and are ethical within the Latin therapeutic community and within the larger Latin culture. First, I will discuss and give examples of when therapists and clients are involved in other professional roles, then I will attend to the mix of social and therapeutic roles in Latin culture, and finally I will discuss collegial cooperation with the clients.

The Extension of Professional Expertise of the Therapist

The combining of different roles between therapists and clients is nor-mal in and congruent with the Latin culture. In addition to formal psychotherapy, there are instances in which a therapist might serve as an instructor in sports, music, driving, self-defense, court hearings (as an expert in psychology), and other activities. He or she might coauthor a paper or book with a patient, or serve as an advisor for a doctoral dissertation.

I, for example, have cured water phobias and taught swimming in Panama, as well as given driving instruction, self-defense training, and musical improvisation lessons to different clients. (In most cases, my limited skills served mainly to provide impetus and motivation for the client to proceed beyond the initial stages.) It seems self-evident to me that the therapeutic bond is omnipresent, and one may shift back and forth between two or more roles. The inverse situation can also occur, when the client functions as an instructor. In one case, I enjoyed a *threefold* relationship with an architect, who was my patient in a group, computer instructor outside the group, and also a graphic designer for our university. Sometimes he was surprised by my limitations for learning computer languages, compared to my expertise as a therapist. I told him that, in transactional analysis terms, one of my "games" is "stupid," both in computational and visual orientation areas. This had no discernibly negative impact on his respect for my clinical skills and the outcome of therapy was the successful attainment of all his goals. Recognition of personal difficulties by the therapist as a demonstration of nonperfectionist self-esteem serves a good model for clients. Now our relationship is confined only to his role as a designer. We no longer discuss any personal issues. Nevertheless, he has indicated that if the need ever arose, he would feel quite comfortable in resuming our doctor-patient relationship—as would I.

The Mix of Therapeutic and Social Roles

Initiating the therapist to social functions with their clients is the norm in the Latin culture. Invitations from clients arise regularly to visit their houses and offices, or to have lunch or dinner. Other dual relationship issues involve family events such as marriages, birthdays, vigils, traveling together, sharing sports, going to shows, and so forth. Latin clients see invitations of this kind as normal exchanges and expect therapists to attend the functions.

Recently, a woman in a group invited me to the 15th birthday party of her stepdaughter. As I had played a significant role in her decision to marry (she and her partner had been living together for several years and had two children together), she stated that she was grateful for my encouragement and support and wanted to share her new family status with me and my wife. I attended and enjoyed the birthday party. In another case a young man invited me to his wedding. Of course, I accepted. Unfortunately, my wife came down with the flu and we could not attend. The young husband was offended and skipped his sessions for 2 months, until he and his wife forgave me. In this case, this young man's parents divorced when he was 6 and his father behaved rather distantly toward him, so we had to work this out in therapy until we arrived at a win-win solution. I explained that I was not going to leave my wife ill and alone, but regretted that my absence had disappointed him. My wife and I gave them a nice present and resumed our positive therapeutic relationship. Obviously, self-disclosure is part of the mixing of social and professional roles in Latin culture.

On the negative side, I have known lonely professionals who frequently participate in social events with their clients to satisfy their own needs, thereby blurring their main relationship. It is also interesting to notice that *dual relationships of a social nature* occur frequently between *members* who attend therapeutic groups. I do not discourage these private interactions, despite the fact that in the course of these meetings many personal issues are usually discussed outside the group, from which other members and the leader are excluded. Nevertheless, the main intent of the group is to enable them to acquire the necessary skills to establish friendships outside of the group. After all, the "friendship training" I provide is intended to transcend the capacity of group members to merely rehearse friendship skills inside the group. Lazarus (1981) has underscored a similar point.

Collegial Cooperation with the Client

Another type of multiple relationship in Latin culture is when outside of therapy, the practitioner shares work roles with the client: giving lectures, providing consultation, doing conjoint research, and even working at the same facility. Here the same rules apply: The welfare of the client has precedence over the other roles, and the shifts between different bonds have to be dealt with in a rational and flexible way. However, as imperfect human beings, we can make mistakes or emit emotional responses that present the risk of weakening our rapport. A client may discover some of our faults! The financial aspects present another factor. How will we bill the common client, or share our fees? Once again, let us remember that the "therapeutic mirror" is always present.

In the 1960s I was in psychoanalytic therapy with Enrique Pichon Riviére, one of the most outstanding psychiatrists in Argentina. He introduced social psychology, the systemic approach to psychotherapy, the Kleinian concepts, and even electroshock into this country, and since his death more than 30 years ago his followers have graduated over 15,000 students in their "social psychology" schools. When I was still his patient, he invited me to assume the role of subdirector of his small psychiatric clinic. Consequently, I had two types of bonds with him, client-therapist and colleague. I admired this man very much and still do admire his teachings, but in our shared work in the clinic I began to disagree with him on aspects that were invisible in the therapeutic setting. So, gradually our link changed and I decided to terminate both relationships. Nevertheless, I learned a lot in both roles and I am glad to have experienced them.

More recently, I asked one of my patients, a 52-year-old lawyer who graduated during his therapy a year ago, to cooperate with me in the divorce and property negotiation case of another patient of the group, a 47-year-old woman with an auto-immune disease. It was—and still is—a stormy case, but finally an agreement was reached early in this year. The divorce is still in litigation and it is hoped will be terminated in a few months' time. During the process, on several occasions, unfinished businesses of the lawyer's own divorce came to the surface, and this had to be dealt with in therapy. Moreover, I also had a dual relationship with the woman—as part of her divorce team.

All these transactions, while normal in the Latin culture, still required clear-cut contracts among the different roles, a great degree of flexibility, and congruence between what was said and done. Personally, I enjoyed these responsibilities because they added a stimulating challenge to my longtime therapeutic work. It also afforded me a greater degree of control and appreciation about the whole case.

FURTHER REFLECTIONS ON DUAL RELATIONSHIPS IN THE LATIN CULTURE

As I read the foregoing paragraphs, I realized not only the inherent link between my Latin culture, therapy, and dual relationships, but also how demanding these multiple relationships can become. I know it is worthwhile, however, to exert the effort and assume the burdens and risks. Multiple relationships foster authenticity as well as provide great opportunities for us to grow and recognize our assets as well as our limitations.

We must always remember that whether or not we extend our boundaries, we constitute role models for our patients and have to gain and maintain their trust. Relatives and friends have disappointed many of them, and we have a chance to remedy these disillusioned feelings and perceptions, and as Eric Berne stated, "help our clients to trust the human race" (E. Berne, personal communication, January 11, 1969).

It is important to note that in several countries of Latin America, especially Argentina, Uruguay, and parts of Brazil, the psychoanalytic approach is predominant, and its rigid framework precludes the establishment of bonds other than the therapeutic. In my opinion, this limits the spectrum of the resources at the reach of the professional, and thereby diminishes his or her effectiveness. This leads to another ethical issue. Are we offering the best possible services to clients, who might need dual relationships for their improvement, by limiting ourselves to the single, antiseptic modus operandi? Or is it at the service and the safety of the professional, who is not willing to take calculated risks to benefit the client? According to the Multimodal model proposed by Lazarus (1981, 1997), the best approach is to adapt our ministrations to the particular situations and needs of each patient. This flexible yet demanding stance has demonstrated its advantages over more rigid or limited approaches (Kertész, 1985).

In my case, it is not only the culture that plays a role in my embrace of multiple relationships with clients, but also my hobby, jazz improvisation in combos. Other musicians prefer to play only written music, following the composer's lead, whereas I elect to add my personal touch to the performances. Indubitably, the personality of the therapist is closely related to his or her choice of the number of roles that he can assume with different clients. Whether inspired by culture, personality, or music, I find that multiple relationships with my clients increase my effectiveness as a therapist and my humanity as a person.

REFERENCES

Kertész, R. (1985). *Evaluación clínica de tratamientos psicofarmacológicos y psicotera-peuticos. (Clinical evaluation of psychopharmacological and psychotherapeutic treatments.)* Unpublished doctoral dissertation, Buenos Aires National University School of Medicine.

Lazarus, A. A. (1981). *The practice of Multimodal therapy.* New York: McGraw-Hill.

Lazarus, A. A. (1997). *Brief but comprehensive psychotherapy.* New York: Springer.

PART 6

Dual Relationships in University Counseling Centers

P art 6 describes some unique boundary issues that pertain to work in university counseling centers where the protagonists often have to juggle and integrate several different roles and functions. Chapter 23 introduces us to some of the complexities in this community as Harris discusses a provocative case that called for an appreciation of sensitive dualities and creative boundary crossings. In chapter 24, Hyman examines the vicissitudes of chance meetings with clients on and off the college campus, and he makes an interesting case against a restrictive one-size-fits-all type of reasoning or response pattern when dealing with extratherapeutic encounters. Finally, in chapter 25, Iosupovici and Luke offer a tour de force, a poignant and erudite account that examines broad, fundamental, and critical components of dual relationships in student counseling centers.

CHAPTER 23

Dual Relationships and University Counseling Center Environments

Rafael S. Harris, Jr., PsyD

> It is not the power itself that corrupts, it is the disposition to corruption (or lack of personal responsibility) that is amplified by the power.
>
> —Tomm, 1993, p. 11

This chapter will explore the complexities of dual relationships as they pertain to university counseling centers. These centers are most typically housed within the student affairs division of university systems. Their role is to address the emotional well-being of the students in order to facilitate their academic progression for the term of their schooling. Dual relationships between therapists and clients at these centers are often unavoidable due to the nature and size of university campuses and the population served (i.e., students), most of which are housed on campus. Counselors at these centers are presented with ethical and clinical challenges that will be discussed in this chapter.

The controversy over the issue of dual relationships has perplexed and bothered me for many years. From being intimidated in graduate training, to further finger cautioning during my preparation for licensure, I have been at philosophical odds with the dogma that dual relationships equal horror. As a young graduate student, I can still remember feeling unethical, ashamed, unprofessional, and alone in ethics classes for just thinking that the professor was perhaps being

337

overly strict in the comments made over the absolute no-no of dual relationships. And so as a good student I both backed off and remained curious about such an extreme position.

This extreme position, evident in my training, was put to practice one afternoon when a fellow trainee of mine left the softball field. We were taking part in an intramural softball league at the university, and another colleague of ours had invited a football intramural team member to join us on the softball team. This person was my fellow trainee's client at the university's counseling center. My colleague's supervisor told him that if the client showed up at the game, that he (the therapist-in-training and my colleague) were to leave the field and not return to the team. Some said that was a valuable lesson for my colleague, a hands-on look at resolving an ethical dilemma. But to my mind, no dilemma yet existed. It was a premature decision at best. It is such thoughtless, blanket proscriptions that trouble me.

Dual relationships in university counseling centers are often unavoidable. Following are examples of how dual relationships as an ethical issue are particularly relevant to university counseling center environments, based on my experience in three counseling centers (Ohio, North Carolina, and Florida):

- teaching a class and having a client in the class
- interacting with clients on campus outside the therapy room
- becoming friends or being social with predoctoral interns whom therapists also supervise
- serving as counseling center consultant to various campus groups and departments (e.g., residence life, athletes, fraternities, etc.), and seeing a member who is a therapy client as well
- being the advisor to a campus organization (e.g., Hispanic Student Association, International Students Association) and seeing a member of such an association in therapy
- being a staff member who requires supervision; this staff member and the supervisor trade favors outside of the supervisory role (e.g., baby-sitting)
- working part-time outside of the university counseling center in an environment in which a client is also employed

SOME PERTINENT REPORTS

Without exception, immersion into the outcome studies literature has always led to the same conclusion: the therapeutic relationship is one of the better (if not the best) predictors of clinical effectiveness (e.g., Bergin & Garfield, 1994; Frank, 1973; Goldfried & Padawer, 1982; Lambert, 1992; Miller, Duncan, & Hubble, 1997). I am not suggesting that therapeutic relationships and dual relationships are the same thing—they are not. However, they are also not two opposite points on a continuum, as so many therapists seem to hold. And so, I have always thought (and frequently practiced) that elements of a dual relationship can be therapeutic if devoid of any form of exploitation or harm; thus, dual relationships are not inherently unethical, but commendable if practiced responsibly.

The issue of dual relationships is not foreign in university counseling center environments. An article in the *Journal of College Student Development* (Malley, Gallagher, & Brown, 1992) identified dual relationships as one of three main clusters of ethical problems encountered by counseling center personnel. Examples include:

- counselors who "take over" clients' problems in ways that encourage clients to become overly dependent on them
- counselors who use the counseling setting or relationship to become emotionally involved with their clients
- counselors who fail to recognize how their needs are being met through their clients and, thus, misuse the relationship
- counselors who have sexual relationships with their clients
- counselors who confuse "advocacy" for counseling (i.e., feminism, racism, sexism)

A study by Hayman and Cover (1986) on ethical dilemmas in college counseling centers found that role conflict occurred 17% of the time. Role conflict was defined as the counselor functioning in multiple roles vis-à-vis the client, as counselor and personal friend, counselor and evaluator, or counselor and supervisor. When faced with ethical dilemmas in general (including dual relationships), college counselors sampled for this study used "common sense" 93% of the time as a way of resolving the dilemma. Consultation with colleagues occurred 81% of the time and following published standards or guidelines 31% of the time.

Sherry, Teschendorf, Anderson, and Guzman (1991) found that university counseling center clinicians generally behave in ways consistent with their ethical beliefs. This study asked the respondents for both the frequency of occurrence of each behavior and the ethicalness of that behavior as perceived by the respondent. Thirteen of the 49 behaviors involved elements of what could be characterized as a dual relationship.

Borys (Borys & Pope, 1989) identified 10 training implications specific to the issue of dual relationships based on the results of her research, which indicated that a sample of psychologists, psychiatrists, and social workers believed dual relationships to be unethical "under most conditions" (p. 283). This is a critical piece of the literature on dual relationships relevant to the present paradigm that asserts that dual relationships are taboo.

For some time up to and after the date of the Borys and Pope (1989) article, there was increasing evidence that students entering the counseling profession needed to be more knowledgeable about the ethical parameters of counseling (Jagmin, Wittman, & Noll, 1978). The premise of the Borys and Pope article had been previously addressed by Baldich (1980), who showed that greater exposure to ethical problems through discussion and case presentation increased the ability of students to make appropriate ethical judgments.

PROFESSIONAL GUIDELINES

The American Psychological Association (APA) does not make any comments on the issue of dual relationships specific to university counseling centers. It duly alerts all psychologists (including counseling center psychologists) " . . . from entering into or promising another personal, scientific, professional, financial, or other relationship with such persons if it appears likely that such a relationship reasonably might impair the psychologist's objectivity or otherwise interfere with the psychologist's effectively performing his or her functions as a psychologist, or might harm or exploit the other party" (APA, 1992, p. 47).

The phrases "appears likely" and "reasonably might" offer very little certainty of harm or exploitation. This wording is vague and thus seems to offer maximum protection to the potentially exploited party or their attorney, but it offers very little in terms of guidelines or protection to the therapist.

The American College Personnel Association (APCA, under which university counseling centers would fall), however, does include a statement on dual relationships as part of their ethical standards in Principle 2.2—"Avoid dual relationships with students (e.g., counselor/employer, supervisor/best friend, or faculty/sexual partner) that may involve incompatible roles and conflicting responsibilities" (ACPA, 1996, p. 408).

Notably this statement is also vague and offers little direction other than the typical avoidance suggestion.

The following case example illustrates the complexity and opportunity of a dual relationship at a university counseling center. It is an example of a dual relationship consistent with the notion of dual relationships due to "community connections" (Zur, 2001, p. 98). The community in this case is both the university and the small town in which it is located. By all available evidence, I judge this dual relationship to have been therapeutic and ethical.

Case Study

I saw "Radu" at a counseling center in which I worked for several months. He was transferred to me after his therapist of 5 months left the center. Radu came into therapy following a very nearly successful suicide attempt. He indicated feeling afraid that without some form of support (in this case therapy), he would fall into the despair that led to the attempt and would try it again (this time, successfully). I remembered Radu from 2 years previously when as a predoc intern I saw him on intake. He self-referred wanting a professional perspective on the potential harm of his heavy marijuana use. He made the type of impression on me that lingered; Radu hooked me more than my typical client. Radu presented with a fairly typical profile of someone with existential woes; he did not understand the purpose of his life and was experiencing meaningless and confusion.

Radu was an internalized human being in that he processed his life within the confines of his own prison—this exacerbated his depression and kept him trapped. It is what led to the suicide attempt, which he reiterated time and again was an effort to find peace. Radu's main coping mechanism was smoking marijuana. Initially, he spoke of the practice as soothing, relaxing, and otherwise calming to his perplexing, conflicted thoughts. He came to understand the notion of self-medicating with pot yet continued the habit as one of the few things he enjoyed—he would do this with others, but also alone (a sign of the extent of his depressogenic mind-set, as smoking marijuana is more typically a social practice among university students) (Ray & Ksir, 1999).

I liked Radu. I had seen him at a local restaurant we both frequented for lunch. He was in therapy with my colleague at that time. Radu was typically alone, reading science fiction, dungeons and dragons, or other fantasy books. I came to discover that this was a way for him to check out of a world in which he felt so out of place. I would see him struggle as he attempted to make interpersonal contacts with fellow students or the staff at the restaurant. Some days he did a better job at this than others.

Different psychologists will no doubt draw different conclusions about what I did with those observations. I decided to tell my coworker about my observations of Radu, with the intent of utilizing what Lambert (1992) identified as the single most potent influence on the outcome of therapy—extratherapeutic factors. These factors are elements of someone's life that occur outside of the therapy room—a significant portion given that there are 168 hours in a week, only one of which is typically spent in the therapist's office. University counseling centers offer therapists the unique opportunity to observe and interact with clients outside the therapy room. While this is not precisely a dual relationship, the dynamics of this case validate the notion that information collected outside of therapy's four walls can be just as helpful as that disclosed within. We would otherwise call this "consultation," and while I am unsure as to how exactly Radu's therapist applied the information, he was receptive to it and would often ask me about the latest encounter with Radu.

Radu recognized me at the restaurant from our previous contact 2 years earlier, as well as from seeing me when he came into the center for therapy with my colleague. During such lunches, I began to say hello to him, and from time to time have a short conversation. I suppose this is when our dual relationship began. In any event, he responded to me, and both as a fellow human being and someone who knew he was in therapy at least in part to improve his interpersonal style, and I was pleased by this reciprocity.

Soon thereafter my colleague had made the decision to leave the center and came into my office to consult about referring Radu to me. He had spoken with Radu about it, and Radu was comfortable about entering into therapy with me. And so now I was formally his therapist. About the same time that Radu began to see me, he gained employment in that same restaurant we both frequented for lunch.

I began our first session with a conversation about what it had been like for him to speak with me outside the therapy situation. He reacted without any of the perplexed looks or comments that I had received from some of my colleagues (not from the counseling center) when discussing the circumstances of this referral. I understood that such mental health professionals were considering the ethics of the relationship based on the dogma of dual relationships. Yet, I also understood that clinical effectiveness sometimes demands that we give precedence to what a client tells us about their unique situation more than what the profession dictates, so I proceeded with Radu without hesitation or concern. Radu had been in therapy before and understood the ethical guideline involved.

I now had a client who not only made my sandwiches and refilled my drinks, but also would openly talk to me at the restaurant (in front of other customers and his employers) in ways revealing of our therapeutic relationship. The premise that this constitutes a breach of confidentiality holds no water— Radu did it, not I. It was not uncommon for me to have Radu make my lunch at noon and then for him to see me in therapy 2 hours later. Is this weird? Is it unethical? Is it unprofessional? No, no, and no—mainly because Radu was pleased and comfortable about it. No doubt a professor during an ethics class, before a licensing board, or when forewarning one about the dangers of lawsuits would disagree.

Was our therapeutic relationship enhanced by my knowledge and interactions of Radu outside of therapy? Yes, he clearly said so. I did not need objective test results for me to use my clinician's savvy in determining whether or not our dual relationship was therapeutic. Radu was my best source for that information, and so I simply asked him from time to time. He was privy to the subtleties of how seeing him during such times was beneficial to my understanding and treatment of the depressogenic mind-set. I came to believe that Radu would have been bewildered by my refusing to engage with him outside of the office due to a professional prohibition on dual relationships. We developed a camaraderie that Lazarus (2000) has described as sometimes forming when stepping outside the "bounds of a sanctioned healer" (p. 16). Further, I strongly suspect that avoiding him would have compromised our therapeutic relationship, and that the discrepancy of intimacy within the office and avoidance outside would have added more to his confusion, sense of isolation, and proclivity to see his relationships as sterile and superficial.

On one occasion when I was ordering, I asked for his input on which side dish to choose. He looked at me after I remarked that he had not shaven and said something to the effect of, 'how about a side of meaning and identity out of which randomness and confusion about the world gets eradicated.' Although I don't remember the exact words, I was struck by the poetic delivery and the significance of the message embedded in the communication that was occurring on at least two different levels. This became an important comment for our therapy.

Obviously, not all cases are like Radu's. This is not at all intended to be an argument toward creating dual relationships with all, or even most, clients. In consulting with my counseling center colleagues and my own exploration regarding other clients, I was fully aware that many prefer to keep the counseling completely private and would feel extreme discomfort at playing multiple roles. Dual relationships can indeed be tricky and volatile, so a careful cost-benefit analysis is in the best interest of the therapy. The avoidance of dual relationships is in an attempt to avoid exploitation and harm, neither of which happened with Radu. Instead, our dual relationship enhanced his therapy—both by his judgment and my own.

The most compelling piece of evidence that therapy was enhanced by our interactions outside of my office came from his comment that seeing me at the restaurant (especially when I went in with my partner) "made you more human." Reminding myself that it is more effective to make my theory fit my client than vice versa, I quickly moved into conceptualizing Radu within the humanistic school of thought. This comment by Radu outside of the therapy room taught me how to treat him quicker and better than any textbook in graduate school ever could.

DUAL RELATIONSHIPS BETWEEN FULL-TIME STAFF AND PREDOCS

As I have stated, not all cases and scenarios are like Radu's. Forming personal friendships between full-time staff and predoctoral interns is another major form of potentially problematic dual relationships. Two of the three counseling centers in which I have worked have developed an APA-approved internship site during my tenure with them. Several counseling center staff members advocated more collegial relationships with the predoc interns than might be promulgated by ethical guidelines. It was considered too cold and aloof to exclude the interns from any social outlets in which the faculty and staff of the center participated simply for the sake of following an ethical principle that is ambiguous at best. Thus, a formal decision was made to include predoctoral interns, knowing that this would probably lead to dual relationships.

Most internship sites begin with funding and structure for one intern, and if they seek APA approval, proceed to the three required for eligibility. Both of the counseling centers where I was employed are located in small university towns, rather isolated in their distance from any large metropolitan areas. One reason for extending social invitations to the interns was to offset the potential for further isolation.

Another consideration was overall staff morale and teamwork, a critical piece of any organization. It also served as a model of organizational development skills and how to navigate institutional politics. Furthermore, interns were coming from farther and farther away, making it increasingly difficult for their social and familial contacts to remain intact, as was the case when they were in graduate school. The implementation of strict boundaries, which vigilantly avoid any extension or crossings thereof, would surely only serve to destabilize morale and create problems that are easily avoided by implementing humane transactions.

This description of the humane treatment of predoctoral interns is a good example of a cost-benefit analysis when thinking about entering into multiple relationships, in this case between predocs and the full-time staff supervising their internship. As counseling center psychologists with an APA-approved internship program, we are mindful of the potential conflicts as a very function of our consideration of the issue.

CONCLUSION

By the time this is published I hope to have resolved yet another dual relationship scenario facing me as I write. I am in my second year of being the consultant to one of the residence life communities at Appalachian State University. As such, I attend the resident director's staff meetings where the staff for my community discuss mental health issues relevant to what may be happening with some of the residents. It serves as a conduit of information that, among other things, may encourage and facilitate a resident life staff member to refer a resident to the counseling center for services.

One of the resident directors for my area has hinted for some time that he wanted to come into the counseling center to see me professionally. "Sam's" hints have become more and more obvious, to the point that they have become direct requests. He was present at the resident director's training which I cofacilitated, when I commented that despite the seeming conflict of interest for resident directors themselves to engage in services at the counseling center, we make efforts to ensure confidentiality and overall comfort.

Sam has directly told me that he wishes to see me because of his assumptions of what I must be like as a therapist, based on his perceptions of me from our interactions in the consultation role. Whether a peer review process matching clients and therapists would maximize Sam's treatment is in my professional opinion less relevant than respecting his judgment in seeking out a therapist who he believes would be good for him. Therapists often speak about word of mouth as the best form of advertising and discourage *Yellow Pages* shopping. I believe there is merit in respecting Sam's request to go to someone whom he thinks can help. My experience has strengthened my belief that clinical effectiveness should take precedence over a one-size-fits-all approach to following ethical constructs.

Dual relationships per se are neither bad nor unethical. I challenge my counseling center and psychology profession colleagues to be more proactive in their thinking regarding this issue. We are mental health professionals driven by the desire to be of help. Let's use the empirical and ethical components of our profession, but neither rigidly nor at the expense of sound clinical judgment.

REFERENCES

American College Personnel Association. (1996). *Statement of ethical principles and standards*. Washington, DC: Author.

American Psychological Association. (1992). *Ethical principles for psychologists*. Washington, DC: Author.

Baldich, T. (1980). Ethical discrimination ability of psychologists: A function of training in ethics. *Professional Psychology, 11*, 276–282.

Bergin, A. E., & Garfield, S. L. (Eds.). (1994). *Handbook of psychotherapy and behavior change* (4th ed.). New York: Wiley.

Borys, D. S., & Pope, K. S. (1989). Dual relationships between therapist and client: A national study of psychologists, psychiatrists, and social workers. *Professional Psychology: Research and Practice, 20*, 283–293.

Frank, J. D. (1973). *Persuasion and healing: A comparative study of psychotherapy*. Baltimore: The Johns Hopkins University Press.

Goldfried, M. R., & Padawer, W. (1982). Current status and future directions in psychotherapy. In M. R. Goldfried (Ed.), *Converging themes in psychotherapy* (pp. 3–50). New York: Springer.

Hayman, P. M., & Cover, J. A. (1986). Ethical dilemmas in college counseling centers. *Journal of Counseling and Development, 64*, 318–320.

Jagmin, R. D., Wittman, W. D., & Noll, J. D. (1978). Mental health professionals' attitudes toward confidentiality, privilege, and third-party disclosure. *Professional Psychology: Research and Practice, 9*, 458–466.

Lambert, M. J. (1992). Implications of outcome research for psychotherapy integration. In J. C. Norcross & M. R. Goldfried (Eds.), *Handbook of psychotherapy integration* (pp. 94–129). New York: Basic.

Lazarus, A. (2000). Not all 'dual relationships' are taboo; some tend to enhance treatment outcomes. *The National Psychologist, 10*, 16.

Malley, P., Gallagher, R., & Brown, S. (1992). Ethical problems in university and college counseling centers: A delphi study. *Journal of College Student Development, 33*, 238–244.

Miller, S. D., Duncan, B. L., & Hubble, M. A. (1997). *Escape from babel: Toward a unifying language for psychotherapy practice*. New York: Norton.

Ray, O., & Ksir, C. (1999). *Drugs, society, and human behavior* (8th ed.). Boston: WCB/McGraw-Hill.

Sherry, P., Teschendorf, R., Anderson, S., & Guzman, F. (1991). Ethical beliefs and behaviors of college counseling center professionals. *Journal of College Student Development, 32*, 350–358.

Tomm, K. (1993). The ethics of dual relationships. *The California Therapist,* *January/February,* 7–19.

Zur, O. (2001). Out-of-office experience: When crossing office boundaries and engaging in dual relationships are clinically beneficial and ethically sound. *The Independent Practitioner, 21,* 96–100.

CHAPTER 24

The Shirtless Jock Therapist and the Bikini-Clad Client

An Exploration of Chance Extratherapeutic Encounters

Scott M. Hyman, MS

T he deep interpersonal exchange that can transpire between client and therapist typically arises from a highly structured encounter. They meet at a designated location, at a specific time, and with the common goal of alleviating the client's emotional suffering. The therapist dresses professionally, places personal issues aside, and mentally prepares to engage the client from a therapeutic stance. The client, in turn, prepares to disclose highly affective personal information that would otherwise remain hidden. Although the two meet briefly, usually for no more than an hour per week, this meaningful connection is important for the emotional well-being of the client. If one adheres to psychoanalytic or psychodynamic precepts, this special professional

I gratefully thank Dr. Eugene May for introducing me to the knowledge of humanistic-existential psychology and for assisting the preparation of this manuscript. Further, I want to acknowledge the editorial comments of Dr. Steven N. Gold, Dr. Robert C. Lane, and Raquel C. Andres.

relationship will not intentionally or ethically extend to the real world. They will not plan to meet for lunch, nor will they continue their conversations while watching a sporting event. In essence, they will not become friends.

Again, if one subscribes to psychodynamic proscriptions, questions may arise when therapist and client experience a chance contact out of the consulting room. These two individuals usually have never encountered each other outside of therapy. Their conversations have never been trivial, nor have they ever interacted outside of the roles of client and therapist. The unplanned contact adds a new dimension to the relationship as the client views the therapist outside the structured therapeutic environment, a situation that may implicitly reveal personal information about the therapist. This can be an awkward experience for therapist and client and may lead to avoidance behavior on the part of both of them. Thus, it is a clinical issue that merits increased attention.

The extent of the psychoanalytic sensitivity to this issue is exemplified by Tarnower (1966) who discussed the symptomatic behavior that can arise in therapist and client from chance meetings. He explains that the client may wish to avoid the contact so that fantasies about the therapist's omnipotence are not contaminated, and also to protect the satisfactory relationship that exists in therapy. The therapist justifies the wish to avoid the contact by claiming concern for protecting the transference and for avoiding intruding on the client's life. The therapist may also be tempted to know about the client's functioning in the real world to obtain reassurance that the therapy has been beneficial, to experience pride and pleasure from the client's improvement, or to fulfill fantasies of omnipotence. Thus, avoidance defends the therapist from experiencing anxiety.

Similarly, Gody (1996) discussed the unintentional self-disclosure that arises during chance encounters and the anxiety that this creates in therapists. She states that the therapist may have a wish to be known and to act normally, which causes anxiety because it is in conflict with the wish to remain the object of therapy. As a result, the therapist may respond highly formally, a distance may be maintained, or avoidance of the contact may be pursued altogether.

According to Strean (1981), another psychoanalytically oriented writer, therapist and client may be fearful of expressing voyeuristic and exhibitionistic wishes and of losing their therapeutic image, which can result in anxious reactions to the contact. Further, the extratherapeutic contact may provoke transference and countertransference fantasies and effects such as oedipal desires and sadistic urges. As a result, therapists may take steps to avoid extratherapeutic contacts.

While the psychoanalytic literature takes note of and suggests possible reasons for mutual therapist-client avoidance of chance extratherapeutic contacts, discussion of therapist behavior and communication toward the client during chance contacts and its impact on the therapeutic alliance are rare. For instance, Tarnower (1966) provides four case examples of chance extratherapeutic contacts. In three of the four, we have no knowledge of the therapist's behavior. All that is described is the client's avoidance behavior during the contact. It is unclear as to whether the therapist may have behaved in a manner that fostered his client's avoidance. Therapist behavior that elicited a negative reaction in the client was mentioned in the fourth case. The therapist walked out of the clinic building as the patient was coming in 10 minutes before her appointment. He smiled as he passed and continued walking in the opposite direction in order to conduct business in his free time. This made his client angry because she interpreted his smile as hypocritical.

It is interesting that in three of the four cases, there is no description of the therapist's behavior. No acknowledgment is made that the therapist may have been somewhat responsible for behaving in a manner that caused the manifestation of the client's anger in the fourth case. I say responsible because the therapist should be sensitive to the types of behaviors that the client is likely to interpret negatively. During the postcontact analysis, the therapist interpreted the client's reaction as a transference reaction in which the therapist came to represent the client's mother. However, considering the intimate nature of their real relationship, it is understandable that she might be angry that her therapist did not take a moment to engage her in a brief dialogue. This encounter may have proceeded much more smoothly if the therapist had stopped for a moment, shaken the client's hand, and explained that he was on his way to run an errand and was looking forward to their session. Thus, the client would have felt acknowledged, would have been provided with an explanation for the therapist's behavior, and would likely have looked forward to the session. Had the client become angry following this acknowledgment, then the evidence would have been much stronger that she experienced a transference reaction.

The point I am addressing ties in perfectly with many of the chapters throughout this book calling for flexible, respectful, and humane treatment of clients. Although an out-of-the-office encounter does not constitute a dual relationship per se, the fact that it is literally outside the confines of the ongoing therapeutic transaction places it in the realm of a boundary extension that calls for intelligent management.

In the case presented by Strean (1981), there is mention of no more than a smile and a greeting on the part of the therapist toward his client when encountered unexpectedly at the theater. This client, who was in her fourth year of therapy, was with a male companion and volunteered a comment on the show, demonstrating that at the least a brief conversation was welcome. I would find it interesting to know if Strean's lack of engagement, possibly because he was with his wife, had any effect on the therapeutic relationship. This was never discussed, however.

Gody (1996) described a chance encounter she had with her client at a park. She did nothing more than wave to her client from a distance of 50 feet, although she felt certain that the client looked directly at her. She also described an encounter at the grocery store while with her children. Gody described that she was angry with her children and, in view of her client, appeared as if she was losing control. Gody felt embarrassed to be revealed in this moment. The client communicated that she was relieved that Gody was a regular person. However, we have no knowledge of any intentional communication on behalf of the therapist to the client.

In almost all these cases, analyses of the contacts were initiated during subsequent therapy sessions. Any discussion of the possibly positive or negative influences of the therapists' behavior was ignored. Of course, this may be due to the theoretical orientation of the authors and a focus on interpreting all reactions as transference reactions.

The common stance, whether intentional or not, seems to be avoidance of full human contact (i.e., not approaching the client, not initiating a conversation) during the encounters and detailed analysis of the interaction during subsequent therapy sessions. The reason for this may be a history of opacity and neutrality on the part of the analyst and the advocating of the role of the therapist as a blank screen that was deemed by many as essential to the analytic situation (Gody, 1996; Lane & Storch, 1986). One can imagine, however, the distress that the client may feel during the time between the contact and the ensuing therapy session.

Should therapists avoid human behavior and communication toward their clients during the contacts only to analyze them later in session? Maybe there would be nothing about the contact to analyze if therapists behaved humanely toward their clients. Perhaps therapists unnecessarily create an awkward situation that seems to necessitate analysis of their clients' reactions. It should be noted that while the analysts are most stringent about avoiding any interactions during chance encounters with clients, similar thinking seems to guide therapist behavior during unexpected extratherapeutic contacts across several other orientations (although it is not written strictly into their therapeutic mandates). Sharkin and Birky (1992), who refer to chance encounters as incidental encounters, found that 60% of therapists from various orientations were concerned about confidentiality violations, and 73% were concerned about violating therapeutic boundaries; 87% reacted to the contacts with surprise—87% with uncertainty and 83% with discomfort.

Borenstein and Fintzy (1980) advocate a human openness rather than aloofness as a catalyst of growth and development of the client only during postanalytic encounters. It is difficult to see why the same approach should not hold for chance extratherapeutic contacts that occur at any time and at any place throughout the course of therapy. As Greenson and Wexler (1969) state, neglecting the real relationship and focusing overly much on transference interpretation reduces all life to explanation, which is not the objective of therapy.

Avoiding clients or giving superficial smiles and waves negate all that therapy attempts to accomplish. Modeling avoidance behavior for the client is not beneficial to the therapy or to the client's social functioning. It is easy to imagine how therapist avoidance of natural behavior and communication during the contact could cause clients to question the authenticity of therapist communication during the therapy hour. For this reason, it seems appropriate that therapists acknowledge their clients as they would anyone with whom they had an intense relationship. However, it is best to take cues from the client.

I have studied my own behavior during chance extratherapeutic contacts and their effect on the therapeutic relationship. I will describe my thoughts and feelings, the manner in which I have behaved during these encounters, and the perceived effects of my behavior on the therapeutic relationship. I hope to demonstrate that therapist awkwardness may come from expectations of how the chance encounter can disrupt therapy and the therapist's desire to appear infallible to the client. I will also provide examples of behavior that have both disturbed and benefited the therapeutic relationship. Although most literature examines the chance contact from an analytic perspective, the present explanation and discussion is grounded in a humanistic-existential paradigm.

THE STUDENT THERAPIST

As a third-year graduate student I experienced a plethora of unplanned encounters early in my career. My clinical placement during this year of training was in the student-counseling center of a university. I was required to conduct 20 hours of weekly therapy with undergraduate and graduate students in the schools of dentistry, medicine, law, physical therapy, pharmacology, and marine biology. Many of my clients lived near or close to campus and participated in campus and off-campus activities. I, too, was a student and, much like my clients, I had an interest in similar activities. Unless I was to hide from life, extratherapeutic client contact was inevitable.

HUMANISTIC-EXISTENTIAL EXPLANATION AND EXAMPLE OF THERAPIST AVOIDANCE

Yalom (1980) contends that a belief in personal specialness is a defense against our own mortality. He believes that many therapists avoid their fears and sense of limitation by inflating their sense of self and their spheres of control in the therapy room. They expect their clients to look to them as omnipotent guides. To many clients, therapists appear to be more than human. They do not express emotional pain, they seem to have conquered life, and they may appear to be self-actualized. In effect, they are all that their clients aspire to be. In this way, clients may view their therapists as ultimate rescuers, which as Yalom states is a second way to defend against fears of finitude. The result is a circle of unrealistic beliefs that can only be maintained in the therapy room. From this perspective, it stands to reason that therapists attempt to preserve these beliefs by avoiding clients outside of therapy.

I was initially seduced by these beliefs, and I behaved accordingly when I encountered my clients in a social setting; however, I soon experienced the devastating effects of avoiding clients and ending conversations with them prematurely. They could sense that I was uncomfortable seeing them, and this appears to have weakened the therapeutic relationship.

This is best illustrated by an encounter I had with Jamie, a client whom I had been treating for relational problems and test anxiety. I had seen her regularly for 10 sessions, and we had a well-established relationship. I had just finished eating my lunch in the school dining hall and wandered outside where I chose to finish my drink. I was leaning against the wall wearing blue jeans and a T-shirt, sucking on my straw. A minute later, someone called my name and I turned to see Jamie standing there with a friend. I immediately became anxious when I saw her. I was worried that seeing me as I was, casually dressed and absent-mindedly sipping on my drink, would harm the relationship. The fantasy of myself as the all-knowing helper would be destroyed. As a result of my fear, I carefully censored what I said to Jamie and avoided answering personal questions. I could not find a place for my hands; my eyes darted away from hers awkwardly. I wanted to ask how she was feeling but wanted to avoid a therapeutic discussion. I was not the caring, thoughtful, and inquiring person that I was in the therapy room. Ultimately, I cut our conversation short by stating that I had a meeting to go to. This, I am now sorry to say, was a lie.

Jamie arrived late, canceled, did not show, or was quiet for weeks after the outside contact. Finally, I questioned her about her poor participation in therapy, even though I suspected that I already knew the answer. She replied, "I don't know why you acted so strange when I saw you at the dining hall." I did not attempt to defend myself because I knew she was right; I did behave awkwardly in her presence. I was not my typical self, friendly and warm. Instead, I behaved as if I was relating to someone less than human. When confronted with the ugly truth in therapy, I decided to own my mistake. I admitted that I was worried that my physical presentation would hurt the therapy. She responded that she knew full well that I was a student and had not expected me to wear my shirt and tie all the time. She explained that she did not feel awkward during the meeting until my aloofness became apparent to her.

Even though we were able to discuss the contact and the associated feelings at length, the relationship was never fully remedied, and Jamie soon dropped out of therapy. It was I who was responsible for the breakdown of the relationship. My false expectations of the encounter, my false belief that my patient saw me as a nonsocial, problem-free being, and my desire to maintain my specialness led to my fear of being human. As a result, my avoidance and awkwardness may have contributed to my client ending therapy.

THE END OF PERSONAL SPECIALNESS AND AN EXAMPLE OF POSITIVE THERAPIST ENGAGEMENT

The negative impact of this experience prompted me to question the expectations that many of us have of ourselves and our clients. Further, I began to challenge the distortions that created the fear of unexpected encounters with them. I no longer believe that my clients fantasize that I am omnipotent, problem-free, and without a desire to enjoy social interaction. If they do, reinforcing their belief is certainly not beneficial to them. They need to see that there is no "ultimate rescuer." Further, I accept my own ordinariness. I am not special. I am an ordinary human being relating to and helping another.

I no longer feel the need to avoid clients outside of therapy. Locking myself at home in fear that I may encounter a client is not the answer to anticipated awkwardness. The answer is to abandon unfounded expectations and the defense of maintaining an illusion of specialness. I treat my clients as human beings when encountered outside of therapy. I do not rely on artificial gimmicks or situational guidelines. Rather, I am myself, and I treat my clients as people.

I have had many unplanned contacts with clients since changing my belief system, and in every instance I was able to avoid fear and awkwardness. Consequently the therapeutic relationship did not suffer; in many instances it was enhanced. Rather than describe every encounter, I will describe the most potentially awkward contact to vividly illustrate my point.

On a Saturday morning, I met friends to play a pickup basketball game on the school courts. After the game, we decided to cool off in the pool adjacent to the court. Just as I removed my sneakers and shirt, I made eye contact with Maria, a client that I had seen for five sessions. I was treating her for stresses associated with the end of an 8-year relationship, the sickness of a family member, and school pressures. She was lying on a lounge chair a few yards away, wearing a bikini, and studying class notes. She reacted with shock and a big smile when she caught sight of me. She stood up from her chair and began to walk in my direction. I, the shirtless jock therapist, was face to face with my bikini-clad client! I had only seconds to react.

At first, I felt extremely embarrassed that my half-naked client could see me shirtless. I asked myself, "How will this negatively affect the relationship?" Before my therapeutic failure with Jamie, I would have been convinced that as an inevitable result of this encounter, Maria would never benefit from continued therapy with me. She would never take my words seriously again. She would never accept guidance and understanding from a shirtless therapist. However, in this instance, my answer was that the relationship might not be affected negatively at all. Rather, I considered the possibility that the relationship might benefit from the recognition of her as an equal rather than solely as a troubled client. Further, I no longer fantasized of myself as special. This diminished my fear of disclosure and enabled my humanity to surface. My new belief system allowed my anxiety to subside, and the newfound relaxation enabled natural human behavior in the face of my client.

I proceeded to move toward Maria with a friendly smile. I did not put on my shirt because that would imply that there was something about her that created a need to hide myself. We greeted each other casually and conversed about trivial things. I asked how she was feeling since we touched upon sensitive topics in therapy the week before. She stated that her week went pretty well but that she had some concerns that she would like to bring up in therapy. She then introduced me to her friend and I shook her friend's hand. I inquired as to what they were studying, and a conversation about their class began. We spoke altogether for about 10 minutes and I ended the conversation by saying that it was nice to see her enjoying herself at the pool. We said good-bye to each other, and I submerged myself in the pool. She and her friend left about 20 minutes later and waved a good-bye.

It is important to note that had Maria not initiated the contact by smiling, I would not have advanced toward her. I believe that it is important to get clues from clients during chance encounters, especially when they are with others. They may not want others to know that they are in therapy, and approaching them when uncertain of their wishes can cause them conflict and anxiety.

When I saw her in therapy the next week, we continued to talk about those things that brought her to therapy. The contact at the pool was not mentioned by either of us. If she mentioned it, we certainly would have processed the contact. However, since she did not, I saw no reason to bring it up; I no longer felt that it was strange to encounter my clients outside of therapy. It was not an abnormal event anymore. She was a person just like myself, and I was a person just like her.

Maria will be ending her therapy in 3 weeks to go on internship. Presently she is on her 13th session, and she has made tremendous progress in therapy. She is actively able to challenge and reframe cognitive distortions that exacerbate her depression related to her ended relationship, and therapeutic support resulted in an increased ability to survive her final exams and grandmother's sickness. This is in sharp contrast to the lack of progress related to Jamie's premature departure from therapy. By changing my beliefs about unplanned client contacts, I was able to avoid behaving awkwardly outside of therapy, the relationship was not damaged, and the client's treatment goals were achieved.

DISCUSSION

Therapists may falsely assume that all clients will develop a belief in an ultimate rescuer, which exacerbates therapists' maintenance of their beliefs in personal specialness. It can be appealing to have clients place their hope in one's omnipotent guidance and tempting to accept the role of being greater than human.

When therapist and client meet during an unplanned contact, there is a disruption of the therapist's illusion. The therapist becomes fearful that ordinary self-presentation will destroy the client's fantasy of him or her as the ultimate rescuer. As a result, the therapist desperately tries to preserve this image by avoiding being human, behaving awkwardly and inhumanly, contributing to the breakdown of the therapeutic alliance. The irony is that this is precisely that which therapists attempt to avoid.

For the therapist to prevent this pattern from occurring following an extratherapeutic contact, the therapist must overcome the belief in personal specialness and must relinquish the assumption that the client regards the therapist as the ultimate rescuer. By doing this, client and therapist are freed to develop more realistic views of each other; no drastic expectations of destroying therapy will exist and a positive relationship built on pure human interaction can flourish.

In psychoanalysis, the extratherapeutic contacts are often considered an intrusion on the analytic situation, and unexpected encounters early in therapy are seen as a potential cause of premature client termination (Weiss, 1975). However, Weiss maintains that the contacts may prove beneficial to the therapeutic alliance if the contact is interpreted properly by highlighting and clarifying transference phenomena. Strean (1981) adds that whether the contact is valuable or hazardous depends on how the analyst and patient feel about the meeting and how the contact is utilized in therapy.

It is proposed here that it is not the event itself that causes the breakdown of the therapy, nor is the analysis the crucial element in maintaining the therapeutic alliance. Rather, it seems that the manner in which the therapist behaves during the contact is of overriding importance. If the client is acknowledged humanely by the therapist and avoidance is not present, the client will feel at ease and cared for. Consequently, postcontact analysis will be rendered unnecessary unless the client makes a reference to the event.

In line with the experiences of Zur (2001), humane behavior with clients outside the office can prove to be a highly valuable intervention. For the analysts fearful of chance encounters, meeting outside the office makes "the transference more reality-based and just provides more 'grist' for the transference mill" (p. 100).

According to Tarnower (1966), the client may desire to engage the therapist in conversation or shake his or her hand. However, at the same time there may be a reluctance to do so, resulting in behavior that indicates confusion, embarrassment, or indecision. Smith (1980) argues that the onus is on the therapist to place the client at ease. The therapist should approach the client and acknowledge the client as a person, modeling that it is perfectly normal to shake another caring human's hand.

Some therapists create an agreement with clients during the initial therapy session that dictates rules of behavior that each will abide by during a chance extratherapeutic contact. This may involve short acknowledgments of the other or rules of total avoidance. I believe that initiating the agreement is a mistake, because setting rules may communicate to the client that the relationship is not real and that the client is only important in the therapy room. However, if the client introduces the topic of developing guidelines about handling unexpected extratherapeutic encounters because of concerns about privacy, then the therapist should respect this and behave accordingly. Therapists may choose to discuss the possibility of chance contacts. If clients express concern, then an agreement, such as having the client wave if contact is welcomed, can be formulated.

CONCLUSION

Student therapists serving student populations and therapists residing in small communities are very likely to experience unplanned client contacts outside of therapy. The topic has not been sufficiently researched and existing commentary is scarce. This chapter explores the issue from the personal perspective of a student therapist.

Although the observations described and the recommendations made are based solely on subjective experience, I believe they provide some insight as to why unplanned client contacts outside of therapy are perceived by therapists as an awkward experience. Further, and more important, the information can be utilized to prevent the avoidance of clients and can perpetuate therapeutically beneficial therapist behavior.

It is not uncommon for people to confuse chance encounters with dual relationships. A dual relationship is established when therapists actively assume a role with clients that is additional to that of a clinician (Zur, 2001). By contrast, chance encounters are not actively pursued and do not result in a change of the therapist's role toward the client. The contacts, however, can cause adverse reactions that may interfere with the therapeutic relationship. Thus, additional discussion and study is needed.

The fact that the handling of incidental extratherapeutic encounters warrants discussion is somewhat of an indictment of the profession. It is difficult to believe that medical doctors, lawyers, accountants, or any other professionals would experience a conflict when encountering patients or clients unexpectedly. Even priests who hear the penetrating confessions of their parishioners will behave humanely during chance encounters. Psychologists' obsessions with and fears of chance encounters signify a problem in a profession where client care and genuineness is of utmost importance.

Future research can focus on empirically identifying therapists' expectations of the encounters, reactions to the encounters, behaviors during the encounters, and the effect of each on therapeutic outcome. In addition, empirical study should include identifying clients' experience of unplanned contacts and their effects on therapy.

REFERENCES

Borenstein, D. B., & Fintzy, R. T. (1981). Postanalytic encounters. *International Journal of Psychoanalytic Psychotherapy, 8,* 149–164.

Gody, D. S. (1996). Chance encounters: Unintentional therapist disclosure. *Psychoanalytic Psychology, 13* (4), 495–511.

Greenson, R. R., & Wexler, M. (1969). The nontransference relationship in the psychoanalytic situation. *International Journal of Psychoanalysis, 50,* 27–39.

Lane, R. C., & Storch, R. S. (1986). A fortuitous extra-analytic event: Countertransference, hindrance or benefit. *Current Issues in Psychoanalytic Practice, 2* (3), 33–43.

Sharkin, B. S., & Birky, I. (1992). Incidental encounters between therapists and their clients. *Professional Psychology: Research and Practice, 23* (4), 326–328.

Smith, V. A. (1980). Patient contacts outside therapy. *Canadian Journal of Psychiatry, 25* (4), 297–302.

Strean, H. S. (1981). Extra-analytic contacts: Theoretical and clinical considerations. *Psychoanalytic Quarterly, 56,* 238–257.

Tarnower, W. (1966). Extra-analytic contacts between the psychoanalyst and the patient. *Psychoanalytic Quarterly, 35,* 399–413.

Weiss, S. S. (1975). The effect on the transference of 'special events' occurring during psychoanalysis. *International Journal of Psychoanalysis, 56,* 69–75.

Yalom, I. D. (1980). *Existential psychotherapy.* New York: Basic.

Zur, O. (2001). Out-of-office experience: When crossing office boundaries and engaging in dual relationships are clinically beneficial and ethically sound. *Independent Practitioner, 21* (1), 96–100.

CHAPTER 25

College and University Student Counseling Centers

Inevitable Boundary Shifts and Dual Roles

Miriam Iosupovici, MSW and Equilla Luke, PhD

The developmental, preventive, and remedial emphasis in college counseling is inclusive of mentoring, teaching, and counseling students. Sequential, and sometimes concurrent, nonsexual and nonexploitative dual roles and relationships will occur. Although there is considerable literature on ethical decision making (see Cottone & Claus, 2000, for an excellent review of models), and many issues are generic to all settings, our focus remains on issues highlighted in college practice. Not fond of prescriptive models, we assert that close attention to multiple factors will lead responsible therapists to clinically sound decision making.

It is noted, moreover, that the current view that dual roles and dual relationships inevitably represent problematic boundary crossings is steeped in a limiting cultural and theoretical perspective (Lazarus, 1994; Zur, 2000). Counseling centers have been in the vanguard of multi-

This chapter is dedicated to Miriam Polster, who taught me—not only by knitting a hooded red sweater for my newborn son—so much about the ethic of giving just what is needed, daring to make caring into visible form.

cultural counseling, recognizing the impact of the university environment on their diverse clients with regard not only to academic performance, but as a causal factor in student mental health problems. Multiple pressures arising from cultural value systems in conflict have a significant impact on dual roles and relationship decision-making for counselors who are members of or work with multicultural populations (see vignette: Drs. Powers and Thoughtful). Pederson (1997) notes that standards of practice of most professional mental health organizations emphasize individualistic values and inadvertently ignore the perspective of collectivist cultures:

> When ethical decisions are implicit, the counselors will base their thinking on those ethical philosophical principles most familiar to them and mistakenly presume that they are maintaining a high level of ethical standards. When those standards of accepted practice are themselves culturally encapsulated, they do not provide an adequate basis for an independent ethical judgment but rather tend to reinforce the ethical validity of the standard quo practices. (p. 26)

Additionally, feminist theorists have emphasized empowerment (Miller & Stiver, 1997), a concept similar to the promotion of self-efficacy. In our experience client empowerment may be enhanced by various kinds of dual relationships (see vignette: Helen B. Goode).

COUNSELING CENTERS IN CONTEXT

Historically, an in loco parentis model of nurturing students required close attention to all aspects of student living. Students were treated more like unemancipated minors than young adults, with close monitoring of student academic and social progress. One-to-one mentoring relationships with faculty and social contact with faculty and deans of students occurred commonly and have been considered a normal part of the learning process.

At a minimum, today's social contact characteristically includes opening year activities, midyear, and end-of-year celebrations, plus special events. As student growth and development are central to the educational mission, engaging in multiple relationships at many levels of university life is seen as beneficial for the student, staff, and faculty. In the helping professions, faculty within academic departments are responsible for educating and socializing trainees, and they also may encourage student participation in social and political aspects of university life. New forms of faculty-student relationship occur during joint projects. Studies have repeatedly demonstrated a wide range of pragmatic and academic benefits resulting from additional mentoring and programmatic attention to student needs (McGrath, 2001).

Within this constructed social environment, the counseling center exists to provide counseling and psychotherapy to undergraduate and graduate students, teach social skills, build self-esteem, and reduce emotional suffering (Berk, 1983). As college and universities have unique cultures and special missions, counseling centers vary in size, focus, and services. Aside from the provision of psychotherapy, the mission may include consultation with faculty and staff, along with university-wide outreach (Guinee & Ness, 2000). At many universities, counselors hold joint appointments and/or work part-time in teaching positions. Moreover, increasing their already complex role functioning, these same counseling center staff may serve in other campus roles such as directors and/or staff of other on-campus student or staff service departments such as employee assistance programs, services for students with disabilities, tutoring and remedial assistance, career development, testing and assessment, women's centers, and/or services to gay, lesbian, bisexual, and transgender populations.

From the inception of the college and university counseling center during the early years of the 20th century, services have grown and changed to reflect changing societal conditions and available resources (Archer & Cooper, 1998). Many counseling centers are comprehensive campus mental health services where clinical treatment is provided along with consultation, campus outreach, and training of psychologists, social workers, and other mental health professionals. Most counseling centers provide primary treatment through brief individual psychodynamic or cognitive behavior therapy, workshop and support models, group treatment, and couples counseling. Multifunction centers may also provide varying combinations of academic advising, testing, and career counseling; disability determination and services; peer counseling programs; specialized services to students of color, and the lesbian, gay, bisexual, and transgender (LGBT) communities; leadership training; and prevention programs (Archer & Cooper, 1998). Other centers are within a health services complex and have levels of administrative and staff interface with medical personnel. Counseling centers may be one-person operations or up to 20 professional staff (Gallagher, Gill, & Sysko, 2000). Because of their significant utilization in the practicum and internship models of mental health training, counseling centers have an enormous impact on the professional and ethical development of future practitioners (Stone, Vespia, & Kanz, 2000).

Although college and university counseling center staff maintain the highest professional and ethical standards as defined by the pertinent ethical code requirements, the staff is systemically linked to the university. Expected to be active participants in campus life, the functioning of the service may be at risk if the staff is not integrated into the campus community (Archer & Cooper, 1998). Avoiding marginalization that will tend to undermine the counseling center and therapist effectiveness is critical, particularly in crucial student advocacy roles, according to Archer and Cooper.

It is interesting to note that the exploitative relationship is a rarely reported event at college and university counseling centers (Gallagher et al., 2000). Traditional private practice models, supporting conventional long-term dynamic therapies in settings where most dual relationships may be preventable, may often be inappropriate to the circumstances of the university counselor and students who are quite likely to engage outside of the therapy setting.

ETHICAL DECISION-MAKING ISSUES

Decision-making, incorporating therapeutic and systemic concerns arising from ethically acceptable dual relationships, must be processed in a manner mindful of why such relationships exist, how they can best be scrutinized, and what rationale is used to determine the feasibility of engagement.

In discussing factors in dual-relationship decision-making, definitional clarity is necessary. The principles of beneficence, nonmaleficence, fidelity, responsibility, integrity, justice, self-determination, and autonomy, called "aspirational ethics" in the proposed American Psychological Association (APA) *Ethical Principles of Psychologists and Code of Conduct* (2001), are more significant than those instituted within codes. As Jordan and Meara (1990) noted, ethical practice requires responding in relation to the question "Who shall I be?" When making clinical decisions, the counselor attempts to balance competing ethical values, a dilemma requiring a thorough knowledge of professional codes and applicable laws. No matter which decision-making model is utilized, this process requires self-knowledge and personal integrity on the part of the therapist.

When looking specifically at the multitude of roles counseling center staff may occupy within a university, it is important to have definitional clarity as to the difference between dual or multiple roles themselves, dual or multiple relationships, and boundary. Anderson and Kitchener (1998) define relationship as "... an ongoing interaction containing the presumption of mutual and reciprocal involvement with another person or persons" (p. 92). According to Section 3.05a of the upcoming APA Ethics Code (2001), multiple relationship occurs when:

> a psychologist is in a professional role with a person and (a) at the same time is in another role with the same person, (b) at the same time is in a relationship with a person closely associated with or related to the person with whom they have the professional relationship, or (c) promises to enter into another relationship in the future with the person or a person closely associated with or related to the person. (Multiple Relationships section, para. 1)

An important element of counseling relationships and varying by theoretical systems, a boundary is defined as "a therapeutic frame which defines a set of roles for the participants in the therapeutic process" (Smith & Fitzpatrick, cited in Bersoff, 1999, p. 1). Typical university examples of boundary variations from traditional models might include the following: Meeting after hours, appointments held outside the office (lab, dorm, off-campus setting), gifts to or from therapist, decision whether or not to use first names, self-disclosure, physical contact (hug initiated by student client and accepted by therapist), and movement from client to peer counselor and/or trainee.

Barnett (2000) states it is imperative "... to differentiate between boundary *crossings*, which are not harmful and which may not only be appropriate at times, but even necessary for providing effective and caring treatment; and boundary *violations*, which are harmful and should be avoided" (p. 1 [emphasis added]).

When decisions regarding dual or multiple relationships arise, the therapist must initiate mutual exploration of ethical issues so that the client is an informed and discriminating consumer. Clearly, the ethical principle of autonomy may be in conflict with other principles when the therapist and client jointly make decisions at any stage of treatment (see Bersoff, 1999, p. 244). In the university and college context, the development of autonomous decision-making on the part of student clients may be either a direct or indirect goal of therapy.

DUAL ROLES

The occurrence of simultaneous ongoing dual relationships between counselor-client pairs is the exception and not the rule in college counseling centers. Partly attributable to relatively short-term counseling models utilized on campus, the resultant development of less intense attachments due to time-limited treatment may make concurrent dual relationship decision-making a less complex process. However, clients in focused group programs (e.g., eating disorders, LGBT, abuse survivors), who may then become peer counselors, do have a relatively high likelihood of multiple relationship events requiring thoughtful management.

It is not uncommon for clients or former clients to become peer counselors, precisely because the seeking of therapy is not considered prima facie evidence of pathology. Some may move into sequential roles as practicum students and interns. And within this group, some may become temporary or permanent staff members. Selection issues may arise and can be handled by thoughtful attention to boundaries and confidentiality. Those who are inappropriate are usually weeded out in the screening and interview process. Care must be taken to keep their records separate while on site (director or clinical director locked files), and primary supervision should be with someone other than the former therapist (see Burian & O'Connor-Slimp, 2000).

Confidentiality

Common confidentiality strains on campus are incidental or chance encounters, third-party inquiries, and entangled relationships (Sharkin, 1995).

Incidental Encounters

Chance encounters between therapist and client have not been well researched and counselors are not trained to handle out-of-therapy casual or brief contact (Pulakos, 1994). Counselors regularly encounter student clients in unpredictable situations, by chance, and relate to them in dual roles with low potential to cause harm and high potential to serve as role models. Pulakos found that students wanted more, not less, interaction with their therapists when they accidentally came in contact with one another. Sharkin (1995) points out that beyond the expected sensitivity to students who may be concerned about stigmatization for client status, avoiding interaction may inadvertently reveal rather than protect confidentiality.

Third-Party Inquiries

Counselors encounter an expectation to share information, a dynamic requiring careful management. Referral sources and on-campus personnel are not under professional confidentiality requirements and have different standards of information sharing than therapists. Their frustration with denial of information requires that counseling center staff be proactive in explaining the protections of confidentiality and find alternatives to give information that is truly needed. Parental requests can be handled with gracious limit setting, including an explanation of their son's and daughter's right to confidentiality, and information they wish to give the counselor should be invited (Sharkin, 1995). These conversations are then communicated to clients. This may open the door to clinically valuable family work.

Entangled Relationships

On campus, as in rural areas and other semi-enclosed settings, clients who are known to one another will emerge in a caseload of individual, couples, and group clients. This requires careful handling of confidentiality strains, as information utilized for intervention could come from another source, and clear explanations to clients when this occurs (see Sharkin, 1995, for an excellent discussion).

VIGNETTES

We present three constructed vignettes, representing typical clinical dilemmas, disguised to protect privacy and confidentiality.

Drs. Powers and Thoughtful: Ethnicity, Client Preference, and Therapist Choice

The African American student population at a large, selective public research university is small. Only 35 new African American students are in the first-year class. Upper-class and graduate African American student numbers are around 200. Many of the students know one another and most are acquainted with the two African American psychologists at the counseling center: Dr. Teddy Powers is the advisor to the African American student organization, while the other counselor, Dr. Lena

Thoughtful, typically avoids any out-of-office contact with the students and maintains what she describes as "professional distance." The students love Dr. Powers because he is actively involved in their college lives. Dr. Thoughtful is admired by some, but not trusted by others, because her boundaries are sometimes misread as a lack of involvement.

Both counselors cofacilitate a counseling center–sponsored support group. The support group meets weekly throughout the year and, although the group is planned for students, African American faculty and staff drop in, their participation helping the students feel more at home on campus. The group, like other support groups sponsored by the counseling center, is not considered therapy or counseling (although led by professional staff and/or peer counselors).

At the beginning or end of each term, the counselors invite the students to a party at the home of Dr. Powers. During the party, people share home-cooked food, play board games, chat, and listen to music. Students use formal names when addressing staff and faculty and maintain culturally due deference for age and role.

At the office, the receptionist informs Dr. Thoughtful that a new intake appointment has been scheduled. She immediately recognizes the student as one of the African Americans from the party and support group. Dr. Thoughtful also knows that this student is a leader in the Black Student Union. The student's presenting problems involve race, culture, and class. Raised in an affluent beach town, the client is having trouble gaining acceptance from some of her working- and middle-class student peers. She is in a relationship she wishes to continue with a male from a working-class background whose parents are not comfortable with her. Since the African American women significantly outnumber the men, she is also afraid that if he breaks up with her she will have few choices.

As Dr. Thoughtful begins to discuss the treatment contract with the student, the client tells her that she chose her as her therapist because she does not want to see her therapist everywhere she goes. She specifically tells Dr. Thoughtful that she will feel uncomfortable if she has to sit in support groups with her or attend parties where she is present. The student also says she needs an African American female therapist at this time in her life because she has not had many role models other than her mother, because her father is Caucasian and she grew up in a White community. Although she says she knows she is biracial, she identifies herself as African American.

At the next session, the student says she and her boyfriend have discussed their conflicts and have decided that he needs to talk to someone about his parents. He feels more comfortable talking with Dr. Powers because he is a male and seems more accessible and involved. Her boyfriend, she says, thinks that counselors who are distant are not as culturally sensitive as those who are involved in your life. She said that he wonders how you can really know someone just in the context of the counseling session.

Differing Strategies

This vignette exemplifies differing strategies for managing dual role and relationship issues. Dr. Powers intentionally engages students in therapy, advising, and socializing. This is an acceptable, indeed much honored, manner to relate to many of the African American students. Dr. Thoughtful intentionally attempts to avoid engaging in dual relationships, yet does play a dual role by virtue of her identification as a member of this ethnic group and by her willingness to participate in carefully chosen social events (such as African American graduation and presentations to ethnically oriented sororities) in order to be known to students as supportive and available. Regardless of their differences in the management of dual relationships, it is quite possible that either of these counselors would find themselves in a dual relationship that might have unpredictable, positive or negative, treatment consequences.

Relationship Expectations During Treatment

The relationship expectations were clearly elucidated by the client because of her desire for secure boundaries between her campus life and therapy. If the counselor agrees to the client's stipulations, she risks alienating more students. Those who already perceive her as inaccessible and aloof, and who see boundary crossing as normal and culturally consonant, are unlikely to understand the thought and effort that goes into such a choice. For Dr. Thoughtful, it is more important to be concerned about the needs of the current client and not speculate about potential clients.

Given a preexisting commitment to the support group, she must work with the student about adapting to her coleadership and presence at the group. They would need to pay attention to specific dynamics raised for the client, role-play scenarios, and plan for uncomfortable situations. Therapist self-monitoring to decrease the likelihood of special treatment may be needed. They can decide how to address each other, if at all, outside the therapy session. Dr. Thoughtful can also decide to keep a very "low profile" in the group during the first phase of treatment, hoping to revisit the issue when the relationship has matured and trust has been built.

The Depth of the Psychotherapy Relationship

Although this is a new relationship, given the client's request for a same gender and similar ethnicity therapist, the potential for building a deep and intense bond exists. Since the client has requested that the counselor not cross boundaries, we believe efforts to honor the client's request are important. The therapist may choose to risk being misunderstood by some to protect and facilitate the treatment of one client.

New Proposed Relationship

Although there is a desire by the client to keep boundaries clear, fairly often college student clients will return for treatment, apply for jobs on campus, and/or hold a high-profile student position (e.g., a peer counselor, residence advisor, or student leader). The counselor who provides the therapy may also be the trainer-teacher for the particular peer program or campus organization. In a perfect world, the counselor informs each client that he or she may develop into roles leading to seeing the counselor in another capacity. However, over the course of an academic year, any counselor may see 75 to 95 clients individually or in groups and many more in workshops and prevention models. Identifying students with whom they may later have a different relationship with is difficult, if not impossible. Until they see a face, many therapists do not remember working with a given student. Similarly, students are frequently unable to identify, at least by name, the therapist they saw during previous treatment. Ethical guidelines and clinical assessment of boundary crossings deserve examination within the variance and complexities existing in subcommunities, situations affecting counselors and clients alike.

Reasons for Boundary Crossings

In this vignette, boundary crossings are an accepted norm in this segment of the African American culture. Since African American students are a small group on a large campus, extra effort is made to attract and retain them; sometimes these efforts lead to multiple relationships.

Counselors who work with or identify with this particular group develop creative strategies to manage the dual relationships while maintaining ethical practice.

Attention must be paid to the uniquely permeable community boundary to ensure ethical choice-making when engaging students in insular ethnic, religious, or gender groups. We do not endorse the development of intimate, social, nonsexual relationships in this context, although significant closeness in mentoring relationships might ensue with no harm as long as professional boundaries are scrupulously maintained.

Helen B. Goode, Committee Member

Helen B. Goode, a counseling center staff therapist receives a letter of invitation from the university president to sit on the campus-wide Committee on the Status of Lesbian, Gay, Bisexual, and Transgender Persons. This prestigious committee makes policy recommendations to the president. A mentor to female students in nontraditional majors and a consultant to the Women's Resource Center, Helen has been recommended for this committee because of her advocacy for LGBT and women's issues. Helen accepts the invitation to join the committee, receives a membership roster and a meeting agenda, and reviews names of three student members of the committee; none of the names are familiar to her.

When Helen arrives at the scheduled meeting, she recognizes a woman in attendance that she is currently treating. Presenting problem was parental divorce. Helen looks around the room and does not acknowledge the client in any special manner. She sits through the meeting and learns that her client is a newly appointed replacement committee member. Helen experiences some discomfort because this particular client has not presented any material about sexuality in treatment and she momentarily wonders whether this is significant or not.

Following the committee meeting, Helen returns to the counseling center and immediately consults with a colleague. The colleague reassures Helen that this was not a predictable event and this dual role has little potential to cause harm. This, he tells her, is most likely an uncomplicated dual role. Since the client will see her for an appointment this week, the matter can be discussed and in case there are unknown issues, reexamined. Helen discusses the issue of being in a dual role with her client, who expresses feeling very good about seeing Helen at the meeting. The client tells her she is a good role model for students, and no one need know about the therapy relationship. She asserts that even if they did know, it would not be much of a problem because all her friends know she is seeing a "shrink" and all her friends are clients of the counseling center. "No one is ashamed of being in therapy!" she tells Helen.

Continuing to follow established policy, Helen tells the counseling center director that a current client is on the LGBT university committee. The director cautiously reminds Helen of proper documentation and discusses strategies to manage the dual roles, including addressing the issue in subsequent counseling sessions. He also encourages Helen to consider the amount of time left in treatment against time to be served on the committee, as he cautions that too much additional role contact may change the nature of the therapeutic relationship. Helen tells him that the committee meets three times a semester. When she leaves this consult, Helen feels her decision is correct: she can serve on the committee and continue a healthy therapy relationship with her client.

Unpredictable Dual Relationship

This vignette is an example of an unpredictable and chance encounter. Subsequent encounters, however, are under the direct control of the therapist and client. The current decision is subject to change should new material surface in psychotherapy or some key event take place on the committee or on the campus. On the university campus, the relationship between therapist and client, although confidential, does not occur in isolation due to the complexity of the system which encourages staff/student interaction.

Relationship Expectations During Treatment

In this particular vignette, the culture of the college or university campus has direct influences on the way mental health professionals work. In this instance, discussing the nature of the relationship and the likelihood of contact on campus is a useful strategy and is frequently done because professionals can anticipate incidental encounters, especially on residential campuses and within special multicultural populations. Many college counseling centers may treat 5 to 20% of the student body, so many students may know someone in treatment if they are not themselves in treatment.

What we learn about Helen and her client based on this aspect of the model is that the counseling relationship was not terminated. Based on this aspect alone, some might recommend that Helen resign without comment from the committee. However, given a presenting problem of parental divorce, we believe that although Helen is in a dual role with her client, she is managing this role in a responsible and ethical manner.

The Depth of the Psychotherapy Relationship

There is some susceptibility in this dimension as the empathic relationship between client and therapist in this vignette could potentially be intense. Both Helen and her client are members of a small cultural community and, given the therapist's importance as a role model, the potential for the client developing a strong attachment to the therapist is apparent. We would advise maintaining the therapy contracts of working on the parental divorce issue. In the event that sexual identity issues arise, we might recommend referral to another therapist to work on this issue. Compartmentalizing therapy issues and working with multiple therapists is one method of practice in college counseling centers.

New Proposed Relationship

Helen will engage in a dual role with her client. She will see her client in committee meetings on occasion and weekly for psychotherapy. But it is just as likely that Helen will see her client at campus events and in the grocery store and maybe at key social events if Helen is asked to attend.

Reasons for Boundary Crossings

Helen's motivations are not known; however, given her willingness to immediately consult, it is obvious that ethical practice was her most important consideration. Perhaps Helen considers this committee appointment a potential career boost and would be reluctant to give it up if requested to do so. If she and the client are able to monitor this dual role as it develops, should Helen have to choose between transferring her client to another therapist and serving on a prestigious committee? If Helen is considering her career while she thinks about her client, is she practicing unethical behavior? To the contrary, we believe she is not required to unilaterally choose between client and career. However, should Helen and her client have a strong disagreement during committee service, they may either decide to reconsider their therapy relationship or work this through. Referral to another therapist may or may not be indicated.

Joan Besafe, Sexual Assault Prevention Counselor

Joan Besafe is the Sexual Assault Prevention counselor and has a joint appointment in the counseling center and the dean of students' office at a small university. As a licensed mental health professional, her job includes crisis intervention and counseling of victims of violent crimes, prevention, education, intern and peer counselor training, and supervision. For the other half of her position, Joan is responsible for sexual assault policy development and implementation, collaboration with campus police department staff, and advising the dean of students on campus violence issues. She and Dr. Close, the counseling center director, are members of the campus crisis team comprised of a representative from the police department, dean of students, director of residence life, and chief judicial officer. Dr. Close and the chief judicial officer are long-time friends as well as colleagues, while Joan has only a professional relationship with the two of them.

Over the summer months, the daughter of the chief judicial officer (JO) has been in self-referred, time-limited treatment with Joan. The client and Joan agreed to a treatment plan including referral to an outside provider before the beginning of the fall term. The client is a survivor of multiple date rapes beginning when she was age 16. Because the daughter and the staff member do not have the same last name, Joan did not know of the family connection until session number 6 when the client revealed that her mother was the college judicial officer. Without disclosing the student's name, Joan informed Dr. Close of the familial connection and the treatment status of the student. The director recognized the difficulty immediately, having dealt with this issue before, since she has directed this small center for many years and treated children of acquaintances while referring children of close friends to her two half-time staff members. Joan and Dr. Close agreed that Joan should consult with the other campus mental health provider to protect confidentiality of the client.

As the treatment continues, the difficult issue of having a high-profile college administrator as her mother is discussed. The client states that although she loves her parents, they have not been supportive of her.

The client believes her parents blame her for the date rapes because she was drinking when they happened. She admits she may have a drinking problem and believes her father, who lives in another state, is a high-functioning alcoholic. She says her mother and stepfather believe she is promiscuous, and they frequently, when angry, blame her for being like her biological father. Joan recommends family therapy for her client and they discuss finding a group practice to facilitate individual and family therapy if she is able to talk her parents into participating. Joan terminates with her client at the end of summer term and schedules a brief follow-up appointment in 3 weeks to monitor the referral process.

At follow-up, the client reports that she has had an initial appointment with the new therapist and feels they can work together. However, when she asked her parents to go to counseling, her mother expressed concern about her standing in the community. Joan's client expresses worry that her mother will learn of her counseling relationship at the on-campus counseling center. Joan reassures her client that under no circumstances will she divulge any information about her therapy.

The fall term begins the following week, and Joan attends a meeting of the campus crisis team to discuss an alcohol-poisoning incident that resulted in a hospitalization. During the meeting, Joan notices the chief judicial officer frequently glancing in her direction. When Dr. Close and Joan debrief later, the director states that the JO seemed very odd in the meeting today. She tells Joan that she noticed the JO seemed to be watching her very closely. The director asks if Joan and the JO had some disagreement over the resolution of a particular case. Joan says she has not and chooses the response that she noticed nothing out of the ordinary at the meeting.

Relationship Expectations During Treatment

The counselor is a specialist whose practice brings her into close working relationships with nonmental health professionals who at times seek privileged information. As holders of privilege, counselors are required to maintain confidentiality. However, when the counselor is treating clients and advising administrators about critical incidents, threats to confidentiality are real. Counselors may have to assert their clinical roles as more significant than any other they may have in the campus community.

Although the vignette relationship has recently terminated, Joan is mired in a multiple-relationship dilemma that includes the client, the counseling center director, and the campus judicial officer. Since Joan's client failed to disclose exactly who her mother was during the early stages of treatment, the counselor could not predict or prevent the outcome. Informed consent does not help us much in this instance either because students are not asked to routinely disclose the names of all family members. In a private practice model, this information would be secured if the client were a minor. However, in the college population, most students are over 18 and treated as adults in the counseling contract.

The client was referred for additional treatment, and termination was completed with follow-up to determine satisfaction with the new therapist. The client does not plan to return to the college counseling center, so her relationship to Joan is over.

The Depth of the Psychotherapy Relationship

Assuming Joan has formed a working therapeutic alliance that helped her begin to work on her relationship and alcohol problems and to avoid self-injurious situations, the bond between therapist and client could be quite strong. However, since the therapist does not plan to enter a dual relationship with the client, the dynamics of this relationship are not central to the posttherapy complexities.

An uncontrollable outcome of the treatment could be that the client discloses to her mother that she has good feelings about her counseling center therapist. While Joan may always maintain confidentiality and behave in the highest ethical manner, she is still mired in a multiple relationship situation.

New Proposed Relationship

Joan must decide how to handle both her boss, Dr. Close, and the campus judicial officer in the aftermath of this role strain. In ongoing work relationships, Joan might act as if nothing has transpired. However, we are all aware when there has been a change in the dynamics of a relationship, even those at the office, so the outcome may be unpredictable. An easy answer is not available to Joan. She cannot simply resign from the crisis team or stop advising the dean of students on matters of import. Joan must endure the discomfort of this multiple relationship dynamic and act as if nothing has happened.

Reasons for Boundary Crossings

Joan seems motivated to do her job well. She intentionally works in a high-profile position and accepts multiple relationships as a natural part of her work life. One might recommend that Joan find an environment where anonymity can be more easily protected; yet these options may not be available or desirable to some counselors.

In this vignette, therapist self-awareness and self-monitoring is crucial. The experience of the college counselor, working as a therapist in a small closed community, is often one of "living in a fish bowl." The milieu inevitably involves multiple relationships, yet they need not lead to ethical violations. Therapists working in small closed communities may be at risk for dealing with stress and isolation resulting from their efforts to provide ethical care for their clients. Proper clinical support, self-care, and a nurturing community are important.

CONCLUSION

The authors, and many colleagues who were consulted in preparing this chapter, all noted that they would not be helping professionals without significant relationships with therapists, supervisors, and professors in educational settings. These pivotal, career-influencing associations exemplify the positive outcomes of nonharmful, nonexploitative dual relationships. Certainly, some therapists may choose to keep therapy experiences private (see Pope & Tabachnick, 1994). However, the dual relationships that frequently are an outgrowth of counseling the future or current professional often call for extended boundaries. Due to the present climate, this counternarrative of good outcome (and those with student clients choosing other professions) is not memorialized. This consigns an important practice to invisibility, resulting in an underresearched process.

When counseling center staff experience ethical dilemmas, decision-making models can be applied utilizing committee and consultative structures already in place or created for this purpose. Before entering into a supervisory or consultative relationship with an off-campus resource or faculty member, confidentiality issues must be adequately addressed.

In the end, therapist integrity is the sine qua non. Consultation, additional training, and/or therapy may be helpful if a therapist is experiencing confusion. For a crucial subcategory of professionals, particularly males with sexual abuse histories, research suggests a need for additional oversight. Jackson and Nuttall (2001), utilizing a nationally drawn and randomized sample, researched male and female therapists with sexual abuse histories. Three of five *male* therapist respondents reporting *severe childhood sexual abuse combined with "high degrees of psychological distress" admitted* to sexual boundary violation with clients (emphasis added).

Intake materials and informed consent can properly prepare clients for the inevitable contact that occurs in the university setting. With both counselor and client involved in decision-making, revisiting informed consent throughout the therapy process is likely to greatly reduce the discomfort of dual-role contact. Moreover, we recommend case records designed to track ongoing client-counselor dual relationship processes clinically. These could be accessed for research data and might include exit and follow-up forms containing questions about the type, frequency, and outcomes of multiple roles and relationships from the viewpoint of both client and therapist.

Funding to conduct empirically based research on college counseling center issues is required (Cottone & Claus, 2000; Stone et al., 2000). As we study the impact on therapeutic practice of dual role and dual relationships, we can further delineate acceptable forms of multiple relationships from those that we all agree should never occur between counselor and client. It is the undisclosed issue, the matter not discussed, and the situation unexamined that undermines our understanding of what it means to engage in nonsexual, nonexploitative dual relationships, whether on campus or in the wider community.

REFERENCES

American Psychological Association. (1992). Ethical principles of psychologists and code of conduct. *American Psychologist, 47,* 1597–1611.

American Psychological Association. (2001, June 24). Proposed revision to *Ethical principles of psychologists and code of conduct.* Retrieved August 2, 2001, from http://www.apa.org

Anderson, S. K., & Kitchener, K. S. (1998). Nonsexual post therapy relationships: A conceptual framework to assess ethical risks. *Professional Psychology: Research and Practice, 29,* 91–99.

Archer, J. A., Jr., & Cooper, S. (1998). *Counseling and mental health services on campus: A handbook of contemporary practices and challenges.* San Francisco: Jossey-Bass.

Barnett, J. E. (2000). *Must some boundaries be crossed?* Retrieved June 20, 2001, from http://www.division42.org

Berk, S. E. (1983). Origins and historical development of university and college counseling. In P. J. Gallagher & G. D. Demos (Eds.), *Handbook of counseling in higher education* (pp. 50–71). New York: Praeger Scientific.

Bersoff, D. N. (Ed.). (1999). *Ethical conflicts in psychology* (2nd ed.). Washington, DC: American Psychological Association.

Burian, B. K., & O'Connor-Slimp, A. (2000). Social dual-role relationships during internship: A decision-making model. *Professional Psychology: Research and Practice, 31,* 332–338.

Cottone, R. R., & Claus, R. E. (2000). Ethical decision-making models: A review of the literature. *Journal of Counseling and Development, 78,* 276–283.

Gallagher, R. P., Gill, A. M., & Sysko, H. B. (2000). *National survey of counseling center directors.* Alexandria, VA: International Association of Counseling Services, Inc., Monograph Series No. 8 J.

Guinee, J. P., & Ness, M. E. (2000). Counseling centers of the 1990s: Challenges and changes. *The Counseling Psychologist, 20,* 267–280.

Jackson, H., & Nuttall, R. L. (2001). A relationship between childhood sexual abuse and professional misconduct. *Professional Psychology: Research and Practice, 32,* 200–204.

Jordan, A. E., & Meara, N. M. (1990). Ethics and the professional practitioner: The role of virtues and principles. *Professional Psychology: Research and Practice, 21,* 107–114.

Lazarus, A. A. (1994). How certain boundaries and ethics diminish therapeutic effectiveness. *Ethics and Behavior, 4,* 255–261.

McGrath, E. (2001, September 10). Colleges of the year: Welcome, freshmen! *Time Magazine, 158,* 64–77.

Miller, J. B., & Stiver, I. P. (1997). *The healing connection: How women form relationships in therapy and in life.* Boston: Beacon.

Pederson, P. (1997). The cultural context of the American Counseling Association code of ethics. *Journal of Counseling and Development, 76,* 23–28.

Pope, K. S., & Tabachnick, B. G. (1994). Therapists as patients: A national survey of psychologists' experiences, problems, and beliefs. *Professional Psychology: Research and Practice, 25,* 247–258.

Pulakos, J. (1994). Incidental encounters between therapists and clients: The client's perspective. *Professional Psychology, 25,* 300–303.

Sharkin, B. S. (1995). Strains on confidentiality in college student psychotherapy: Entangled therapeutic relationships, incidental encounters, and third-party inquiries. *Professional Psychology: Research and Practice, 26,* 184–189.

Stone, G. L., Vespia, K. M., & Kanz, J. E. (2000). How good is mental health care on college campuses? *Journal of Counseling Psychology, 47,* 498–510.

Zur, O. (2000). In celebration of dual relationships: How prohibition of nonsexual dual relationships increases the chance of exploitation and harm. *The Independent Practitioner, 20* (3), 97–100.

PART 7

Special Dual Relationships

Part 7 consists of two chapters that fall outside the usual purview of most dual relationships and one that delves deeply into the vicissitudes of a profound friendship between a therapist and a client. First, Clifford Lazarus (chapter 26) discusses a boundary crossing that goes beyond the customary functions and expectations that typically entail what psychotherapists address. He inquires if a psychotherapist may, can, and should step out of role on occasion and perform the functions of a matchmaker? He discusses the dual relationship of therapist and matchmaker, its pros and cons, and provides a responsible modus operandi for implementing it. In chapter 27, Thomas discusses bartering in lieu of monetary or customary fees. This is a provocative and insightful chapter in which he describes how to meet one's client's needs first and foremost, and how to avoid the pitfalls of creating excessive gratitude in impecunious clients. Finally, in chapter 28, Goldin describes what enticed her to cross a therapeutic boundary, and the emotional journey that ensued when she and her client developed a profound friendship. She regards the way it finally turned out as one of the most powerful and greatest accomplishments of her career.

CHAPTER 26

The Therapist as Matchmaker

Clifford N. Lazarus, PhD

T his chapter presents the rationale for a therapeutic duality that goes beyond the customary functions and expectations that typically entail what psychotherapists address. May one, can one, should one step out of role on occasion and perform the functions of a *matchmaker*? What follows is an argument in favor of the dual relationship of therapist and matchmaker, its pros and cons, as well as a responsible modus operandi for implementing it.

BACKGROUND

Sally, a single, 31-year-old assistant editor for a large publishing company originally sought therapy for panic disorder that responded very well to cognitive-behavior therapy (CBT). Indeed, after 12 sessions over approximately 6 months, she was panic-free and well equipped to implement her newly acquired anxiety-management skills. During one of her last sessions, Sally expressed appreciation for the successful therapy and semi-jokingly said, "Now if only you could fix me up with a nice, employed guy, my life would be just about perfect."

Bill, a 35-year-old, single, school administrator came for therapy to learn to master his fear of heights, because his parents had recently moved into an apartment on the 23rd floor of a modern high-rise. After

15 sessions of CBT, he had conquered his phobia and happily reported that he had visited his parents, stood out on their balcony, and, while admittedly aware of some autonomic arousal, felt very much in control of his anxiety. "I feel great," he remarked at his last session. "Conquering that phobia really boosted my confidence." "Now," he continued, "if only I could find a nice, emotionally together girlfriend, I'd be happy as a clam."

As therapists, we have both the privilege and the responsibility of helping people cope with and even master a wide range of life's challenges. It is extremely gratifying to help people recover from debilitating depressions, conquer crippling anxieties, resolve traumatic events, and deal with relationship difficulties, to name only a few of the therapeutic missions we routinely undertake. To do so, we have at our disposal a truly effective array of methods, techniques, strategies, and procedures (especially if we employ the empirically supported and evidence-based approaches of CBT). Nevertheless, there is a specific intervention, a therapeutic maneuver of potentially unparalleled power that, ironically, most therapists are loath to consider, let alone employ, and that many regard as the penultimate boundary violation, second only to sexual exploitation. That is, the "matchmaking method"—a clearly thought out, calculated, therapeutic stratagem. By arranging for two seemingly compatible people to meet each other, the traditional benefits of psychological treatment can be vastly enhanced.

Healthy human beings are highly social animals evolutionarily adapted to forming intimate pair-bonds. Thus, in some instances beating back depression, conquering anxiety, overcoming panic, and/or mastering phobic avoidance can be seen as merely the starting point of comprehensive psychosocial therapy rather than its endpoint. The finish line can be viewed as enabling specific clients to enter into a stable, intimate relationship that brings with it the chance for a lifelong and loving partnership. Personal ads, dating services, and more recently, matchmaking web sites are used by literally millions of people as avenues for meeting potential partners. This reflects the enormous importance that people place on seeking companionship. Yet, despite their mass appeal and popularity, these mechanisms for meeting people are very crude insofar as even high-end personal introduction services do a superficial job in psychological screening and compatibility assessments. Alternatively, trained, experienced therapists are in a far better position to objectively assess the psychological status and potential compatibility of two people—without the intrinsic conflict of interest that most dating services have, namely a financial concern in making a certain number of personal introductions or dating referrals. Hence, who better than a qualified mental health professional to arrange such meetings when appropriate?

It may be argued that the blanket prohibition and out-of-hand rejection of therapists acting as matchmakers is a mistake and that the idea requires, at the very least, a critical analysis and serious consideration. After all, at the core of the matter is the fundamental principle in clinical decision-making of weighing the benefits of a treatment with the risks of that treatment. When a clinician decides to implement a therapeutic method, he or she has, presumably, ascertained that the benefits considerably outweigh the risks. Indeed, all clinical decision making ostensibly takes a direction from the compass of risks and rewards and rests on the foundation of informed consent that, itself, is a crucial dimension of the therapeutic relationship (e.g., C. Lazarus, 2001; Lazarus & Fay, 1984). Thus, a conceptual launching pad for a critical analysis of the "matchmaking method" is to consider its potential benefits and risks, pros and cons, advantages and disadvantages. To do this, the most cogent questions raised by the process will be addressed and discussed. Because the very nature of the therapeutic relationship lies at the core of this matter, before examining the matchmaker method under a higher magnification, we will first discuss the foundations of informed consent.

INFORMED CONSENT

In previous eras, clinicians were viewed as beneficent healers who were presumed to know what was best for a client and had no obligation to explain decisions or ask permission to perform actions. Hence, in the traditional model of the doctor-patient or clinician-client relationship, the doctor treated the patient as a caring parent would treat a child, and the patient had no fundamental right to informed consent, truth telling, or confidentiality. Today, based on the writings of Immanuel Kant, the doctor-patient relationship is conceptualized as [more] egalitarian. Thus, patients are treated as responsible, rational, and self-governing with rights of self-determination that must be respected even if they make decisions that work against them (e.g., the right to refuse treatment). At the very heart of this autonomy-based model of patient care is the process of informed consent.

Many clinicians, especially prescribers, tend to think of informed consent as a single event that has the sole purpose of informing the patient about the risks of a particular treatment. (As an interesting aside, consider that much of psychopharmacology, and especially clinical research, is driven by consent forms that would baffle the editors of most scientific journals. Indeed, most informed consent forms are designed by hospital or drug company lawyers and are court-tested, boilerplate documents that are intended to protect prescribers from litigation, rather than inform patients about treatments. Ironically, even the most carefully constructed consent form has little chance of standing up in court since almost any attorney can shred the most meticulously crafted document. In addition, all a patient has to say is "I didn't understand a word of it, but the doctor told me I had to sign it." Furthermore, there is an intrinsic paradox of consent forms—if they're complete enough to be comprehensive they're incomprehensible, and if they're short enough to be comprehensible they're invariably incomplete.)

It is best to conceptualize informed consent neither as a single event nor only in terms of information. It is not a document nor a signature on a document. Rather, in its purest form, informed consent is a moral and ethical dimension of the therapeutic relationship that starts with the first moment of eye contact and evolves throughout the entire duration of treatment. Conceptualized in this way, informed consent is an ongoing and evolving process of discussion and information exchange that forms the very foundation of the therapeutic alliance. In addition to being an excellent method from the standpoint of information exchange, this way of construing informed consent also serves as a powerful risk-management tool because the degree of relatedness engendered by this kind of process is virtually incompatible with litigation (see Gutheil, 1994; Gutheil & Gabbard, 1998). Clients who see themselves as part of a solid therapeutic alliance almost never sue their providers. (As has been underscored previously in this book, it is a great pity that most risk-management seminars teach clinicians to see their clients as potential litigants. This impels them to adopt rigid boundaries that adversarialize the relationship and ironically renders them more susceptible to litigation. See A. Lazarus [1994] for an earlier and provocative discussion of boundaries in psychotherapy.)

In evolving the informed consent process, there are three technical aspects that must be considered: information, voluntariness, and competency (e.g., Arnott, 1998). Information is the "informed" aspect of informed consent and must be presented in clear and understandable language. Therefore, instead of shoving a bolus of technical facts down the client's throat, the clinician and the client collaborate in exploring the scope of available information about the treatment being considered. Voluntariness refers to the "consent" dimension and implies that the client can say "no" as easily as "yes," thus indicating the absence of coercion and fostering consensual therapeutic decisions. Hence, informed consent can be withdrawn if the client changes his or her mind. The final aspect of informed consent is competency, which is defined as the capacity to take in, process, and weigh information and then make a rational decision based on the facts supplied. Again, it is a mistake to think that a document is a good informed-consent mechanism; at best it is a formality, literally. A client cannot have a relationship with a document, and it is the relationship that is the very heart of the informed consent process. Nevertheless, there are some settings where informed consent is a document-driven procedure (e.g., hospitals and research facilities) and in those settings one must use the forms; provided they are used only as an adjunct to the process we are advocating here, not in lieu of it.

To extend this framework to the "matchmaker method," the clinician-client discussion would first explore the available options: the matchmaker method (proposed treatment), traditional methods or dating services (alternative treatments), and doing nothing proactively (no treatment). A serious risk of the proposed treatment (matchmaker method) might be that the client likes but is rejected by his or her intended partner. This can have potential repercussions not only for the rejected individual personally, but also for the clinician-client relationship (a point we will discuss further below). Serious risks of alternative treatments (e.g., dating services and/or the personal ads) include spending significant amounts of money yet not meeting a compatible partner, in addition to the rejection possibilities. A serious risk of no treatment is chronic loneliness and general dissatisfaction.

A common risk of the matchmaker method might involve the couple simply failing to hit it off, despite the therapist's rational sense that the two people share many compatible attributes. A common risk of alternative methods might be devoting a lot of time to the process to no avail. And ongoing romantic frustration might be a common risk of doing nothing. Specifically relevant risks might include a socially anxious person having to deal with various components of anticipatory apprehension and performance concerns (matchmaker method), a person working two jobs to make ends meet spending a lot of time and money that he or she really can't afford (alternative interventions), and heightened vulnerability to relapse in a person with a history of recurrent depression (no treatment).

In essence, regardless of the client's condition or complaints and the mode or method of treatment, all therapeutic interventions necessarily rest on the foundation of informed consent which itself is an integral, moral, and ethical dimension of the clinician-client relationship. As long as a clinician uses the relationship in an egalitarian, noncoercive, nonexploitative, collaborative way to openly explore and discuss the range of therapy options vis-à-vis benefits and risks, no matter what method is ultimately agreed to, the relationship and its boundaries will not necessarily be undermined.

Now that I have provided the conceptual context of how all therapy methods ideally emanate from the collaborative alliance of an informed-consent process, which is a crucial cornerstone in the foundation of the therapeutic relationship, I will address some specific concerns that the "matchmaker method" calls into question. At the outset, I want to underscore that the method involves very judicious selectivity, that is arranging introductions only between two generally high-functioning people who do not have any significant Axis II pathology.

SOME IMPORTANT QUESTIONS AND ANSWERS

Q: Wouldn't the "matchmaking method" be a clear violation of client confidentiality?
A: Obviously, for a therapist to surreptitiously arrange an introduction wherein only one person is aware of the fact that both members of the pair are in therapy with the matchmaker is a clear and egregious violation of confidentiality. Alternatively, in keeping with the spirit of true informed consent, if the therapist discusses the approach with both members of the prospective couple individually while protecting their privacy, and through such a process it is agreed by all that a meeting is desirable, confidentiality has not been compromised. Of course, the therapist must consider the broader social context of the individuals lives to avoid potential conflicts should the couple prove incompatible, for example, they work for the same company, attend the same church or synagogue, or share some other common factor that might prove problematic if the two do not succeed as a couple.

Q: Since therapists are not trained to be matchmakers, wouldn't doing so constitute an ethical violation in that it is practicing beyond the scope of the therapists legitimate expertise?
A: While not specifically instructed in matchmaking, per se, most currently practicing therapists describe themselves as "eclectic" (i.e.,

they draw from diverse sources in formulating client problems and devising treatment plans). Hence, most eclectic therapists often use methods and techniques in which they have not received formal training, but rather learn to implement through reading, observation, practice, and experience. In other instances, a therapist might attend a seminar that emphasizes a particular method or approach (e.g., eye movement desensitization and reprocessing) and then hones his or her skills through clinical application and experience. With respect to the "matchmaking method," most therapists already possess the knowledge, experience, and skills necessary to successfully carry out the technique (i.e., relationship building, information gathering, clinical assessment, treatment planning, and technique implementation). It is simply a matter of using their knowledge and skills in a creative, "out of the box" and controversial manner.

Q: Wouldn't playing matchmaker be a personal boundary violation in that it extends the focus of therapy beyond the therapeutic relationship? **A:** As the basic premise of this book argues, there are many valid reasons to extend the therapeutic relationship beyond the confines of the consulting room. For example, behavior therapists have been conducting in vivo desensitization across a wide range of settings for more than 3 decades (e.g., A. Lazarus, 1971). Indeed, it seems to be a regrettable residue of traditional, analytic psychotherapy that the relationship is still seen by many practitioners as a rarefied, sacrosanct entity from which all therapeutic powers flow. Thus, doing anything that might obfuscate the pristine clarity of transferential phenomena is tantamount to committing therapeutic sacrilege. Fortunately for the mental health consumer, more recent, and perhaps more enlightened, ways of construing the therapeutic relationship see it as [merely] the vehicle through which interventions and methods are effectively delivered. That is, relationship components are necessary but not sufficient to produce therapeutic change. As Lazarus and Fay (1984) have metaphorically stated, the relationship is the soil that enables the specific technique to take root. Therefore, it is our view that if one has established a fertile enough relationship, any rational, noncoercive, nonexploitative, nonsexual boundary extension that is based on the elements of informed consent and collaborative decision making would in no way constitute a boundary violation.

Q: Wouldn't serving as a matchmaker jeopardize the therapeutic relationships if the prospective coupling doesn't work out?

A: While there is always the chance that a failed pairing might have an adverse impact on the therapeutic relationship, this is also the case with any intervention a therapist might propose. That is, on the one hand, if a treatment fails to produce the desired results a client might "fire" the therapist. On the other hand, if the treatment was selected through the collaborative process of informed consent that has been outlined above, the client's reaction to failure might be very accepting, reflecting a healthy "well, we gave it a try," attitude. Thus, as mentioned previously, all therapeutic choices are best made within the context of informed consent and collaborative decision-making. This not only empowers the client, but also has him or her implicitly agreeing to assume a degree of personal responsibility for the selection of the method. Hence, if the method fails, the client will be less likely to blame the therapist.

Q: Isn't the method an abuse of the therapeutic relationship since its intrinsic power disparity and "demand characteristics" makes it almost impossible for the client to say "no" or run the risk of displeasing the therapist?
A: Within the context of the morally and ethically egalitarian relationship that lies at the heart of all positive therapeutic alliances, there really is no power disparity, per se. Rather, there is a knowledge and skills disparity that the very purpose of therapy aims to reduce. What's more, no matter what the intervention, clients face the challenge of saying "no" to their therapists. By engaging in the honest and open, alliance-based process of informed consent, clients become active decision makers in their therapy and not simply passive recipients of treatments. Indeed, at the core of informed consent is voluntariness, which means the client can in fact say "no" as easily as "yes." Thus there is no coercion and the therapeutic decision is consensual.

Q: Aren't there possibly significant, unforeseen problems that might come to light only after the couple has met, such as one person being in serious conflict with a member of the other person's family or social circle?
A: As with any intervention, there are always possible unforeseen complications. The hope is that during the implementation of the method vis-à-vis exploring the potential benefits and risks, various scenarios will be discussed. In the worst case, if such a conflict is discovered to exist, the couple may simply decide not to pursue the relationship further. Alternatively, if they really hit it off, they can make an effort to resolve the conflict or merely cope with it as many couples do.

Q: What happens if only one person is eager to deepen the relationship? How will this affect the course of their individual therapies vis-à-vis the therapist's bias or disappointment?

A: If the method is engaged in properly, there will be no bias on the part of the therapist who (we hope) is competent enough to avoid letting personal feelings cloud his or her therapeutic judgment. In addition, it is possible that a failed pairing can provide important material for the therapy. For example, if one member of the pair rejects the other person based on either capriciousness or superficial considerations, the therapy can focus on issues such as unreasonable expectations or questionable priorities. Moreover, if it comes to light that there is a more significant reason why person A rejects person B (e.g., poor manners), with appropriate authorization in place, the therapy can focus on person B's heretofore unknown social skills deficits.

Q: If the method involves very judicious selectivity, that is arranging introductions only between two generally high psychosocially functioning people, why should such individuals need such an intervention? Wouldn't their failure to have found suitable partners through traditional methods reflect a deeper degree of social maladjustment than is appropriate for the method?

A: Not necessarily. Many high-functioning and generally well-adjusted people experience considerable trouble finding suitable romantic partners for long-term relationships. To purport that only socially maladjusted people fail to find compatible partners through traditional methods (i.e., meeting at school, through friends, at work, or random encounters at various venues) is a great disservice to the millions of people who use the personals, web sites, and dating services. What's more, one need only to consider the disturbingly high divorce rate to call into question the long-term effectiveness of most [traditional] couplings. Indeed as stated earlier, who is better qualified than an experienced mental health professional to rule out serious (Axis II) psychopathology and once done make personal introductions when appropriate?

AN ILLUSTRATIVE DIALOGUE

To illustrate how the matchmaker method might unfold, let's return to the couple the chapter started with, Sally and Bill.

S = Sally; T = Therapist.

S: Now if only you could fix me up with a nice, employed guy, my life would be just about perfect.

T: Are you serious about that, Sally?

S: Sure! As long as he's not a nutcase.

T: Tell me more about your expectations. If you were to describe an ideal partner, what characteristics would you mention?

S: Well, okay . . . I'd want a guy in his thirties, who has a decent education and a career. I think he'd have to be honest, you know, not into silly macho game playing, and as I said before not be a nutcase.

T: What do you think of as a "nutcase?"

S: You know, not crazy, like either an alcoholic or drug addict. Also not violent, or a liar. And able to communicate and express his feelings, not hold stuff in too much.

T: What about physical characteristics? And other things like religion?

S: I'd like a guy who takes care of himself, but he doesn't have to be especially athletic. Also, I hate to say it because it sounds so superficial, but I really don't go for the short, heavy, and bald type. As for religion, it really doesn't matter as long as he believes in God.

T: How would you feel about me introducing you to a fellow who seems to satisfy all of your criteria?

S: Are you serious?

T: Yes. But, there are a few issues we'd need to discuss up front before we explore the possibility any further. For one thing, I'd have to confirm that the guy I have in mind is okay with the idea, too. Assuming he is, let's talk about how this meeting can take place. We need to discuss a variety of pros and cons because there is no guarantee that the two of you will hit it off. Do you have any concerns, so far?

S: Is this guy one of your clients?

T: Yes. Is that a problem for you?

S: What is he seeing you for?

T: I can't share that with you right now, but I'm confident he's not a "nutcase" and, like you, he's a very high-functioning person who's in therapy only to get a little help with achieving a rather straightforward objective. In fact, he's met his goals, and we, too, are in the process of finishing up his treatment.

S: Well, I trust you, so I'm sure you wouldn't steer me wrong.

T: I would never steer you wrong on purpose, but as I was saying there are no guarantees that you'll like him, or that he'll like you, for that matter.

S: There are no guarantees in any relationship!

T: Right. So, let's discuss the options. How have you approached dating in the past?

S: You know, I just sort of met people. I dated a guy in college for about two years, but that didn't work out. I met a guy where I work and we dated for a few years, but it turned out he wasn't the committed type. Other than that, I've just gone on random dates.

T: Have you considered the personals or a dating service?

S: I've answered a few personals. The guys sounded good on paper but there was no chemistry with any of them. A couple didn't even have real jobs. I've never tried a dating service, but a few of my friends have suggested that I try one. What do you think?

T: I think that it's like rolling the dice, a numbers game dealing with the law of averages. Given enough rolls, you're bound to come up with some winning numbers. The problem is mostly time and money. Reputable dating services are pretty expensive. Around this area, it can cost several thousand dollars for a handful of introductions.

S: Wow!

T: Another shortcoming with dating services is that, as far as I know, they really don't have the resources to screen applicants and clients for potentially serious psychological difficulties. Mostly they focus on demographics, not mental health.

S: Well, I sure don't need to pay a service to line me up with some nutcases, I've done fine finding some of those on my own.

T: (Laughs) I'm sure many of the guys aren't "nutcases," but my point is there is usually no filter to screen out psychologically unhealthy people and you may have to kiss a lot of frogs before you find a prince. And that can take a lot of time and money. On plus side, you would be dealing with pretty serious men. I mean if a guy is plunking down a few thousand bucks himself, I'd think he was highly motivated to find a meaningful relationship and not very likely to be just messing around or wasting time.

S: That makes sense.

T: So, there are some pros and cons with either approach.

S: I think I'd like to met the guy you told me about, can you tell me more about him?

T: Let me bounce the idea of an introduction off him and get back to you with the details. First, let's talk about what can go wrong.

S: Huh? What do you mean?

T: Well, as I touched on before, you might not like him or he may not be into you. How do you think something like that might affect our relationship?

S: I don't think that would be a problem for me either way. Just as long as you try not to schedule us with back-to-back appointments if things don't work out (chuckles)!

T: Fair enough. If things don't work out, and I think it would be helpful, would you consider giving me permission to do a "post-mortem" on the date? That is, to discuss some of his impressions of you with you and some of your impressions of him with him? Assuming, of course, he also feels it's okay to do so?

S: I guess so, but I'd like to take a wait-and-see on that.

T: No problem. Do you have any specific concerns about going forward with this plan?

S: Do you really think it will work out?

T: Well, as I said before I can't promise anything. I can assure you, though, that he is a well adjusted, educated professional who has no serious problems that I've picked up with my psychological radar and I've gotten to know him about as well as I've gotten to know you. I'm also confident that the worst thing that could happen is that you two just wouldn't hit it off for whatever reasons, but I really think it's worth the risk.

S: Hey, what have I got to lose? Let's give it a try. At least I'll be meeting a guy who has been "pre-shrunk" (laughs).

After a similar dialogue with Bill, it was agreed that it would be worthwhile to arrange an introduction. If Bill had not consented, Sally would have simply been told the meeting is a "no go."

CONCLUDING REMARKS

To reiterate, while we are not necessarily strongly advocating the widespread adoption and routine use of the "matchmaker method," we do firmly believe that under the right circumstances it can prove to be extremely helpful. Just as sometimes the single most important intervention a therapist can perform is getting a neurochemically imbalanced client to agree to a trial of a psychotropic medication (C. Lazarus, 2001), facilitating the union of two souls, each in search of a life partner, can be almost as crucial. We hope this brief introduction to the "matchmaker method" will have provided a valuable peek through the keyhole, and at the very least stimulated some objective thought and discussion about the subject.

REFERENCES

Arnott, S. (1998). Medicolegal issues in clinical practice. *Hospital Medicine, 59* (2), 149–153.

Gutheil, T. G. (1994). Risk management at the margins: Less-familiar topics in psychiatric malpractice. *Harvard Review of Psychiatry, 2* (4), 214–221.

Gutheil, T. G., & Gabbard, G. O. (1998). Misuses and misunderstanding of boundary theory in clinical and regulatory settings. *American Journal of Psychiatry, 155* (3), 409–414.

Lazarus, A. A. (1971). *Behavior therapy and beyond.* New York: McGraw-Hill. (Reissued 1996, Northvale, NJ: Jason Aronson.)

Lazarus, A. A. (1994). How certain boundaries and ethics diminish therapeutic effectiveness. *Ethics and Behavior, 4,* 255–261.

Lazarus, A. A., & Fay, A. (1984). Behavior therapy. In T. B. Karasu (Ed.), *The psychiatric therapies* (pp. 485–538). Washington, DC: American Psychiatric Association.

Lazarus, C. N. (2001). Foundations of pharmacopsychology. In S. Cullari (Ed.), *Counseling and psychotherapy: A practical guidebook for trainees and new professionals* (pp. 246–288). Boston: Allyn and Bacon.

CHAPTER 27

Bartering

J. Lawrence Thomas, PhD

A few times over the last 2 decades as a private practice psychologist, specializing in neuropsychology, I have entered into barter arrangements with patients. I have never felt completely comfortable about it, but in each case it seemed to be the best alternative. The major issue hinges around the following question: How should we act and what should we do when a patient has little or no money?

I find it curious that the meager literature on bartering in American Psychological Association (APA) journals (e.g., Sonne, 1994; Woody, 1998) makes little mention of bartering as a means of helping the needy but poor patient. It can serve as a relatively dignified way for the patient to compensate the therapist for professional work. It seems as if the compassion that psychotherapy professes has been forgotten under the scepter of potential lawsuits. According to several authors, this is in fact the main reason barter arrangements should not be made: it opens the therapist up to liability. So far I have found only one article (Hill, 1999) that discusses bartering as a legitimate means of helping out a poor person, which seems the most obvious reason to enter into such an arrangement.

My view, in common with others articulated throughout this book, is that if we do not take some risks on a regular basis, as psychotherapy professionals we are not worthy of the job. A second and complementary theme I support is that venturing into any dual relationship requires careful, thoughtful judgment, which varies considerably from situation to situation. To preclude whole categories of arrangements because of legalistic or doctrinaire reasons (e.g., psychoanalytic views of the therapy relationship) serves only to narrow our work and contributes to an artificial and sterile context of psychotherapy.

There is an elephant in the room that no one is speaking about regarding the private practice of psychotherapy. And it is simply that many people who need our services cannot afford our fees. In recent years there has been less and less insurance coverage for psychotherapy, particularly if there is no "medical necessity," which is most of the time. Currently in New York State, the official rate (No-Fault/Workers Compensation) for a psychotherapy session by a psychologist is $120; neuropsychological and psychological testing is $140 per hour. How many people can write out checks for a full neuropsychological evaluation (15 to 20 hours) or for psychotherapy week after week? Not many.

Thus, bartering should become *more* prevalent because of these cost considerations. I have rarely been challenged on the session fee per se. Clients often just don't have the necessary funds. But the countervailing prospect of enduring a lawsuit, as Woody (1998) and others predict, outweighs making services possible by way of bartering.

A HIGHER STANDARD

An issue that must take salience in any discussion about dual relationships and the profession of psychotherapy is the "higher standard" that psychotherapists should strive for, and by this I only mean that the welfare of the patient should be paramount. Focusing on this higher standard as a basic stance in professional commitment is different *in kind* than most other principles we are asked to uphold as professionals. While this higher standard is mentioned in the preamble of the ethic manual of the APA (APA, 1992), it is a prelude to the many things we should *not* do in order to protect ourselves. If bartering can be justified as a consideration for helping the patient by virtue of a higher standard, this should carry significant weight as to whether such an arrangement should be acceptable. A bartering arrangement should not be precluded because there is a slim chance that the patient may sue the therapist, but I do agree that it should occur infrequently. The vast majority of our professional work should be paid by the usual monetary means, if only for practical reasons. But when this is not possible because of the economic situation of the patient, some allowance should be made so that our services can be available. This has become salient in my own particular specialty of neuropsychology, because brain damaged people sometimes have a hard time earning a living.

I will present a few of my own cases and some situations from colleagues to describe some successful barter arrangements.

THE RELEVANCE OF MY SPECIALTY

A main reason I have been occasionally involved in barter situations is that my particular treatment methods are not commonly available. I specialize in assessing and treating patients with mild brain dysfunction, and they frequently are not able to work in competitive society well enough to earn a living. Having *mild* brain dysfunction can be worse, in some ways, than having a severe head injury, because the funding for their support and health care can be quite problematic. A severely injured person stands out, and there is often no question that support in the usual arenas is needed—rehabilitation, medical and hospital care, follow up health care, and vocational training. Patients with mild brain dysfunction, however, often look quite normal, and a common view is that if they tried hard enough, they could overcome their problems. Little sympathy is elicited. Family members are confused, because their loved one is both the "same" and "different," in the case of head injury. Funding for treatment is difficult. Justification for treatment to insurance companies can become torturous.

Patients with these and other mild brain dysfunction diagnoses are repeatedly misdiagnosed and poorly treated over the course of their problems. Generally, this is a "difficult" patient who is lumped into a familiar category by the doctor or therapist, with the response less than optimal. Through my experience with this population, I have developed a number of ways to address the problems of mild brain dysfunction.

Case # 1: George

George met me at an Adult Attention Deficit Disorder (ADD) Support Group in Manhattan and arranged to see me in consultation. Although he had attended an adult ADD therapy group of mine for a few sessions, he chose another direction—to get a complete neuropsychological evaluation to clarify the diagnostic picture. It was at this point that the barter system began.

I first performed an extensive neuropsychological and learning disability evaluation, including assessment of psychopathology. I then administered neurofeedback with him for what I understood to be his partial complex seizure disorder. The detailed neuropsychological and personality evaluation took *about 20 hours of professional time by itself. The neurofeedback treatment, which is still ongoing, I estimate to be about 70 to 100 sessions. All this adds up to approximately $15,000 worth of services—for someone on public assistance. The fact that he had a profession (cabinetry) that was of value to me made it convenient for my professional services to be provided. Let me present this case of a barter arrangement more completely.*

History.   *George is single and currently 43 years old. He has regularly sought help from a number of professionals over the last 20 years. He has an enormously large dossier of medical records. He related his history to me in some detail, and it included a number of strange experiences as a child and throughout his life, with varying degrees of frequency. These experiences could alternately be interpreted as psychotic, borderline, or symptoms consistent with subclinical temporal lobe partial complex seizure phenomena. When the SCID was administered (Structured Clinical Interview for DSM–IV), the results indicated that he satisfied the diagnostic criteria of almost every disorder. He has in fact had all of these diagnoses given to him over the years.*

Testing.   *Neuropsychological testing was done in order to clarify his diagnostic picture with the goal of determining the degree and nature of brain dysfunction, and, in this case, to distinguish this from a long-standing learning disability. It was also important to determine the degree of psychopathology. This took about 20 hours of professional time. The results revealed that George appeared to have some degree of brain dysfunction and showed impairment on several measures. He used this report that was written to get psychopharmacological treatment and in obtaining the proper treatment. He also seemed to have some kind of subclinical seizure disorder,* absence status epilepticus. *This means he has blanking out periods that can last as long as a few hours.*

As a cabinetmaker, he had been inhaling lacquer and lacquer thinner in his nonventilated wood shop regularly for more than 15 years. Toxins such as these (and there were others) can be harmful to cerebral functioning (Hartman, 1988), and he was completely unaware that these fumes probably made his condition worse.

Treatment.   *Because George had a history of not responding well to medications, I decided to use neurofeedback with him to help stabilize his brain physiology. Very briefly, this involves biofeedback of one's own brain waves. One's electrophysiological information, or brain wave information, is displayed on a computer screen. The patient is asked to raise or lower certain waves, and over time, the patient learns how to do this. This is experimental work,* and it is unlikely George could find this help in a low-cost clinic that would accept his public assistance insurance; insurance companies have also been very reluctant to pay for this treatment. A popular book (Robbins, 2000) and a text (Evans & Abarbanel, 1999) are recommended for those interested in learning more about this area.

A major problem in utilizing neurofeedback for diagnoses such as seizure disorders and ADD is that 20 to 40 sessions are recommended, preferably twice per week, for 10 to 20 weeks in a row. For more complex cases, 40 to 100 sessions are often required. George was a complex case, and my estimate was that he needed at least 100 neurofeedback sessions. We agreed upon a schedule and the exchange rate, and we began the sessions. We agreed on a retail-to-retail exchange, meaning that he and I would use the usual fees in a proportionate exchange of hours. He would build me designs in exchange for my professional time. We would keep track of our hours and see where we stood every month or two.

Within a few sessions, George reported that his seizure problems were getting better. Each week he stated that his periods of being able to function were longer and he was more productive. He appears to be improving, and I have a few possessions I have wanted to have built. We both benefited from this arrangement.

The Three-Way Barter.   When I began to entertain the idea of barter as a way to provide services, I also arranged to provide some of my professional services to my chiropractor, Dr. Lewis, who was treating me. Dr. Lewis (not his real name) wanted a desk and cabinet for his office, and we agreed to barter retail-to-retail for this. As part of my former profession (architecture), I have designed cabinets, bookcases, and similar items for many years. In this situation, I designed a special cabinet for Dr. Lewis, showed him the drawing, and we discussed the design. I then asked George to build it as part of our barter arrangement. I still have some misgivings about this arrangement, particularly involving a third party in the barter, even though it eventually worked out. The reason is that George was very slow in completing this cabinet (over a year late), much to my embarrassment. However, this awkward situation finally turned out well.

The Benefits and Problems with George's Bartering Arrangement.   This case illuminates some potential problems with the bartering situation that other authors have mentioned. What happens if patients do not live up to their part of the bargain? How do you treat lapses on the patient's part? Similar to a missed payment? Or do you consider this as "water under the bridge," and simply take it as a loss? My recommendation is to take it as a loss. First, *however, the snag in the arrangement should be discussed because this often signals a more general problem in the patient's life. Indeed, it is safe to assume that the problems patients have in their lives are going to be reflected in the bartering arrangement between therapist and client. Discussing and resolving as much as possible the "barter snags" is a unique side benefit to these kind of arrangements: the therapist can experience first hand the frustrations of relating to this patient! The idea of using the barter arrangement as integral to the therapeutic work has been developed to a significant degree by Rappoport (1983), and is discussed next.*

Case #2: Rachel

Rachel, aged 32, was a highly skilled graphic artist prior to her head injury. She was walking out of a subway entrance in New York City when a large, heavy object fell on her head. In fact, it bounced three times on her head. To make matters worse, it bounced on her right parietal-occipital area—the worst possible place for a graphic artist to sustain an injury. I performed the neuropsychological evaluation and followed up with treatment. After about a year, the insurance company cut off payments to me, but I decided to continue treatment.

Rachel desperately needed someone to talk to who believed in her complaints; many health professionals dismissed her symptoms as "psychological" as there was no hard evidence of her brain damage in magnetic resonance imaging or computed tomography scans. Later, when a single-proton emission computed tomography scan showed that there was a brain injury and a deterioration in her right hemisphere, her complaints were more respected. But she had to endure a few years being labeled hysterical or having psychological problems as explanations for her neurological symptoms. I was the only health professional who believed her and was willing to explain her symptoms to her. In addition, since I had been a visual designer (architect) in an earlier career, I believed I was especially well qualified to understand and help her.

During the time of treatment, the insurance company cut off payments to Rachel for lost wages, and she was desperately poor. She came from rural Idaho, and her parents were also of modest means. No help from her family was available. During this 2-year period, I recall Rachel going to her church and getting emergency money to pay the rent. But this could be done only a few times, and she was desperate.

Now to my "bad deed"—the act of bartering. During Rachel's very poor period, I hired her and paid her money to help me with some of my office matters, for a day or two per week. She readily admitted when she was having cognitive problems in doing some things, and I understood these processing problems when they occurred. The work was therapeutic for her, even though she did it poorly, which enabled me to see another side of her. I saw how she functioned in "real world office tasks." It became painfully obvious why she was not able to function in the competitive marketplace—she could not process directions rapidly enough to make her abilities accessible, and therefore valuable. She could not function as a professional graphic artist for the time being. Or perhaps ever.

The Job Trial. In the field of rehabilitation it is common for a patient recovering from a head injury to go on a "job trial." When I worked at the Head Injury Program at NYU Medical Center, the patient volunteered in some part of the hospital complex and was supervised carefully by a head injury program staff member, usually the vocational counselor. Real work would get done, but the level of productivity would often be understandably low.

Having a patient perform real work-related tasks can be a way to assess how they would function in the real world of employment. Thus, one might see gaps in memory that might not have been apparent in the ordinary therapy sessions. As a neuropsychologist, I can see the cognitive problems better than an ordinary employer, and I can obtain a multilayered impression of the possible impact of these deficits on work performance.

The strategy of doing a job trials is well-known in the world of rehabilitation. But it is essentially bartering. Regardless of whether I paid Rachel or not, I would consider this arrangement as bartering. In both Rachel's case and in traditional job trials, the patient gives time and energy in exchange for a head injury professional's assessment as to the quality of work performed. Even in the protected environment of a hospital-based situation, however, I am sure there are a number of ethical snags. For example, a classic one is that it is hard to fire a volunteer. What if the work is far below a satisfactory level? What if the therapeutic agenda (of helping the patient's self-esteem, for example) conflicts with the workplace standards? Even with these caveats, it does not take much persuasion to convince caring family members and professionals that going through this kind of experience is likely to be in the best interests of the patient. Also, in my years of working with job trials, I have never heard a complaint that the patient was being exploited.

Rachel is doing much better now. She eventually won a modest settlement, moved back to Idaho, and recovered slowly. She has changed the direction of her career and is doing fine artwork, but at a slower pace. And her artwork is beautiful. The commercial world of being a graphic artist is too fast paced for her.

Case #3: Jane

Jane is an artist, and had problems in her relationships with men. We worked well together, but after a year and a half she ran out of money. Over time, I mistakenly allowed the bill to amount to several thousand dollars. She offered to pay off some of her bill with one of her paintings. I saw the painting, and agreed, and I have it today over my couch. I am still not sure whether this was the best thing to do, but it appeared to be reasonable at the time. My guess is that many therapists receive artwork from patients for professional services, but no one knows about it other than the active parties.

CASES FROM COLLEAGUES

I asked a few colleagues about bartering, under the assumption that trade-offs happened much more than is reported, especially with professionals who have been in practice for many years. Every one admitted that they occasionally bartered services with a patient, but they have been hesitant to reveal these arrangements to colleagues. Most of the time, the bartering emerged out of a previously established relationship. Every story was different and had a special twist to it. Nicholas Cummings (N. A. Cummings, personal communication, July 11, 2001) states that all bartering arrangements he has had over the years were benign, with no negative effects. Along with founding a number of organizations (more than 10) in the field of psychology over a span of more than 40 years (Thomas, Cummings, & O'Donohue, 2002), he has had a private practice for more than 50 years. It was his custom to always see some patients pro bono, and this was his arrangement with a man we will call Henry, who was in one of Cummings's therapy groups in the 1950s. Henry felt he wanted to "give back" something, and Cummings relates this story below:

> I do not remember too much about the patients who bartered their fee, as they were all straightforward with no negative effects. In my private practice I always reserved some slots for patients who could not pay. Most of these volunteered bartering, stating they would feel better about it. I remember one patient who was in one of my agoraphobia groups, and I will call him Henry Sturgeon. Because of his agoraphobia, Henry had not been able to work for several years and was accepted on a no-fee basis. At this point I should describe the building I owned for over 20 years on Judah Street in San Francisco. It was one-story and faced on three sides a classic city courtyard paved in antique bricks. On the fourth side was the blank wall of the three-

story building next door. The group room not only faced the courtyard as did most of the offices, but French doors allowed the group to go into the courtyard on nice days for the group session. The only handicap was that to enter the courtyard one had to go through the building. Therefore, I had no regular gardener for obvious reasons, and periodically had someone go into the courtyard to trim and clean.

Well, Henry decided he would redo the courtyard, arranged it with my receptionist, and over a 2-week period transformed it into a showplace. He got several of the patients to chip in for new plants and trees, unbeknown to me. The group had a bronze plaque made stating the date and "Garden by Henry Sturgeon." They held a dedication ceremony during the group meeting and declared Sturgeon's agoraphobia gone forever, and embraced the new Henry Sturgeon who subsequently created his own successful landscaping business. The bronze plaque remained for several years, and Henry maintained the courtyard regularly on his own time and expense, stating his usual fee should go to another worthy no-fee patient. In 1987 I sold the building and it was torn down and replaced with a multistory building. Henry called me in tears, but stated his agoraphobia never returned and he no longer needed the "Garden by Henry Sturgeon." (N. A. Cummings, personal communication, July 11, 2001)

According to the APA ethics committee, I am not sure whether this would be considered bartering, since Dr. Cummings never asked that these services be performed. But if we assume at some point a quid pro quo was understood between them, would the therapist be obliged to terminate the activity? I would assert that the patient's "giving back" was of therapeutic benefit in this case and similar ones.

Arnold Lazarus (A. A. Lazarus, personal communication, August 5, 2001), shortly before this book was sent to press, was invited by a professional group to talk about dual relationships. It was revealed that the licensing board in this state was going to prohibit bartering in their newly revised state code. Lazarus wrote to them:

This troubles me for several reasons. Let's assume that an impecunious man in need of therapy consults me. I could refer him to a clinic, or treat him pro bono, but I believe that this would only hurt his pride and render him inappropriately beholden to me. He happens to be a good carpenter, and so I strike up a deal. I will buy some wood, and he will build me a bookcase that I need. In that way, although he is unable to pay me, he will have given me a "fee" for service. He derives benefit from my professional ministrations and feels happy that he was not a "taker."

The board gets wind of this and I am censured. This harks back, in my opinion, to the McCarthy era. The harsh penalties that are often meted out by the board to psychologists who may be completely innocent, or have committed a minor infraction, have totalitarian overtones.

This raises an important point about the effects of bartering: What is the likelihood that the vast majority of bartering is benign? That is, both parties are satisfied (or at least the patient is), and there is little likelihood of a lawsuit. Only when the arrangement goes awry does the ethical principle appear to come into play. The APA (1992) supposedly represents a profession guided by evidence in human behavior. Where is the evidence to support their discouragement of bartering? How often does bartering turn sour? Is there any hard evidence that this is a bad thing to do? Should the stories and commentaries of Koocher and Keith-Spiegel (1998) and others guide our behavior?

Apparently a number of bizarre stories of ethical violations have been reported to state and APA officials, and these are then published in volumes about our ethical principles (Canter, Bennett, Jones, & Nagy, 1994; Koocher & Keith-Spiegel, 1998). These probably represent a tiny fraction of the professional activities of psychologists (probably similar to other professions). Even admitting that bartering is risky for professional psychologists, I doubt that other professions have the degree of sanctions that we do. Are we being held to standard that is much higher than other professions, and which is therefore unfair?

LITERATURE REVIEW

The APA is in the process of revising its Code of Ethics, but at present the quote related to bartering (from the 1992 APA *Ethical Principles*), is noted below:

> Psychologists refrain from accepting goods, services, or other nonmonetary remuneration from patients or clients in return for psychological services because such arrangements create inherent potential for conflicts, exploitation, and distortion of the professional relationship. A psychologist may participate in bartering only if 1) it is not clinically contraindicated, and 2) the relationship is not exploitive. (APA, 1992, p. 1062)

This passage says almost nothing. In other words, you should not do bartering if it is contraindicated or if it is unfair. But no precise circumstances or criteria are stated. Nevertheless, as has been pointed out in some articles on bartering (Sonne, 1994; Woody, 1998), psychologists *have* been punished for bartering, with our vague ethics code being used as a weapon against them. Incidentally, those of us who have entered into these arrangements often find that if anyone is exploited in a bartering arrangement, it is likely to be the therapist.

There is another fundamental area that merits some consideration. If a group in the name of a profession puts a code in writing, everything in that code can be taken quite literally, and can be taken out of context—to the detriment of someone in a circumstance for whom that particular interpretation was never imagined. I would assert that psychotherapists are bad lawyers, as a general rule, and should not try and put into words what essentially is a simple moral stance of trying to do the right thing. When we write down a lot of conditions, often ambiguously worded, we open ourselves up to all kinds of possible abuse. This is because someone skilled at doing this (e.g., lawyers) can use each sentence as a weapon against us. Every time we write down a rule, recommendation, principle, or aspiration, we fashion a noose for ourselves. In recent times, the APA (1992) Ethics Code has been used to prosecute psychologists for violations in dual relationships, with nooses of our own making.

The literature on bartering in psychotherapy is sparse. There seem to be two main issues. First, barter can be an avenue for the poor but needy patient to obtain psychological services. I found only one article that discusses this in depth (Hill, 1999), plus one book on the subject (Rappoport, 1983). The second issue is whether bartering opens up the professional to possible sanctions from either a lawsuit or an ethics complaint. These two broad issues are in conflict with each other, and most writers agree that caution is the watchword. Although bartering might be a last resort, it is worth keeping in mind that this may take place more than one might suspect if it is seen as a possibility by the patient. Thus, the writers who advocate avoiding bartering at almost all costs have some moral obligation, in my opinion, to provide an alternative.

In Woody's 1998 article, the examples he points out about the problems psychologists have gotten into with respect to bartering appear to rest on strikingly bad judgment. One psychologist, he reports, concludes his justification for bartering with " . . . besides I needed another car for my teenager" (p. 174). Another example was a psychologist who invested in a patient's business, but the business had troubles, and the psychologist sued the patient and his partner. In my opinion, the barter was foolish and the lawsuit was even more ill considered. Woody comes to the conclusion that bartering should be avoided, despite his providing guidelines for bartering. Since Woody is both an attorney and a psychologist, it is not surprising that he errs on the side of caution. But there is no evidence presented as to what percentage of the time bartering situations go awry. My guess is that bartering happens far more than is admitted and that the vast majority of the situations are benign, with no ill effects. Professionals get themselves into jams when they do not think through the pros and cons and subsequently mishandle the arrangement.

What is disturbing about Woody's article is that he opens it by discussing the fact that since many people cannot afford therapy in the current era of managed care, bartering might be considered. He goes over all of the problems of getting involved with bartering but has no solution for the poor person who cannot afford therapy. He then advises the therapist not to engage in this kind of arrangement. What happens to the prospective patient, besides being told that the therapist cannot see them because of a remote possibility of a lawsuit? Where are the values that psychotherapy professes? Woody offers no solution, leaves the therapist helpless, and the patient adrift—an arid solution, and ultimately irresponsible.

In an article by Marcia Hill (1999), however, much more discussion is given to trying to help poor people who need therapy. Bartering is considered a viable, if cautious, alternative. This article is one of the most sympathetic articles about bartering. Hill writes about barter in the context of feminist therapy, and she is one of the few to deal extensively with the fact that many people needing or wanting therapy may simply not have the money. Hill reviews the pros and cons, as well as going over in some detail the considerations as to whether one would engage in a barter arrangement in the first place. For example, she and Lazarus (1994) would agree that getting involved in dual relationships with borderline or histrionic patients is best avoided. If the barter appears to reach a "threshold of consideration," then other concerns emerge. These could be whether one is bartering goods or services, with the latter being inherently more problematic because providing services suggests a new relationship, which is commercial and evaluative.

In addition, Hill (1999) explores whether the particular relationship is appropriate for barter, whether there is a power differential, which may end up tilting the barter too much in favor of the therapist, thereby increasing the potential for exploitation. She also discusses a number of psychodynamic considerations, such as transference and the possible symbolic aspects of such arrangement. I would recommend any professional considering bartering with a patient to study this article, because she discusses a number of issues in detail; reviewing these could save a therapist a great deal of discomfort.

The Koocher and Keith-Spiegel book *Ethics in Psychology* (1998) has a chapter entitled "Multiple Role Relationships and Conflicts of Interest," and there is a section on bartering. For some reason, these authors insist on giving silly names to all of the (asserted) true stories of ethical violations reported to the APA and state licensing boards. For example, a psychologist named Alan Groupie went into business with a famous rock star and billed him $150 per hour for 24 hours a day, 7 days a week. It is as if Koocher and Keith-Spiegel were treating as a joke that psychologists sometimes act stupidly or end up with ruined careers. The problem is that these bizarre and presumably true stories are the foundations for those writing the ethics code. Besides Koocher and Keith-Spiegel's bad taste (or conflict of grammar), however, the conclusions reflect mainline APA (1992) Ethics Code reasoning. I wonder if there is another side to these bizarre stories? To base a code of ethics code around extremely untoward stories is unreasonable and is ultimately patronizing to our entire profession.

ETHICAL AND PRACTICAL ISSUES IN BARTERING

1. *The Patient's Welfare Prevails.* Much of the rhetoric about dual relationships is concerned with the exploitation of the patient by the therapist. If this is viewed from another angle, so that the therapist holds to the higher standard of the patient's welfare, then the issue of exploitation is solved. Within the ethical guidelines is the *higher standard*, and that is the meat of our code. If this is not kept in perspective, we invite problems.

2. *That Help Exists.* One issue I have rarely seen raised in our professional ethical principles is whether bartering allows services to be provided at all. In the case of George, the services would not have otherwise been available, because the treatment I was able to provide is relatively obscure. There are additional caveats in modern psychotherapy practices: Besides insurance companies not approving innovative treatments, more and more practitioners are refusing to deal with insurance companies. Bartering is one avenue of providing help outside the insurance reimbursement system for the less affluent.

3. *A Well-Lit Room.* Haas and Malouf (1989, cited in Hill, 1999) have used an illuminating analogy about the prospect of bartering with a patient for psychotherapy. Their phrase conveys the principle that this arrangement should be able to be scrutinized by one's colleagues in "a well-lit room." This honesty with yourself might help shape your decisions and guide your prospective bartering situation.

4. *Review the Dilemma with the Patient.* We can assume that the initial stage of embarking on bartering arrangement is benign and that the

patient is eager to move forward in such an arrangement. Go over the basic issues in creating a barter arrangement, and create a written contract. Specify in the contract a regular period of time in which to review the agreement, particularly in terms of hours spent (my preference) by each party. People sometimes forget their arrangements and tend to let certain matters slide. Having the barter arrangement as part of the therapy, to whatever extent, is an interesting and potentially powerful way to get extra therapeutic mileage out of the arrangement.

5. *Document the Arrangement.* A good way to protect one's self is to make notes about the bartering and discuss the situation at regular intervals with the patient. *These notes go directly in the chart.* Documenting not only helps make the agreement clear, but also could help us defend ourselves if this becomes necessary.

CONCLUSION

Bartering is still a troublesome topic. This chapter has explored some of the potential advantages and disadvantages. This topic confronts us as to where we stand in our contribution to society, specifically helping those who cannot ordinarily afford our services. Our stance in this matter points to our professional character, and asks us if we are doing the right thing. Our Ethics Code (APA, 1992) should support us, not make us to turn away those in need. Thus, some reexamination of the underlying values and implications is needed in our Ethics Code so that the higher standard is the focus.

REFERENCES

American Psychological Association. (1992). Ethical principles of psychologists and code of conduct. *American Psychologist, 47,* 1597–1611.

Canter, M., Bennett, B., Jones, S., & Nagy, T. (1994). *Ethics for psychologists.* Washington, DC: American Psychological Association.

Evans, J., & Abarbanel, A. (1999). *Quantitative EEG and neurofeedback.* San Diego, CA: Academic Press.

Haas, L. J., & Malouf, J. L. (1989). *Keeping up the good work: A practitioner's guide to mental health ethics.* Sarasota, FL: Professional Resources Exchange.

Hartman, D. E. (1988). *Neuropsychological toxicology.* New York: Pergamon.

Hill, M. (1999). Barter: Ethical considerations in psychotherapy. *Women and Therapy, 22* (3), 81–91.

Koocher, G., & Keith-Spiegel, P. (1998). *Ethics in psychology.* New York: Oxford University Press.

Lazarus, A. (1994). How certain boundaries and ethics diminish therapeutic effectiveness. *Ethics and Behavior, 4,* 253–261.

Rappoport, P. S. (1983). *Value for value psychotherapy.* New York: Praeger.

Robbins, J. (2000). *A symphony in the brain.* New York: Atlantic Monthly Press.

Sonne, J. (1994). Multiple relationships: Does the new ethics code answer the right questions? *Professional Psychology: Research and Practice, 25* (4), 336–343.

Thomas, J. L., Cummings, N. A., & O'Donohue, W. (Eds.). (2002). *The entrepreneur in psychology.* Phoenix, AZ: Zeig, Tucker & Theisen.

Woody, R. H. (1998). Bartering for psychological services. *Professional Psychology: Research and Practice, 29* (2), 174–178.

CHAPTER 28

Authorization to Continue

A Posttermination Friendship Evolves

Marjorie Goldin, DSW

Exploring boundary issues has evolved from the broader field of applied and professional ethics. Reamer (2001) distinguishes between boundary violations, wherein the key feature is a conflict of interest that harms clients or colleagues, and boundary crossings, wherein a human service professional enters a dual relationship or crosses traditional boundaries in a manner that is not exploitative, manipulative, deceptive, or coercive but in fact helpful to the client. Boundary violations can involve a breach of ethical standards, while boundary crossings are not inherently unethical. Appropriately handled, boundary crossings, such as judicious self-disclosure, attending a graduation, or consoling a bereaved client with a hug, are helpful (Ramsdell & Ramsdell, 1993).

Dual relationships can be problematic from both an ethical, as well as practice point of view, because role conflict sets up disequilibrium (Corey, Corey, & Callahan, 1988; Kitchener, 1988). A therapeutic relationship involves client vulnerability and practitioner influence, partly because of its uniqueness and partly because it is a fiduciary relationship. When a client and professional enter a second relationship, the dynamics of the therapeutic relationship potentially continue to dominate and the people involved may be under an illusion that they are defining the second relationship around different roles and rules (Kagle & Giebelhausen, 1994).

This issue remains controversial, but some practitioners are going beyond removing the prohibition against dual relationships to advocate continuation after therapy if there is mutual consent between those involved. For this practice to occur, a careful assessment of motives and the potential negative effect on the specific people who will be involved is required. But doing so can provide unique knowledge of the client, facilitate better health and healing by decreasing isolation, and increase treatment outcomes (Lazarus, 2001; Zur, 2001). Within the past 12 years, studies began to appear reporting that more than 20% of respondents in the mental health field acknowledged developing a friendship with a client (Borys, 1988; Jayaratne, Croxton, & Mattison, 1997; Pope, Tabachnick, & Keith-Speigel, 1987; Salisbury & Kinnier, 1996) and equivalent numbers considered this behavior professionally appropriate and ethical.

This chapter is an accounting of my personal experience with crossing therapeutic boundaries. My former patient and I, both women at midlife, did not preplan or spend much time discussing a journey of this kind. Earlier decisions throughout led to the next logical later ones until ending our contact didn't really appear to be an option. I would argue, in fact, that ending it would have been contraindicated. Over time our relationship became more social, our lives more intertwined, and as the professional work wound down it evolved, almost as if predestined, into a posttermination friendship that continues to this day. The descriptive material will show a sampling of how exceptions were made to several commonly accepted clinical ideas and methods during the treatment, followed by the theoretical rationale for doing so. Although unorthodox in many respects, this is the story of a singular therapeutic success, one that resulted in a strengthened patient with an enhanced life and marriage.

In more than 25 years of clinical practice, I had never before attempted to modify the professional contract and become friends, despite many invitations from other patients to do so. If I had thought about it, I would have described myself as a therapist who "played by the rules." Yet more recent closer examination has made me question this self-view. Social work has a rich tradition of practice outside a consultation room. Throughout my career I have made home, hospital, and school visits, collaborated with members of other service delivery systems and involved clients with them, participated in advocacy of all kinds, and once went to a client's funeral.

Although colleagues who have walked this path may have a different tale to tell, I found that supporting conversions of professional relationships into friendship is easier in the abstract than actually attempting it. Against a backdrop of perceived distain, and without prior role models, considerable effort was required on my part for the professional structure to fall away. I had difficulty discontinuing my counseling role, and I revisited basic questions about the differences between listening to other people as a friend and as a professional that I had not addressed since the earliest days of my clinical training. Furthermore, I believed the closeness of the therapeutic encounter could not only continue, but become two way. For this to happen, I intended to balance the dynamics between us such that she would come to know more about me. However, once the patient role was thrown off, she demonstrated that she wanted a different style of relationship. Expectations had to change, adjustments had to be made, and hurt feelings assuaged. Ultimately, this is the very human story of women's friendships, their complexities, disappointments, and triumphs.

THE JOURNEY TO FRIENDSHIP

Vanessa,[1] age 46 and an only child, presented for treatment in a debilitating major depression several weeks after the unexpected death of her father. To further complicate the clinical picture, Vanessa's mother, Ethel, was suffering from a severe reaction to the loss of her husband of more than 50 years. Her parent's marriage had been dependent and symbiotic in nature. Because it operated to the exclusion of other ordinary social systems, there were no close friends and few relatives that could act as a safety net. Consequently, the dependence Ethel had had on her husband instantly shifted to her daughter upon his death. Vanessa, struggling to survive in an unhappy marriage and reeling from her own grief, could not tolerate the burden of being heavily leaned on by her mother.

Furthermore, the preceding several years had been riddled with other stressors. These included a breast cancer diagnosis requiring a lumpectomy, 6 months of chemotherapy, and radiation treatments. Lymph nodes were cancer-free and the prognosis was positive; however, illness seemed to stalk her as many acquaintances and extended family members suffered relapses and deaths. These incidents of bad news

---

[1]Although this piece was written with the permission of those involved, names and identities have been changed to protect privacy.

were always taken with great difficulty and with a renewed fear that she would be next.

Coping with the loss of her father would have been enough of a task, but after returning from the cemetery she was contacted by a technician at the radiologist's office saying her most recent mammogram was "suspicious." In the days following, grief and fear combined their assault, despite the fact that the physicians reassured her they were only seeing scar tissue. She became unable to function at work and required a 1-year disability leave from her employer.

In her childhood home love was commingled with teasing and sarcastic humor, the kind that many adults use with an overriding intent to convey affection. Vanessa did not know how to respond or defend herself. Additionally, while her mom was attentive, she was not empathic, and Vanessa's signals of hurt and insecurity went largely unnoticed. With no one aware when she was in pain, she began to feel unlovable and did not grow fully strong. Being raised within a solid marriage should have instilled security and self-reliance. But because her parents were so wrapped up in each other she felt like an outsider in her own family, which was not fertile ground for developing self-worth. From this beginning has often come a harbored sense of inadequacy and feeling unsure, even in situations where she should have been confident, such as at work.

Throughout her lifetime Vanessa has found relationships painful and unsatisfactory. From elementary school forward the responses she got from others seemed mysterious and unpredictable. In a repeat of her position in the family, she often found herself on the periphery of social circles, wishing to be included more. Kind-hearted and compassionate, she tried hard to establish connections but could not sustain them. When successful at maintaining a few long-term friendships, she did so from afar, always expecting to be hurt.

Vanessa's parents believed they were instilling strength in her when they took the position that they would never give her anything she could obtain for herself. However, as a young child that philosophy backfired when she came to the conclusion that the world was a place where people might claim to love you but couldn't always be counted on to be there for you. Because her early experience lacked sufficient maternal attunement, and attempts at even asking for comfort from other people didn't work, by adulthood she had learned to stifle her feelings and was reluctant to share either her material or her emotional needs. But a repetitive pattern emerged as resentment would build when problems were not addressed, and, at a later time, no longer able to hold back, she would become explosive.

When I first began working with Vanessa, the depth of the depression was a serious concern. There was suicidal ideation without intent or plan, and I was able to obtain authorization from the insurance company to meet with her twice weekly. A course of antidepressant medication was prescribed and monitored by a psychiatrist but did not offer much relief. She worried about "going over the edge" and needing hospitalization.

Our first year together was fairly routine. At regular appointments in my office we addressed the overlaying major depression as the initial focus of the treatment. Vanessa had almost no source of comfort or satisfaction anywhere in her life. But our working alliance, that sense of teamwork between client and professional, was in place almost from the beginning. She developed a strong positive transference with me and responded well to the safety and support offered by the therapy. Likewise, I felt an immediate rapport with her and vowed to myself I would do whatever it took to erase the look of misery in her eyes.

Hers were the most powerfully expressive eyes I had ever seen. When she looked at me I had the sensation that if she could shrink down small and crawl into my lap, she would have. I began strongly reacting to that profound and penetrating look with a powerful and maternal interest to take care of her and protect her.

Because of our unusual bond, early on ordinary boundaries became flexible. Her phone calls to me between sessions became more frequent and lengthy, especially during times of high emotion, and I never set a limit as to how long I would be willing to listen, giving her unrestricted access to me.

During the second year, as the mourning process progressed, the depression continued to lift. We decided she no longer needed twice-weekly therapy and the focus began to shift to the stress in the marriage. I had been heavily involved working on the problems in her life by conducting individual sessions with both her and her husband, now adding conjoint marital sessions as well. I felt confident that if Vanessa were in emotional trouble she would contact me. Coincidentally, when Vanessa went back to work she was assigned to an office near where I was consulting in a clinical program. After we heard the good news that she had been found capable of resuming employment, I invited her to celebrate by having lunch at the local diner.

We both knew that scheduling future sessions would be a challenge. Evening appointments were the most likely possibility but would be a hardship because of her problems driving in the dark. As a solution we made the unusual decision together to continue having weekly appointments at the diner during her lunch hour, even though doing so made me feel like a misbehaving child.

What made me feel like that? I knew that one can be taught the fundamentals of personality organization, psychodynamics, treatment techniques, and the basic helping process, but in many respects psychotherapy is an art form. Each clinician brings their own style and personality to the work, as well as clinical judgment derived from training, years of further study, and self-monitoring. As the therapist listens, he or she learns what material to respond to in a session and when to intervene. With experience one becomes better able to listen and think simultaneously so that the chosen interventions will be most effective. In the last analysis, knowing what to say and when is intuition, based naturally on knowledge of the particular individual and their circumstance and theory. Like snowflakes or fingerprints, no two patients or their situations are ever exactly alike, each offering their own challenges. Meeting with Vanessa in the diner seemed exactly right to me.

Conducting psychotherapy sessions in a diner is different, to say the least. It is harder to focus in such a public place, and some people might feel inhibited discussing personal matters in that informal environment. I never really questioned whether or not what Vanessa chose to discuss was affected by our location. Had we eavesdropped on conversations in other booths, I felt sure that we would have heard much the same topics being discussed by any other two women.

As time went by, these lunches started extending past the traditional 50 minutes. Our conversations began straying beyond the strictly therapeutic, as we talked about mundane life and I started participating more, inaugurating a transition away from the one-sidedness of psychotherapy. I was enjoying her company, and we began to shift into a "hybrid" relationship, one that was partly friendship and partly professional. Just after 2 years from when we met, our professional relationship came to an official end.

Beyond our comfort with each another, perhaps the most striking quality about our relationship was Vanessa's innate ability to "read" my thoughts. Almost from the start, Vanessa was able to see into my spirit, even before I made any efforts to expose it. Likewise, I knew her so well that I could anticipate her reactions and also "read" her. Occasionally she would startle me with her insights, and she could always recognize a bogus statement no matter how well I tried to disguise it. Always very direct and precise about her observations, she'd tell me how I was feeling and I'd think 'has this woman crawled inside my thoughts?' Not even friends of long-standing could do that with me as accurately as

Vanessa, and that was the most tangible thing about my increasing commitment to the friendship. While initially I felt uneasy with this ability, I later came to both respect and expect it, experiencing pressure to be completely honest with her at all times and encouraging me to share more with her. The sensation of being "known," a rare ingredient between people, is almost like seeing a rainbow.

After we instituted regular meetings at the diner, we gradually became more embedded in each other's extended families. Vanessa rented the vacant apartment attached to her home to my son, and I began advising her daughter on a job search. I informally met with Vanessa's mother to help her make some lifestyle decisions. We began exchanging holiday cards and gifts.

As the friendship moved forward and matured, certain other changes became evident. Whereas Vanessa hadn't hesitated to call me at all hours of the day or night when she was my client, as my friend, she seemed reluctant to reach out, taking a more formal approach. It seems that we each held different versions and expectations for our friendship. Ultimately, I had to learn to love her differently and withdraw some of my energy away from the relationship. It almost felt as if I had had to develop a relationship with another Vanessa, someone quite different from the woman who initially consulted me.

THEORETICAL CONSIDERATIONS

As one might do desensitizing a phobic patient, for example, many of the boundary crossings were not preplanned as part of a treatment plan per se. Decisions were made as the circumstances dictated based on the following clinical realities.

Failure to Develop Self-Soothing Techniques

Vanessa's parents did not intend to hurt her, but from her perspective she grew up in an emotionally impoverished environment, which left her vulnerable to feelings of insecurity, abandonment, exclusion, and rejection. She typically responded to emotional situations with one overwhelming uncomfortable distress, an inner experience she described as "drowning." These powerful feelings, which initially she was unable to accurately identify and compartmentalize in herself, were always close to the surface and could be triggered easily. What appeared to others as anger were her attempts to soothe herself and call attention to her pain. Unfortunately, often just when she needed the most shoring up, other people felt the most like recoiling. In therapy, she learned to recognize and talk about the specific underlying effect and find comfort when upset, working hard at finding the "Band-Aids" in her life that would help stop the emotional bloodshed.

The decision to conduct weekly sessions in a diner gratified important empathic needs. Convenient to both our daytime schedules, continuing lunch appointments was a logical choice for someone with poor night vision once she returned to work and provided me with another avenue to demonstrate valuable support. Evening appointments would have been difficult, if not impossible. While not common practice, therapeutic work with clients outside an office setting is not unheard of (Peck, 1978; Lazarus, 2001) but not universally recommended.

In many ways psychotherapy is a "corrective emotional experience," a "developmental second chance" (Greenberg & Mitchell, 1983). Patients can examine early deficits or interpersonal impasses that are problematic in current-day relationships or have an opportunity to repair faulty or poorly developed ego apparatuses. This growth-inducing process is sometimes described as a form of reparenting. At the basis of this construct is the notion that if there is to be healing, then the patient must receive at least a portion of the genuine love, commitment, listening, and exercise of power with humility of which they have been deprived. The "good enough therapist," like the "good enough mother," is being most effective when he or she is attuned to and aware of the patient's authentic needs and feelings (Glickauf-Hughes & Wells, 1997). At times, crossing traditional boundaries is part of what a "good enough therapist" does. Occurring throughout the therapeutic process as the clinician reacts to manifestations of the true self, these experiences begin to help the patient extend them beyond the therapy (Molnos, 1998).

Countertransference

Although my feelings toward Vanessa as a person were caring and warm, from the classic psychoanalytic position, an argument could be made that I had countertransference problems that compromised my ability to work with her. Those who would study this "case" and make such a statement would be implying that my feelings for her were somehow a detriment. They would say that not setting better limits, crossing several traditional boundaries, and establishing dual relationships were thera-peutic errors. This understanding of countertransference holds that the therapist's unconscious has an excessive libidinal (positive) or aggressive (negative) emotional response toward the patient or the patient's trans-ference. Originally regarded as reflecting deficits in the personality of the treating professional, today we understand that the responses of the professional toward the patient cannot be removed from the helping process. Far from being undesirable, these unavoidable feelings become an important source of diagnostic information.

Significantly, the issue of the therapist's feelings for the patient and the importance of boundary crossings have filtered into movies, such as the 1997 film *Good Will Hunting* and the popular literature. In his best-selling book entitled *The Road Less Traveled* (1978), Dr. M. Scott Peck, a psychotherapist, explores love and the concept that therapists reach beyond themselves and take action on behalf of their patients. Far from describing love as a limiting manifestation of positive counter-transference, he takes the position that love is an essential ingredient of the therapeutic alliance and belongs there. I would argue that my strong positive feelings for Vanessa, the boundary crossings, and the dual relationship were ultimately an essential significant factor in the outcome, as I offered her relatedness based on honesty and commit-ment. Our bond became a prototype for what it feels like to trust and be trusted, resolve conflict and be safe.

Establishing and Continuing the Friendship

The friendship between Vanessa and I evolved over time as the relation-ship became more social. Once begun, it gained momentum and we became increasingly involved in each other's extended family. A mutu-ally acceptable arrangement, after the professional relationship officially ended with the discontinuance of insurance payments, there was no question that the relationship would continue. Despite the changes and adaptations that took place over time, continuing our contact cemented and enhanced the therapeutic gains.

Ongoing healthy bonds with other people are emotionally and physi-cally essential for us. While this statement seems basic enough, in some ways it contradicts the position that the path of human relatedness to others begins with emotional dependence or symbiosis and proceeds through various stages to internal psychological and personal indepen-dence. Emanating from the Stone Center of Wellesley College, a quiet theoretical revolution has been taking place as a group of women led by Jean Baker Miller (Jordan, Kaplan, Miller, Stiver, & Surrey, 1991) have been meeting since the late 1970s to reassess prevailing theories. Their papers, contained in *Women's Growth in Connection* (1991) and *Toward a New Psychology of Women* (Miller, 1976) and further developed in *The Healing Connection* (Miller & Stiver, 1997), examine a new way of looking at emotional development, especially that of women, and calling it "self in relation" theory.

"Self in relation" theory suggests that the child becomes differentiated from others and establishes object constancy but at the same time becomes more connected. It is not increasing autonomy but a dynamic process of connection with a person who is involved with them in an ongoing relationship that builds a future adult who is self-reliant, yet attached to friends, family, and community in a healthy manner (Berzoff, 1989; Jordan et al., 1991). An additional vast body of literature contends that women's friendships satisfy emotional hunger, contribute to their well-being, and even support their marriages (see, for example, Eichenbaum & Orbach, 1988; Isaacs, 1999; Oliker, 1989; Rubin, 1985).

The thinking of the Stone Center study group fits a unique niche that modifies and extends object relations theory, especially as it relates to the development of women. They are questioning the ways in which we can be intimate with significant others if it is true that all our developmental tasks are essentially striving along the path toward separation and individuation, the opposite of true intimacy (Miller & Stiver, 1997). Important questions arise from this "central relational paradox" when one tries to apply theory to practice. In situations such as my work with Vanessa, where a treatment focus is on establishing and maintaining relationships, the therapist becomes significant as a person who is authentically present and participating with the client. We foster an investment in a caring bond, and from within it emerges the tools to examine, improve, and cultivate other relationships. Perhaps the greatest paradox of all is that we encourage patients to form connections with us, their therapists, when we know we intend, by and large, to one day end these very connections.

CONCLUSION

With the luxury of retrospect, what conclusions can be drawn? With a structured approach and traditional limit setting, Vanessa would have ultimately become less depressed and would likely have discontinued her sessions when she felt better and was able to return to work. She would probably have used this episode of therapy as many people do, to get past a crisis and return if another crisis were to occur. According to many definitions, she would have done well and the therapy would have been considered a treatment success. Not "brief treatment" in the sense that managed care insurance likes to see, but it would have nonetheless fit their medical model framework. However, I do not believe the fundamental shifts in how she feels about herself and the ways in which she handles her life that are evident today, would be present. There would have been no forum to address her emotional hyperreactivity, to slowly and steadily show her the benefits of identifying one's inner feelings, and to find constructive ways to self-soothe. She would not have learned to be more trusting. Her newfound stability, self-assurance, strength, and ability to more effectively protect herself and problem solve would not have been accomplished. From the insurance company perspective, the goal of reducing depression and returning her to work would have been demonstrated. But the quality of her life, the more subtle changes, would not have happened.

Also, I believe it is questionable whether Vanessa and Bob's marriage would be intact at this time. Because I never lost hope, I often played the role of cheerleader. Left more to their own, many of Vanessa and Bob's fires would have burned out of control and the rickety building that was their marriage would have been a heap of charred remains, even though it stood on a decent foundation. Not that I helped them put out all the fires, but what I offered was a never-ending supply of firefighting equipment of all kinds, and often this led to less damage. No matter what, I encouraged them both to keep working, and keep trying. I was determined not to stop until I found a way to help them successfully stay together. Vanessa often spoke of having fed off of my hope for them. This hope was a sustaining element.

On the other hand, I would say that this level of relating had a downside for me. Caring about Vanessa so much was often costly, as I suffered with her when she was suffering. Many was the night when I lay awake wondering how I could be more helpful, wondering how to handle the many "wars from hell" that arose between her and her husband, second guessing myself and wondering if somehow I could have done something differently. I felt the heavy responsibility of my pivotal role in her life and marriage and it often preoccupied my thoughts. I never denied her and Bob the attention they needed, often at the expense of my own time. In the same way as one would tend to a sick child, I often stayed on the phone or in Vanessa's presence for long periods of time. I did not offer what I could not, or would not, be willing to do, reserving the right to say no to her, something I rarely did. This intense level of support, done consistently and willingly, was the water that put out many superficial fires and was the yarn that slowly and steadily began to knit together the gaping holes in her spirit and soul.

Generalizing to other therapist–former patient friendship pairs is tempting but impossible. I would predict that the problems I had shedding my role might be universal. Though there are similar elements, therapy is a very different manner of listening, commenting, and relating than is friendship. Attempting this conversion would likely have different characteristics with a client who has a different friendship style than Vanessa, however. Some day this will make an interesting study.

So how does this story turn out in the end? In a beautiful contemporary home near the Gulf of Mexico, Vanessa has continued to redefine herself. The ragefulness that was once always so ready to boil over has all but disappeared. Vanessa's new approach to herself and to life has not only helped to improve the quality of her marriage, but also her relationships with the rest of her family as well. Now a grandmother, Vanessa derives great pleasure from a new purpose in her life.

Bob works hard at not overreacting in highly charged situations and tries to ensure that Vanessa feels like she is "number one" in his life. Their marriage no longer represents the ongoing clashing of two fiery people. For all intents and purposes they are living happily-ever-after. A work in progress, Vanessa and Bob continue to grow together to build the solid partnership they both wanted so much.

Today there is an ongoing unbreakable link between Vanessa and me, and we are permanent fixtures in each other's lives. By the effort of extending my limits, love became visible and tangible. Her growth, while simultaneously taking her emotionally further from me, has been a source of personal and professional satisfaction. It is not the relationship I thought it could be, but I now accept its limitations. She is unrecognizable from the beaten-down, temperamental, and depressed woman who came into my life as my patient. I am proud of her and what we have done together, easily the most powerful yet greatest accomplishment of my career. Truly we were involved in "mutual empathy" as per the Stone Center view. In the process a marriage was saved, and both of us were enlarged. I look forward to sharing all that lies ahead with her, whatever that is, the good stuff and the not-so-good. Because we are friends now and that is what friends do for each other.

REFERENCES

Berzoff, J. (1989). The therapeutic value of women's adult friendships. *Smith College Studies in Social Work, 59* (3), 267–279.

Borys, D. S. (1988). *Dual relationships between therapists and clients: A national survey of clinicians' attitudes and practices.* Unpublished doctoral dissertation, UCLA. UMI #8810892.

Corey, G., Corey, M. S., & Callahan, P. (1988). *Issues and ethics in the helping professions* (3rd ed.). Pacific Grove, CA: Brooks/Cole.

Eichenbaum, L., & Orbach, S. (1988). *Between women.* New York: Viking Press.

Glickauf-Hughes, C., & Wells, M. (1997). *Object relations psychotherapy: An individualized and interactive approach to diagnosis and treatment.* Northvale, NJ: Jason Aronson.

Greenberg, J. R., & Mitchell, S. A. (1983). *Object relations in psychoanalytic theory.* Cambridge, MA: Harvard University Press.

Isaacs, F. (1999). *Toxic friends/true friends: How friends can make or break your health, happiness, family and career.* New York: W. Morrow.

Jayaratne, S., Croxton, T., & Mattison, D. (1997). Social work professional standards: An exploratory study. *Social Work, 42* (2), 187–199.

Jordan, J. V., Kaplan, A. G., Miller, J. B., Stiver, I. P., & Surrey, J. L. (1991). *Women's growth in connection: Writings from the stone center.* New York: The Guilford Press.

Kagle, J. D., & Giebelhausen, P. N. (1994). Dual relationships and professional boundaries. *Social Work, 39* (2), 213–220.

Kitchener, K. S. (1988). Dual relationships: What makes them so problematic? *Journal of Counseling and Development, 67,* 217–221.

Lazarus, A. A. (2001). Not all 'dual relationships' are taboo; some tend to enhance treatment outcomes. *The National Psychologist.* Retrieved February 4, 2001, from http://nationalpsychologist.com/articles/art_v9n7_1.htm

Miller, J. B. (1976). *Toward a new psychology of women.* Boston: Beacon Press.

Miller, J. B., & Stiver, I. P. (1997). *The healing connection: How women form relationships in therapy and in life.* Boston: Beacon Press.

Molnos, A. (1998) *A psychotherapist's harvest.* Unpublished manuscript.

Oliker, S. J. (1989). *Best friends and marriage: Exchange among women.* Berkeley, CA: University of California Press.

Peck, M. S. (1978). *The road less traveled.* New York: Simon and Schuster.

Pope, K. S., Tabachnick, B., & Keith-Spiegel, P. (1987). Ethics of practice: The beliefs and behaviors of psychologists as therapists. *American Psychologist, 42,* 993–1006.

Ramsdell, P. S., & Ramsdell, E. R. (1993). Dual relationships: Client perceptions of the effect of client-counselor relationship on the therapeutic process. *Clinical Social Work Journal, 21* (2), 195–212.

Reamer, F. G. (2001). *Tangled relationships: Managing boundary issues in the human services.* New York: Columbia University Press.

Rubin, L. (1985). *Just friends: The role of friendship in our lives.* New York: Harper and Row.

Salisbury, W. A., & Kinnier, R. T. (1996). Posttermination friendship between counselors and clients. *Journal of Counseling and Development, 74,* 495–500.

Zur, O. (2001). Out-of-office experience: When crossing office boundaries and engaging in dual relationships are clinically beneficial and ethically sound. *Independent Practitioner, 21* (1), 96–100.

Feminist Perspective on Dual Relationships

Part 8 outlines how the feminist perspective emphasizes *connections* as the basis of personal empowerment and almost mandates, when appropriate, a type of relationship in which the therapist must cross traditional boundaries and engage in authentic dual relationships with clients. In chapter 29, Greenspan provides a powerful critique of therapists as authoritative distanced experts and the misuse of the term "boundaries" to justify the culturally based, masculine bias in therapy. She emphasizes the importance of compassion, trust, and safe connection to facilitate healing. Next, Walker (chapter 30) presents a series of challenging vignettes in which boundary crossings by the therapist seem essential for the effective therapy with victims of domestic violence, abuse, and other traumas.

CHAPTER 29

Out of Bounds

Miriam Greenspan, MEd, LMHC

A client in psychotherapy tells me that her father repeatedly sexually molested her as a young child, explaining that he had a "problem with boundaries." Another woman informs me that both of her children were the result of marital rape; she describes her husband—a violent alcoholic who battered her—as a man who "violated" her "boundaries." A brochure put out by the Massachusetts House of Representatives Committee on Sexual Misconduct is called "Broken Boundaries: Sexual Misconduct by Physicians, Therapists, and Other Health Professionals."

It seems that everywhere you look, the psychotherapy world is buzzing with talk about boundaries. The term is used by patients and therapists alike, by incest survivors and self-diagnosed "codependents," by psychoanalysts and radical feminists, by individual and family therapists. In this language, good boundaries make for healthy, safe relationships; in therapy, they keep the relationship ethical by creating a safety zone of distance between patient and therapist. Poor boundaries lead to physical, emotional, sexual, or spiritual abuse.

The phrase "poor boundaries" is used to describe all manner of professional conduct and misconduct—from the social worker who hugs a client at the door to the doctor who rapes a patient he has drugged. Just as smoking marijuana is believed by some to be a step on the road

Reprinted by permission. Greenspan, M. (1995). Out of bounds. *Common Boundary Magazine*, July/August, 51–58.

to serious drug addiction, so even the smallest boundary erosion—for example, going over the limits of the sacred 50-minute hour—may be viewed as a temptation that moves the therapist in the direction of overtly abusive boundary violation.

The image of secure boundaries contains an inviolable principle: that of the right to one's own integrity—including the rights to be respected, to defend oneself against exploitation or harm, and to speak out when harm has occurred. But while everyone would agree we need an ethic of nonabuse for professional relationships, the question of whether or not the language of boundaries helps promote such an ethic is debatable. How does the language of boundaries help us understand the complex psychological, ethical, and political dimensions of abuse in psychotherapy? How does it muddle the issues?

To my mind, the language of boundaries is problematic at best. The most serious problem is that it psychologizes the social dimensions of interpersonal violence both in and out of therapy. Both the perpetrators and the victims are viewed as suffering from a psychological impediment that impairs their ability to maintain their border zones. Perpetrators are prone to invading the borders of others; victims have trouble protecting their borders from these onslaughts. By this logic, if only fathers in families would firm up their boundaries, they wouldn't rape or molest their daughters. And if only helping professionals would tighten up their boundaries, they wouldn't sexually abuse their female patients.

The truth is that sexual exploitation and violation in families and in therapy are more than simple lapses in judgment. In the majority of cases, acts of sexual abuse perpetrated by male professionals against female patients exist on a spectrum of male violence against women in general. These acts are particularly likely to occur in relationships with a power hierarchy that replicates the gender hierarchy of our society. Incest in the father-daughter relationship and sex abuse in the therapist-patient relationship are mirrors of each other not because of what therapists call transference and countertransference but because both of these social units—the family and traditional therapy—are patriarchal. That is, they are relationships based on the dominant social power of masculine authority. The language of boundaries, wittingly or unwittingly, camouflages the political dimension of violence against women and dilutes the strong feminist analysis that brought to light the abuses now called "boundary violations."

Personally, I have always chafed at the language of boundaries. The imagery of relationships with hard borders between enclosed individuals does not make me feel safe. On the contrary, it brings up feelings of isolation, exclusion, and disconnection. Perhaps the language of boundaries has little emotional appeal for me because as a child of Holocaust survivors, born and raised for 4 years in a German camp for "displaced persons" after World War II, I experienced boundaries as the borders that kept my family and thousands of other refugees from entering safer havens. For me, the imagery of interconnection, not separation, feels safe.

Boundaries do not exist in reality; we use the imagery of boundaries to help us understand the relation between self and other. But in the helping professions, the language of boundaries has come to dominate the way we think and practice. In recent years, for instance, the "boundaries police" have been installed in the form of increasingly rigid standards on the part of malpractice insurers, boards of licensure, review boards, and professional organizations. In my own practice, I worry that some of the most feminist and innovative aspects of my work are the most likely to be construed as unethical. For example, I am a great believer in the art of therapist self-disclosure as a way of deconstructing the isolation and shame that people experience in an individualistic and emotion-fearing culture. When strict boundaries are used as the litmus test of professional ethical behavior, this art—and therapist authenticity in general—can appear dangerous.

This situation reflects the hegemony of what I call the "distance model"—the reigning psychodynamic paradigm of psychotherapy. In this model, the less the therapist contaminates the therapeutic process with his presence, the better. Distance is enshrined; connection is seen as inherently tainted and untrustworthy. The danger zone is thought to reside in any manner of person-to-person touching—physical, emotional, or spiritual—that might take place in the therapy relationship. In my training, one expert in marital therapy taught us that the therapist should take notes and inform his patients to behave as though he weren't there—as though his absence, rather than his presence, would facilitate their "cure."

But what makes us think that the therapist's absence is more objective than his presence? That emotional withdrawal is more neutral than contact? That distance is more trustworthy than connection? The answer in two words: scientism and patriarchy.

The most appealing quality of the distance model is its appearance of objectivity, which makes it attractive to those who would like therapy to have the absolute authority of hard science. This approach enshrines the cult of the "Expert," whose superior knowledge and power bring cure to the inherently defective, disordered, or sick patient. But the so-called scientific, value-free objectivity of the Expert is, on inspection, the hidden bias of the dominant culture. The neutrality of the Expert is the silent embodiment of our culture's fundamental and unquestioned assumptions.

One such assumption is the patriarchal bias against relationality and connection. The term "boundaries" itself comes from the psychoanalytic concept of "ego boundaries." In this view, the ego presumably develops its boundaries in the course of separating itself from others, starting with the earliest separation from the mother. The norm of healthy development is the attainment of the masterful, autonomous ego, with "rigid" or "firm" (like a phallus?) boundaries between itself and everyone else. Not surprisingly, male ego boundaries more often exhibit this firmness, while women (the apparently more infirm and watery second sex) tend to have more "fluid" or "permeable" ego boundaries. In keeping with the patriarchal nature of this theory, the masculine ego is posited as the norm. It is just this ego that is embodied in our standards of healthy boundaries for the psychotherapy relationship.

Once we remove ourselves from the spell of this masculine bias, we can see that there can be connection without harm, love without power abuse, touching without sexual abuse in psychotherapy—but the language of boundaries doesn't help us see our way clearly into this arena. Rather, it keeps us steeped in the patriarchal model of self—a model that has been contested not only by feminists but also by social critics, new scientists, deep ecologists, Buddhists, and mystics. For example, the Wellesley Stone Center theorists have posited a theory of women's self-development in the context of relationship and connection, not separation. Social critics such as Robert Bellah have written about the dysfunction and pathology of American individualism. Deep ecologists and ecopsychologists like Joanna Macy and Theodore Roszak have described the bounded self as an inherently embattled and conquering ego that has wrought havoc on the earth and from which we must evolve if we are to avert global ecocide. From the Buddhist point of view, the bounded ego is a profound illusion, and our true nature is, to use Thich Nhat Hanh's term, "interbeing." The imagery of boundaries fits with an entrenched Western worldview that sanctifies individualism, private property, and nationalism. The idea that relational safety resides in the defense of one's borders reflects, on a microcosmic level, the social macrocosm.

Why use a language that supports the basic delusion of Western society, that keeps us fixated in the patriarchal ego and stuck in the distance model? Why not let go of this archaic metaphor and use straightforward language to talk about ethical issues in psychotherapy? Abusive therapists don't have problems with boundaries; they have problems behaving ethically, with using their power wisely and well. Boundaries are not violated in therapy; people are. So-called boundary issues in psychotherapy are fundamentally about the misuse of power by professionals.

Ironically, the rigidification of boundaries as a response to abuse by therapists—insofar as it reinforces the distance model—may well produce more, not less, power abuse in therapy. Sexually abusive therapists, for example, in almost all cases manage to convince themselves that their behavior is in the best interests of the patient. It is not that such therapists are not aware of their power; it is that they suffer from the inbred arrogance of the Expert. They have been trained to see their power as curative—and it is just one short skip away from this belief to the belief that their *sexual* power is curative.

Since publicly challenging the distance model, I have received numerous letters and phone calls from women who have spoken eloquently and often heartbreakingly of the damage they have suffered in the course of a well-bounded professional relationship. In my practice, too, I have seen many survivors of therapy who have not been sexually victimized or exploited, whose therapists have followed the distance model to the letter, but who have experienced a particularly virulent erosion of self-esteem during the course of therapy. For these women, the distance model has been neither safe nor trustworthy; it has been a progressive experience of disempowerment that comes from years of being treated in a system that devalues and pathologizes connection.

Therapists trained in the distance model often view their intuitive inclinations toward connection in therapy as "boundary lapses." Sometimes the client's "manipulations" or "seductiveness" are blamed for these outbreaks of authenticity, leading to a kind of emotional abuse that is not likely to be named as such by professional review boards but that has devastating effects on clients nonetheless.

What we need is a clearly stated ethic of nonabuse for therapy that is not based in the language of boundaries and therefore not beholden to the distance model. The healing potential of psychotherapy has less to do with pseudo-objective distance than it does with safe connection. It is not about detached neutrality; it is about passionate but trustworthy engagement. Compassion rather than distance is the prime mover of what is healing about psychotherapy. And compassion—the willingness to identify and suffer with others—is by definition boundless; it crosses the divide between self and other. This is so for any psychotherapy, whatever the theoretical orientation; it is just that the distance model doesn't name or frame it this way.

But what makes connection safe or trustworthy? And how do we cultivate safe connection? For me, the answers are largely a matter of working within the healing paradoxes of the therapeutic situation— cultivating equality in a hierarchical relationship, mutuality in an inherently nonmutual relationship, empowerment in a power-imbalanced relationship. The therapist who sees himself as an all-knowing Expert and his client as a diagnosis is much more likely to abuse his power than the therapist who sees herself as an accountable coequal in therapy and her client as a person with an inherent wisdom that guides the therapeutic process.

A connection model of therapy requires, for starters, that therapists move away from the conditioned role of the Expert. Safe connection is about trustworthy companionship, not superior or omniscient power. And trustworthy companionship starts with an absolute and unshakable respect for the integrity of the person called patient or client.

This respect includes some very specific skills, including the skill of "active listening." This is not about listening for the preordained categories that fit our theories of the patient but rather listening with an ability to surrender one's theoretical understanding into the living presence and self-knowledge of the other person. The moment that we begin to lose sight of the patient as a person and to rely on our notions of expertise to shield us from the sometimes frightening and often exhilarating experience of human encounter in therapy, we are in the danger zone that is likely to produce abuses of power.

Another aspect of a nonabusive ethic for therapy is the fundamental principle of therapist accountability. Some of the worst emotional harm that comes to patients in traditional therapy comes from this lack of accountability, which is built into the distance model's way of interpreting patients' complaints about the therapy or the therapist as matters of transference, resistance, or pathology. If patients do not have the right to question their therapists' work without the risk of being labeled or pathologized, then therapy comes to resemble the closed and well-bounded systems we call cults.

The sanctity of the client's empowerment in therapy is another fundamental feature of safe connection in a nonabuse ethic. Respect for boundaries is meaningless if the patient's power in the psychotherapy relationship is seen as control, manipulation, or pathology. (I remember one of my superiors whose motto was "The question in therapy is who controls whom? Make sure it's you who controls the patient.") In an empowerment model, the client is credited not only with her own inherent wisdom but also with the power to control the agenda—insofar as this meshes with the basic ethics of the therapist.

Perhaps one of the most controversial issues of safe connection is the issue of safe touch in therapy. In the distance model, there is no concept of safe touch. But defining all touch as abusive is rather like considering all talk dangerous because it can lead to emotional abuse. There is no one-size-fits-all rule of safety in psychotherapy; what feels safe to one person would feel traumatizing to another. In my practice, I have a client who has asked me to touch her gently on the arm if she is in the midst of intense traumatic memories. Another client has made me swear I will not touch her. In an empowerment model of work, clients get to have the choice about these matters.

A good number of people in my practice have been emotionally abused by therapists who have blamed their clients for their own shortcoming or confusions. The safe therapist is the self-aware therapist. It is humbling to think how much power we are given in the therapeutic situation and how much we need to work continually on ourselves to use our power well. Our clients are a population at risk—coming to us when they are most vulnerable and trusting in our help. The patient's trust is not something we ought to assume; it is something we must earn. We must be clear that we are not using clients to gratify unconscious or greedy needs of our own—including needs for power or money.

While it is comforting to think that boundaries keep everyone safe, it is clear that the rigid adherence to boundaries can bring harm as well as help in therapy. Safe connection is more likely than rigid boundaries to protect clients from abuse. It is safer to see the therapist as accountable than to see the client as pathological. It is safer to value empathy for the client than to regard it with suspicion as something that makes one lose one's objectivity. The connection model is safer than the distance model. Healing happens when someone feels seen, heard, held, and empowered, not when one is interpreted, held at a distance, and pathologized. Safe connection and healing in therapy are a matter of breaking through old boundaries—including conventional divisions between self and other, patient and Expert—and embracing a more open system of interconnectedness that rests on respectful compassion.

CHAPTER 30

Feminist Ethics, Boundary Crossings, Dual Relationships, and Victims of Violence

Lenore E. A. Walker, EdD, ABPP

Maria, a 35-year-old woman had been a client for 3 years. She had originally sought psychotherapy because she wanted to end a 10-year marriage with a man who physically, sexually, and psychologically abused her. They had two young children who, she felt, made it impossible to sever their relationship. Although she found that his controlling behavior was oppressive, she could not fail to respond to whatever he ordered. Therapy progressed well and within 6 months she had instituted a separation followed by a dissolution of the marriage. She obtained sole legal custody of their children, permitting her to make whatever decisions were necessary on their behalf without having to seek his concurrence. The children needed some therapy to help them adjust to the new situation, which was done together with Maria in my office. After the divorce was final, Maria began dating a man and I saw them together for a few sessions of couple's counseling, mostly around issues that came from her response to a new, nonabusive relationship. After some period of time, they planned to marry. Maria and her husband-to-be invited me to the wedding. Should I attend?

Jennifer is a 7-year-old girl who was seen for psychotherapy after she revealed that her father had been sexually abusing her for the past 2 years. She had gone through the assessment required by the courts, her father admitted the abuse, and the court had ordered them both to be in treatment in order to begin supervised visitation after a period of 1 year of minimal contact. The court asked Jennifer's therapist to work out a schedule with her father's therapist so that Jennifer was protected as best as possible. Should I work with both Jennifer and her father in treatment?

Judy was referred to me for a forensic evaluation during the pendency of her lawsuit against a government agency for discrimination. She had worked for this agency as a professional for more than 20 years and recently her new male supervisor had demoted her and taken away many of her responsibilities. Judy filed a complaint for sexual discrimination and harassment and stated that she was capable of performing her job duties but if she wasn't, it was due to the harassment she experienced from this supervisor. During the evaluation it became clear that Judy had experienced other forms of abuse, including having been raped at age 17. One night, before the evaluation was completed, I received a telephone call from the police stating that Judy had told them to call me. She was barricaded in her house and refused to let them in or come out herself. They asked me to talk to her to make sure she was all right and to persuade her to cooperate with them. Should I take on a new role at this time?

Feminist psychotherapists often treat clients like those described in the previous cases. Maria, Jennifer, and Judy each made a typical request to extend the boundaries of the therapy relationship that may occur when treating clients who have been physically, sexually, or psychologically abused at some point in their lives. Each of these cases raises issues that ethical psychologists must consider before determining whether or not they are acting in a competent manner within the boundaries of their expertise. The requests made by these clients, to enter into another type of relationship with them, has the potential to help or harm the client, no matter what decision is made. It is how the therapist engages in the new relationship that will make the difference. This chapter presents issues and vignettes that reflect boundary crossings, and it will argue for flexibility in this regard. As several contributors to this book have underscored, the differences among boundary crossings, boundary violations, and dual relationships are significant. In essence, a boundary violation refers to an unethical act or acts that are deleterious to the therapeutic relationship and harmful to the client. A boundary crossing (such as spending time with an agoraphobic client in a shopping mall, or having a meal in a restaurant with a recovering anorexic client) is a helpful extension beyond the confines of the consulting room and is the focus of this chapter. A dual relationship refers to some degree of fraternization with a client, the pros and cons of which have been extensively presented in this book.

The current American Psychological Association (APA) Ethics Code (1992) does not forbid boundary extensions, boundary crossings, or dual relationships with a client unless such an association impairs the therapist's objectivity or causes exploitation or other harm to the client. However, most psychologists commonly believe that all multiple relationships are so dangerous that they should be avoided at all costs. Therapists-in-training are taught to avoid any other relationship with a therapy client. Faculty in psychology training programs have been known to insist that it is better to avoid the potential problems than try to teach students how to make appropriate judgments. But is this good therapy practice? It is my professional opinion that psychotherapists must learn how to make such professional judgments without fear that an ethics committee, state licensing board, or malpractice attorney will judge them punitively without understanding the complexities of the issues that often get raised when treating clients.

WHAT DOES FEMINIST THERAPY SAY ABOUT MULTIPLE RELATIONSHIPS AND BOUNDARY CROSSINGS?

Feminist therapists have attempted to deal directly with the decision to cross boundaries and about entering into multiple relationships with a client, using several of the tenets that underlie the theory of feminist therapy (Lerman & Porter, 1990; Rosewater & Walker, 1985). One such tenet insists that therapists understand and carefully monitor the power dynamics between client and therapist (Worell & Johnson, 1997). Exploitation and harm are seen as most likely to occur when the therapist does not hold equal respect for the client's power as well as their own. During the early years when feminist therapy was developing as a specialty area, some women therapists took advantage of other women by entering into multiple relationships with them—sometimes it involved exploitation over money issues, sometimes it involved a sexual relationship. This was in the early 1970s, when sexuality was more freely and casually expressed, and before sex between client and therapist, no matter what gender, was strictly forbidden by ethical, moral, and sometimes legal standards (see Brown & Walker, 1990 for further information around the issue of self-disclosure and potential client exploitation). Often multiple relationships involved barter, especially when each person had a skill or could perform a service needed by the other. The problem here was trying to put an equal financial value on unequal skills or services. For example, a 1-hour therapy session might be considered equal in monetary value to 10 hours of typing, hardly seeming like an equal exchange in terms of time or effort (Berman, 1985).

As the feminist movement matured, the original notion that the client and therapist must be equal because they were both women changed and, instead, the goal for each became reaching an egalitarian relationship (Lerman & Porter, 1990). That meant that both the therapist and the client respected the knowledge and skills that each brought to the therapy session. When attention is paid to developing this kind of respect in therapy, it can be of assistance in making sure that multiple relationships that could cause the therapist to lose objectivity and behave in harmful ways do not occur.

It became important for the feminist therapist to acknowledge and monitor the fact that, at least in the therapy situation, the therapist has more power than the client does. In feminist ethics, the therapist was responsible for monitoring the distribution of power although there were suggestions on how to help the client take more responsibilities, as she was able. For example, if the therapist knew that she held a particular viewpoint that might differ from the client's, on any particular issue, it was important to discuss it with the client at the appropriate time and to ask the client for help in monitoring that she did not overstep her boundaries on that issue. Giving permission to the client to confront the therapist should she become uncomfortable about that particular issue helps empower the client in taking more responsibility for her own mental health.

Feminist theorists dealt with the issue of multiple relationships and possible exploitation or harm to clients while also cautioning that the issues known about the healthy woman's psychological development not be sacrificed for the theory that separation, individuation, and independence be the only standard for healthy emotional development (Green, 1990). The study by Broverman, Broverman, Clarkson, Rosencrantz, and Vogel (1970) helped us understand that there were two different standards by which healthy emotional development was measured—one for men and one for women. The healthy adult was seen as having those characteristics similar to how men develop, favoring rationality over emotionality, individuation over togetherness, and independence over connection.

Understanding the double-bind that holding such a view presented for women, feminist psychotherapy began to deal with ways to better understand men's and women's emotional development (Walker & Dutton-Douglas, 1988). Feminist theorists such as Jean Baker Miller (1976), Judith Jordan, Janet Surrey, Alexandra Kaplan (1983), and others from the Stone Center at Wellesley began to study the psychological strengths that came from women's connectedness. In taking another look at common problems that motivate clients to approach therapists for treatment, Brown and Ballou (1992) suggest that a feminist reappraisal would involve changing our therapy methodology if we are to be helpful. Brown and Root (1990) and Comas-Dias and Greene (1999) studied the impact of different theories of development from a gender and multicultural perspective, again finding that the standard of independence, individuation, and separation are not supported by other cultures or groups where connectedness, especially to extended family and culture, are more highly valued.

Although these theorists did not apply their research directly to boundary crossings or dual or multiple relationships between the client and therapist, it is clear that dealing with interpersonal relationships must be a critical part of feminist multicultural psychotherapy. Dutton-Douglas and Walker (1988) and Worell and Johnson (1997) present ways to integrate both gender and multiculturalism into other therapy theories. It is a logical outgrowth of this knowledge to suggest that an important part of psychotherapy is to learn to deal with complex relationships. Surely working on such relationships with a therapist is one important way to develop and fine-tune such skills.

WHAT DOES TREATING VICTIMS OF VIOLENCE SUGGEST ABOUT BOUNDARIES AND MULTIPLE RELATIONSHIPS?

Dealing with interpersonal relationships and monitoring the power differential between client and therapist become especially important when working with victims of violence. The therapist can help teach the client how to monitor other complex interpersonal relationships by paying attention to the interactions between the therapist and herself. For example, therapists often become uncomfortable when battered women stay in a dangerous relationship with the batterer. Sometimes therapists usurp the client's power and try to manipulate her into leaving the relationship. This can be deadly in some cases, such as if the batterer stalks and kills the woman and the children. It is important to help the client know that an important goal of therapy is to help her find greater safety for herself and her children—not to terminate the relationship. However, sometimes the only way to live in a nonviolent environment is to leave the batterer. This is especially true when the batterer refuses to go into offender-specific therapy or change his violent behavior. Is this advocating for the client or is it advocacy for nonviolence?

In Maria's case that was described earlier, although she came into therapy stating that she wanted to terminate the relationship with her husband, I allowed Maria to take her time in deciding whether that was really what she wanted to do. My role as the therapist was to be Maria's advocate to protect herself and her children as best she could. This was not a neutral stance. Survivor therapy, which is based on a combination of feminist and trauma theory, calls for advocating for nonviolence (Walker, 1994). But it also gives the client the right to choose the timing and the action she will take as long as the children are not in immediate danger. If the children are in danger of abuse, then the therapist is mandated to report it to the proper authorities. Of course, the law mandating child abuse reporting must be discussed with the client at the very first session so that if the client informs the therapist of any danger to the child, she is aware of the consequences.

Advocacy is often considered a boundary violation by those who interpret the admonitions against dual relationships very strictly. In Maria's case, although it was clear that Maria was my primary client, I engaged in therapeutic activities with her children and her husband-to-be. But, did I violate boundaries or was this an appropriate and even necessary intervention on the client's behalf? Had I not engaged in these interventions, would I have been less helpful to Maria?

Therapists need to be advocates for their clients who have been victims of violence. By advocacy I mean that they must take their client's side in the abuse scenario. Victims of violence lose the ability to perceive objectivity and neutrality. Either you are with them or you are considered part of the problem! Validation of the client's pain as she describes the abuse is part of this kind of advocacy. Listening to them without either overtly or subtly blaming them for their victimization is another kind of advocacy. Taking their reports of danger of further abuse seriously is yet another form of advocacy. This can be underscored by putting a safety and crisis intervention plan into action with the client. Knowing that the client is aware of various safety options she can follow should the abuse reported reoccur, also helps the therapist give her the time and space she needs to do it herself.

It is also important to understand the violence victim's difficulty in trusting that anyone can really help her. This is especially true for victims of family violence where the abuser is someone who also may treat the victim-survivor lovingly at other times. Feminist and survivor therapy build on the client's strengths, which helps in reestablishing trust and belief in their own power—reempowerment. In Maria's case, I made the decision to see her together with her children as part of her adjustment to her new status as a single mom with sole responsibility for making decisions in the children's lives. The fact that her children benefited from the sessions is an extra bonus. The same rationale was given for seeing Maria and her new boyfriend in joint sessions. In this case, Maria and I made the decision together to add other family members to Maria's treatment as needed. Those who are untrained in family therapy could make an argument that adding these members to the therapy session became a boundary violation even though it turned out as expected—a positive experience for everyone and helped reach the specific treatment goals negotiated between Maria and myself.

So, in Maria's case, I felt comfortable after discussion with Maria in deciding to attend the wedding. I knew the children and the husband-to-be. The community was small enough that others who would be attending the wedding would know me both personally and in my role as Maria's therapist. Thus, part of the discussion between and Maria and me was to decide how to handle people's inquiries without violating her privilege. Maria felt that my attendance would be a signal to herself, her groom, and her family and friends that she was psychologically okay to enter into this new relationship. While I did not feel my attendance should take on such significance, I did believe that Maria was well prepared to go forward with her new life. I also made it clear, however, that I would not violate Maria's confidentiality by saying or doing anything at the wedding. Whatever Maria chose to tell others was her prerogative, but I suggested that it might be less intrusive for me to simply state I was a friend, should anyone ask. I also stated that I would not acknowledge or discuss Maria's progress in therapy with anyone other than Maria, herself. With these ground rules in place, I did attend the wedding as a guest and as might be expected, everyone had a good time. Thus, this is an example of a carefully considered boundary crossing that was helpful and meaningful for the client and rewarding for me as well.

STRETCHING THE BOUNDARIES WHEN
TREATING ABUSED CHILDREN

Jennifer, a child abused by her father, needed her own independent relationship with her therapist. Although the court imposed intervention with her family, in fact, it is often counterindicated by the child's therapist, and adding the family members to her treatment could be considered a boundary violation if there had not been a court order to do it. Even so, Jennifer's own feelings about a new therapist needed to be taken into account before a final decision was made by the therapist. One of the most important treatment issues is the restoration of an incest survivor's trust after experiencing the fundamental betrayal by a parent. Thus, the therapist must be extremely careful about respecting the child's boundaries. At the same time, the court was insisting she learn to deal with her father's behavior, including his seduction and manipulation. She will need to learn these skills in order for her to be able to protect herself from revictimization. Jennifer was still angry with her mother, who she believed had failed to notice or protect her earlier. Again, this is another indication that this child was not yet ready to deal with complex multiple relationships.

It seemed to me that it would be better for someone else to do the joint counseling sessions at this point in treatment. However, Jennifer's reaction to this suggestion was dramatic—not only did she protest verbally, but she went into a serious panic attack that frightened her. I called Jennifer's lawyer who, based on my information, asked the court for more time before beginning these joint counseling sessions, citing the possible irreparable harm should Jennifer's panic attacks continue.

Six months later, the court once again mandated the counseling as a step toward reunification of the family unit, stating the requirement to do so under the Uniform Children's Code. At this time, the therapist and Jennifer agreed that they would do the counseling sessions together with her father and his therapist. Although this is still a dual relationship, it appeared to be the best compromise position. The fact that her father would have his own therapist to monitor his behavior reduced the need for me to advocate for anyone except Jennifer. Although Jennifer was not told this, the court agreed that I could terminate the session if Jennifer should go into another panic attack irrespective of her father's behavior. Obviously, if her father did not follow the ground rules set up between his therapist and myself, then the session also could be terminated early.

This case illustrates the need for the therapist to be flexible in making boundary decisions, especially when someone with more power, such as the court, was mandating a dual relationship that could harm the child.

THE DUAL ROLE OF FORENSIC EVALUATION AND THERAPEUTIC INTERVENTIONS

Judy's situation illustrates a widespread opinion among forensic experts to avoid any type of dual relationship with the client or her attorney. It would not be unusual for the forensic expert to automatically decline from intervening with the police in trying to calm down the situation and persuade Judy to cooperate. But, would that serve the purpose? Here is an opportunity for the forensic evaluator to observe, first hand, a different repertoire of Judy's behavior. It appeared that Judy was having a major decompensation, perhaps even having gone into a psychotic state at the time the police called. Would talking to her on the telephone and trying to use the relationship already established during the evaluation have biased the ultimate conclusions? Would observation of Judy after she had decompensated, or while it was occurring, been helpful or hurtful to her legal case? How do potential boundary violation decisions need to be made when there is an emergency situation such as the police in Judy's case described?

Yes, it does matter that the forensic evaluator was going to be viewed in an additional role if contact was made with Judy while she was so distressed. However, unless the psychologist observes this behavior for herself, it could not form a basis for a professional opinion. Because Judy was the plaintiff in the lawsuit against her employer, and the evaluator was hired by her attorney to assess for damages, whatever she demonstrated as her current mental state would play a role in developing the forensic opinion. However, it is also known that victims of sexual harassment and discrimination have difficulty in keeping to boundaries between themselves and others that are important in their lives. Thus, it was possible that blurring the boundaries in Judy's case could make her so upset that she literally couldn't tell who was on her side.

In Judy's situation, the issue was quickly resolved when I asked the police officer to offer to hand Judy his cell phone through the window so she could talk directly with me. I then asked her whether she was afraid and if so, of whom? She admitted being afraid of the police officer and stated that she was unsure who he was, given her confusion. As we talked for a while, Judy sounded much better and said she was able to continue working on the project she had taken home from work. She sounded less confused, had more clarity cognitively, and controlled her affective responses. I asked whether she thought she would hurt herself or someone else, and she denied any suicidal, homicidal, or other violent thoughts or behavior.

After finishing my conversation with Judy, who gave me permission, I asked to speak directly with the police officer again and listened while he told me that Judy's boss had called the police with a complaint that Judy was harassing him. When he got to her house, Judy became so frightened that she actually closed up the entire house to avoid contact with the police. By the time I had been called, the police and Judy were at a standoff for approximately 12 hours. Judy decompensated mentally as the police officer became more aggressive in demanding that she come out and let him search her apartment. This increased her paranoia, which is commonly seen in victims of abuse.

My willingness to enter into another role with Judy and make an intervention, as was requested by the police, is an example of boundary crossing, multiple roles and flexibility, which prevented a client from hurting herself.

BOUNDARY VIOLATIONS AND MULTIPLE RELATIONSHIPS

Abuse survivors do have difficulty with boundaries especially if they have to work together with different members of a legal and mental health team. The only possible antidote to this is to try to keep the boundaries simple and clear whenever possible. As demonstrated by these cases, however, it is not always possible or desirable to avoid multiple relationships when working with abuse survivors. For Judy there doesn't appear to be much of a boundary violation given the crisis situation. But in other cases, like the one with Sara, the potential to serve in multiple roles is more problematic.

Sara was a battered woman who lived with her abusive partner for approximately 2 years. She sought therapy for herself and eventually became strong enough to challenge the power and control of her husband, Jim, over her. She had taken a part-time job outside of the home which meant that their two children were not greeted by her any longer when they came home from school. As she spent more time working on a new computer program for her boss, Jim came home and played with her computer, erasing everything on her hard drive. Sara was furious. She confronted Jim and for the first time, he beat her up causing her to have to go to the hospital to treat her broken arm. I got a call from the Emergency Room doctor who wanted to report the incident to the police. Sara refused. When I finally got to speak to her, she pleaded with me to let her come to my house so she would be safe from further abuse that night. What should I do?

What is the issue in Sara's case? Is there ever a time to take home a client? When I taught children in a special program for acting-out and mentally disturbed youth, it was not uncommon to have one or more kids spending a night or two at my home. Again, this was the 1970s and not the 1990s or 2000s. Although some of the children were abuse survivors, this was not a therapeutic maneuver to heal that part of their lives. Sara, by contrast, was hurt and in crisis, and she turned to me, her therapist, for protection. A videotape of these sessions (Walker, 1996) clearly shows that the therapist's responding to Sara's plea would have interfered with the treatment goals of getting her to take responsibility for her own safety. So, instead I had a discussion with Sara, first determining that she was all right and then acknowledging and validating the pain she had experienced. Then, I inquired about the arrangements she had made to have the children in a safe place. She informed me that they were with her sister at her own house.

Finally, I asked her about her own safety and protection. This was when she blurted out that she wanted to come and live with me. I gently told her that living with me was extremely inadvisable and she understood. I further ascertained that she didn't expect her husband back at the home that night as he was supposed to leave on a business trip. But, just to be safe, I gave her some suggestions to stay with her sister because the children would probably be with his sister by then. Sara's high levels of anxiety were getting in the way of her usually careful analysis of situations. Other victims may have been so isolated socially that they would require a refresher course in social skills before they were ready to move on. In addition, I continued to validate the seriousness of the incident by giving her an appointment for early the next morning to come in to see me, which she did. Cases like Sara's can easily trigger a therapist or counselor's "rescue fantasies." It is intended to serve as a reminder of the need to assess when and when not to cross certain boundaries.

NINE STEPS TO HELP THERAPISTS MAKE CRITICAL JUDGMENTS ABOUT DUAL RELATIONSHIPS AND BOUNDARY CROSSINGS IN THESE TYPES OF CASES

It is important to:

1.   Fully understand the legal and kinship networks that help support the client and the impact, if any, of adding or subtracting a major client role. *In Maria's case, it was important to her treatment to include her children and her husband-to-be as part of her therapy and then accept the invitation to attend the family wedding.*

2.   Clarify the legal issues pending for the client by speaking with attorneys. *In Jennifer's case, it was critical to get the judge to understand that it was not in the child's best interests to include her perpetrator father in her therapy. However, it was also important for the therapist to learn what the law stated—reunification, to help make the final decisions about entering into that dual relationship.*

3.   Either be introduced or introduce oneself to the other support persons in the client's life, especially if that person is recovering from abuse. *In each of these cases, the client talked about therapy with support persons so that we were all working on behalf of the client's recovery. In some cultural groups, however, it may not be acceptable to be in therapy, so it is important to discuss this step with the client before making the decision to attend a family event.*

4.   Review the negotiated goals of treatment or evaluation with the client to see if the client's request would fit in with those goals. *It is important to connect all techniques used in treatment with the goals of treatment. For many survivors, engaging in multiple relationships may be a way to strengthen interpersonal relationship skills in complex situations and help to overcome the isolation often caused by victimization.*

5.   Asses what it would take to fulfill the request and how it might impact the therapy relationship. *As was noted in Jennifer's case, I believe that entering into the dual relationship with her and her perpetrator-father was preferable to the impact on the child by not doing so, if the court insisted the joint therapy take place anyhow. In Sara's case, it was considered too much of a boundary violation for me to help provide safety for her after the abuse and counterindicative to her therapy goal to protect herself, while in Judy's case, intervention with the police was deemed appropriate.*

6.   Know what the APA Ethics Code (1992) says about this issue. *Be familiar with the actual standards as written in the APA Ethics Code. Call APA or your state for information if they do not seem clear around the particular*

issue with which you are dealing. The APA Ethics Office suggests psychologists call for an opinion before making a decision, especially if it is a complicated case.

7.   Know what forensic evaluators and other clinicians think about this topic. *Although it is not necessary to follow what others write about a particular issue, it is important to show that you recognize the need to consult (either personally or through the literature) before making a decision. Document your efforts to educate yourself on the issue in your notes.*

8.   Fully understand the risks inherent in complying with the client's request. *It is also a good idea to document the risks that you considered before making a decision to stretch the boundaries or enter into a multiple relationship with a client.*

9.   Ask yourself: "What are the risks to therapy and the client's well-being if I do not honor the request?" *As in Judy's case, the damage of not intervening appeared to have the potential of being more serious than any probable harm from dealing with the police. With Sara, it was clear that acceding to her request to come to the therapist's home would be antithetical to treatment goals and damaging to the therapy relationship in the long run. However, it was important to offer her the early morning therapy appointment, to indicate the seriousness of what had occurred to her.*

CONCLUSION

In conclusion, it is sometimes good psychological practice and enhancing to the therapeutic process to cross boundaries and have more than one kind of relationship with a client. Crossing or stretching boundaries will probably create changes to the already established relationship; it is important to review the steps outlined previously and illustrated in the cases of Maria, Jennifer, Judy, and Sara. Boundary crossings and multiple relationships can be helpful to clients as well as harmful. It is important for therapists working with abuse survivors, most of whom are women who thrive on emotional connectedness, to help their clients establish positive interpersonal relationships. Hopefully, the next revision of the APA Ethics Code will address the issue of how to train practitioners in good decision-making when opportunities for boundary crossings or multiple relationships occur.

REFERENCES

American Psychological Association. (1992). Ethical principles of psychologists and code of conduct. *American Psychologist, 47,* 1597–1611.

Berman, J. S. (1985). Ethical feminist perspectives on dual relationships. In L. B. Rosewater & L. E. A. Walker (Eds.), *Handbook on feminist therapy: Women's issues in psychotherapy*. New York: Springer.

Broverman, I., Broverman, D. M., Clarkson, F. E., Rosencrantz, P. S., & Vogel, S. R. (1970). Sex role stereotypes and clinical judgments of mental health. *Journal of Consulting and Clinical Psychology, 34,* 1–7.

Brown, L. S., & Ballou, M. (Eds.). (1992). *Personality and psychopathology: Feminist reappraisals*. New York: Guilford.

Brown, L. S., & Root, M. P. P. (Eds.). (1990). *Diversity and complexity in feminist therapy*. Binghamton, NY: Haworth Press.

Brown, L. S., & Walker, L. E. A. (1990). Feminist therapy perspectives in self-disclosure. In G. Striker & M. Fisher (Eds.), *Therapy perspectives in self disclosure* (pp. 135–154). New York: Plenum.

Comas-Dias, L., & Greene, B. (Eds.). (1999). *Women of color: Integrating ethnic and gender identities in psychotherapy*. New York: Guilford.

Dutton-Douglas, M. A., & Walker, L. E. A. (Eds.). (1988). *Feminist psychotherapies: Integration of therapeutic and feminist systems*. Norwood, NJ: Ablex.

Green, G. D. (1990). Is separation really so great? In L. S. Brown & M. D. P. Root (Eds.), *Diversity and complexity in feminist therapy* (pp. 87–104). Binghamton, NY: Haworth Press.

Jordan, J. V., Surrey, J. L., & Kaplan, A. G. (1983). *Women and empathy: Implications for psychological development and psychotherapy*. Wellesley, MA: Stone Center for Developmental Studies and Services.

Lerman, H., & Porter, N. (Eds.). (1990). *Ethics in psychotherapy: Feminist perspectives*. New York: Springer.

Miller, J. B. (1976). *Toward a new psychology of women: Treatment toward equality*. Springfield, IL: Charles C Thomas.

Rosewater, L. B., & Walker, L. E. A. (Eds.). (1985). *Handbook on feminist therapy: Women's issues in psychotherapy*. New York: Springer.

Walker, L. E. A. (1994). *Abused women and survivor therapy: A guide for the psychotherapist*. Washington, DC: American Psychological Association.

Walker, L. E. A. (1996). *Survivor therapy and abused women: A video*. New York: Newbridge Communications. Available from Walker & Associates, 915 Middle River Dr., #401, Ft. Lauderdale, FL 33304, drlewalker@aol.com

Walker, L. E. A., & Dutton-Douglas, M. A. (1988). Future directions: Development, application and training of feminist therapies. In M. A. Dutton-Douglas & L. E. A. Walker (Eds.), *Feminist psychotherapies: Integration of therapeutic and feminist systems* (pp. 276–300). Norwood, NJ: Ablex.

Worell, J., & Johnson, N. (Eds.). (1997). *Shaping the future of feminist psychology: Education, research and practice*. Washington, DC: American Psychological Association.

PART 9

A Final Peek Behind
the Scenes

Chapter 31 presents a unique, daring, and cutting-edge analysis of the means and methods by which consent has been manufactured about the putative depravity of dual relationships. Using Chomsky's model of manufacturing consent, Zur presents 11 methods that disseminate, promote, and uphold the faulty belief that dual relationships are essentially unethical and lead to exploitation and harm.

How Consensus Regarding the Prohibition of Dual Relationships Has Been Contrived

Ofer Zur, PhD

T he goal of this chapter is to describe the means that have been used to promote a consensus that dual relationships are ipso facto detrimental. Throughout this book, it has been emphasized that dual relationships are unavoidable in many settings and communities and that judicious boundary crossings can enhance treatment effectiveness. Many of the contributors to this book have documented how the codes of ethics of all major professional psychotherapy associations do not consider dual relationships to be inherently unethical. In this chapter, I will present 11 methods that have been used to manufacture the mistaken view and commonly held belief that dual relationships are essentially unethical, harmful, and dangerous.

For the reader who may be browsing and has not read the preceding chapters, I will state again that dual relationships in psychotherapy refer to any situation wherein multiple roles exist between a therapist and a client. Examples of dual relationships are when the client is also a student, friend, family member, employee, or business associate of the therapist. Like the rest of the book, this chapter focuses only on nonsexual dual relationships. Sexual dual relationships with current clients are always unethical. It must be fully understood that it is imperative to avoid any dual relationship that might impair the therapist or counselor's objectivity, competence, or effectiveness in performing his or her professional duties and functions. Likewise, great care must be exercised to ensure that the dual relationship will not expose the client to any form of exploitation or harm.

As any discerning reader who has perused several sections will undoubtedly have discovered, this book does not offer a blanket endorsement of dual relationships. Instead, the goal is to advocate a message that is consistent with most updated codes of ethics that simply caution therapists to be thoughtful and careful when they engage in dual relationships with their clients. Like any other clinical intervention, dual relationships should be employed as part of a well-articulated, individually tailored treatment plan that is discussed with and agreed upon by the clients.

Noam Chomsky's (1988) model of manufactured consent offers help in understanding how the urban analytic risk-management approach has come to dominate the field of psychotherapy. This domination is true for the field of ethics in general and dual relationships in particular. Manufactured consent has been described as the process whereby a few people in a certain subculture are positioned to have an overwhelming power to influence public opinion, decision-making, and the determination of how such a culture functions. In applying this understanding to the field of psychotherapy and dual relationships, it becomes clear that the profession has been dominated by a handful of people in key positions who disseminate and control the flow and type of information available to the rest of profession. Manufactured consent in the area of psychotherapy is presided over by people who are not necessarily conscious of or conspiratorial in their manipulations. Mostly they are committed professionals with a strong belief in their ideas and great determination to convince the remainder of the field to support them and practice the "right way." The net result, however, is what Hedges (1993) described as the "malignant concept of dual relationships" (p. 47) and the raison d'être throughout this book is to provide a benevolent and balanced account of this significant topic.

THE CORE GROUP OF EXPERTS

The saturation of the professional literature on the depravity of dual relationships and the absence of the supportive view is fueled by the handful of "authorities" who hold, as predicted by Chomsky (1988), significant positions of power. These positions include book and journal editors; chairpersons and members of boards, committees and task forces; professors and department heads at universities and colleges; authors of articles and books and expert consultants and witnesses for courts. Their influence continues to be felt in a wide range of settings, from disciplinary actions by regulatory boards to the formation of codes of professional conduct. Above all, their influence has established and supported a pervasive belief among professionals about the depravity of dual relationships. What will be referred to as "the core group" includes Bersoff (1999); Borys (1992, 1994; Borys & Pope, 1989); Brown (1994); Epstein (Epstein & Simon, 1990); Gabbard and Gutheil (Gutheil & Gabbard, 1993); Kitchener (1988, 1996); Koocher (Keith-Spiegel & Koocher, 1985; Koocher & Keith-Spiegel, 1998); Langs (1974); Pope (1986, 1988, 1989, 1990, 1991); Simon (1989, 1991, 1992, 1995); Sonne (1994); and Strasburger and Jorgenson (Strasburger, Jorgenson, & Sutherland, 1992). These writers and scholars advocate for, disseminate, and preserve the belief that almost all dual relationships are fundamentally unethical and harmful.

HOW CONSENSUS HAS BEEN ACHIEVED

Manufactured consent that dual relationships are basically unethical, clinically ill-advised, exploitative, harmful and often lead to sex has been achieved and fueled through the following means:

1. *Dissemination of the belief that dual relationships are basically and fundamentally unethical.* The propagation of the erroneous idea that dual relationships are almost always unethical has been one of the most powerful tools in manufacturing consent about the presumed destructive nature of dual relationships. The often-quoted ethicist Kitchener (1988) claims that "All dual relationships can be ethically problematic and have the potential for harm" (p. 217). O'Connor-Slimp and Burian (1994) state, "American Psychological Association's (1992) Ethical principles of Psychologists and Code of Conduct mandates that most types of multiple or dual relationships be avoided" (p. 39). Craig (1991) asserts, "Ethical counselors cultivate unambiguous relationships. . . . Unethical counselors cultivate dual relationships" (p. 49). Though giving some lip service and acknowledgment that dual relationships are not always avoidable, the writings of the above-mentioned core group

promote the falsehood that almost all dual relationships are basically unethical. Some of the previously mentioned scholars have served on the task forces that developed several of the codes of ethics cited above. Yet they still disseminate the misinformation that almost all dual relationships are fundamentally unethical.

2. *Overflow in professional literature of the idea that dual relationships are harmful and exploitative.* The aforementioned influential and like-minded core group have been by far the most frequently cited authors on the topic of dual relationships. They quote each other often, incessantly and at times almost exclusively. A few examples may be found in Borys (1994), Gabbard (1994), and Gutheil (1994), in which the writers from the core group comprised 83%, 60%, and 75% of the citations, respectively. In Bersoff's (1996) widely used ethics textbook, 4 (44%) of the 9 entries on dual relationships in therapy are authored or coauthored by Pope, and the remaining 5 (56%) were written by other authors from the above-mentioned list. Such a repetitive and at times exclusive circulation of a set of references creates a sense that it is the only valid position available in the professional literature—cultivating an illusion that dissent does not exist and consent about the depravity of dual relationships is universal.

3. *Lack of acknowledgment of opposing perspectives.* Articles that represent a more inclusive attitude toward nonsexual dual relationships, such as Barnett (1992), Barnett and Yutrzenka (1994), Brown (1991), Hedges (1993), Jennings (1992), Lazarus (1994), Sears (1990), Smith (1990), Stockman (1990), and Tomm (1993), have been generally excluded from most articles and texts on ethics. A few striking examples out of the dozens of books and articles published *after* the above articles appeared that refer to almost none of them (in their supposedly balanced, ethical, and scientific discussion of dual relationships) are: Bersoff (1996), Gabbard and Nadelson (1995), Kitchener (1996), Simon (1995), Sonne (1994), and St. Germaine (1996). Perhaps the most outstanding example lies in the extensive reference list of the text by Pope and Vasquez (1998), in which Pope includes 48 citations of his own work but *none* of the above references. In fairness, it should be noted that Bersoff's second edition (1999) includes an article by Lazarus (1994), who presents a positive view of dual relationships.

4. *Inordinate dependence on psychoanalytic theory to refute the arguments of nonanalytic practitioners who support dual relationships.* The endlessly cited works of analytically oriented writers such as Epstein (Epstein & Simon, 1990), Langs (1974), Lakin (1991), and Simon (1991, 1995) are very common in the articles that demonize dual relationships. Ac-

cording to these authors, almost any deviation from the strict analytic blank screen stance results in the nullification of therapeutic effectiveness and causes harm. The rigid analytic orientation of these authors blinds them and their followers to the fact that *most* practitioners do not adhere to, believe in, or practice analytic theory. The works of these analytically oriented writers have been used to justify the imposition of strict rules and even administrative and civil sanctions on all practitioners, regardless of their orientation (Lazarus, 1994, 2002; Williams, 1997, 2000; Zur, 2001b).

5. *Methodical avoidance of references to nonanalytic clinical practices supportive of dual relationships.* Behavioral, cognitive-behavioral, humanistic, group, family, and existential therapeutic orientations are among the most practiced orientations today. Their practitioners, when appropriate, endorse what are considered clear boundary violations by most ethicists, psychoanalysts, and risk-management advocates. The most influential critics and opponents of dual relationships ignore the works of Bugental (1986) or Yalom (1980), on Existential therapy; Ellis (1977), on Rational Emotive Behavior therapy; Rogers (1942), on Humanistic therapy; and Lazarus (1989, 1997), on Multimodal therapy. For instance, the aforementioned are almost entirely absent in the writings of Bersoff (1996, 1999), Borys and Pope (1989), Brown (1990), Epstein and Simon (1990), Kitchener (1988), Keith-Spiegel and Koocher (1985), Koocher and Keith-Spiegel (1998), Pope (1988, 1989, 1990), Simon (1991), and Strasburger et al. (1992).

6. *Dearth of recognition of beneficial dual relationships.* Most of the professional literature fails to note that dual relationships are not only sometimes unavoidable, but in fact can be beneficial (e.g., Brown, 1991; Hedges, 1993; Herlihy & Corey, 1992; Jennings, 1992; Lazarus, 1994, 1998; Sears, 1990; Smith, 1990; Stockman, 1990; Tomm, 1993; Zur, 2000, 2001a). This type of lacuna is known to be extremely effective in spawning half truths. Here are a few examples: In Keith-Spiegel and Koocher's (1985) classic textbook, and in its second revision (Koocher & Keith-Spiegel, 1998), the chapters on dual relationships include 51 and 55 cases, respectively, of dual relationships. Almost none of these exemplifies a positive outcome. Austin (1998), Borys (1992), Grosso (1997), Nagy (2000), Pepper (1991), Simon (1989), Sonne (1994), and the widely quoted text by Pope and Vasquez (1998) mostly fails to present meaningful documentation about beneficial dual relationships. In fairness, it should be noted that Koocher and Keith-Spiegel (1998) include some references to resources supporting dual relationships. However, the 30-page chapter on dual relationships devotes less than 2 pages to positive views of dual relationships.

7. *Ignoring the inevitability of dual relationships in military, rural and other close-knit communities.* The known fact that not all therapists practice in large urban areas or in communities where therapists' anonymity is possible or desirable has been largely ignored by writers, such as Austin (1998), Epstein and Simon (1990), Langs (1974), and many others. It has been given lip service by writers, such as Bersoff (1999), Koocher and Keith-Spiegel (1998), Pope and Vasquez (1998), and Sonne (1994), but who still maintain a general stance against the incorporation of dual relationships in psychotherapy. Even though all major professional associations have changed their codes to accommodate settings where dual relationships are unavoidable, the literature on dual relationships rarely acknowledges this reality (Hedges, 1993). Absent from the majority of literature on the topic is the inevitability of dual relationships in small, tight-knit, interconnected groups of people such as those found in rural (Barnett, 1996; Barnett & Yutrzenka, 1994; Hargrove, 1986; Jennings, 1992; Schank, 1998; Schank & Skovholt, 1997); church (Geyer, 1994; Montgomery & DeBell, 1997); military (Barnett & Yutrzenka, 1994; Johnson, 1995; Staal & King, 2000); lesbian (Brown, 1989; Smith, 1990); feminist (Brown, 1991; Heyward, 1993; Lerman & Porter, 1990); and ethnic minority communities (Sears, 1990). Most scholars either avoid mentioning this inevitability or minimize it by devoting only a few insignificant statements to the subject.

8. *Equation of dual relationships with exploitation, harm and betrayal.* Most writers present dual relationships not only as essentially unethical but also as harmful and exploitative and highly likely to lead to sex (see Pope, 1990). Austin's (1998) book opens the Dual Relationships chapter with: "Any relationships with a client other than the therapeutic relationships constitute a dual relationship. A client has the right to be treated by a therapist who will not exploit their trust" (p. 450). Kitchener (1996) links dual relationships with lack of integrity, betrayal, and untrustworthiness: "Multiple relationships that cross boundaries and distort the contract between psychologists and those with whom they work further exemplify a lack of integrity since they involve betrayal of trust between a psychologist and the person with whom he or she entered into a relationship" (p. 362). Sonne (1994) equates the resemblance of dual relationships to drunk driving, and Koocher and Keith-Spiegel (1998), like so many other writers, associate most dual relationships with inherent harm and conflict of interest. Literature on the topic is largely devoid of any mention that dual relationships are not synonymous with harm and exploitation, and in fact can strengthen trust, increase clinical effectiveness, and reduce the chance of exploitation

(Herlihy & Corey, 1992; Lazarus, 1994, 1998; Sears, 1990; Tomm, 1993; Williams, 1997; Zur, 2000, 2001a).

9. *Advocating the necessity to avoid dual relationships for the purpose of risk management.* According to popular belief, risk management is a valid reason to avoid dual relationships. Risk management is the process whereby therapists refrain from engaging in certain behaviors and interventions, not because they are clinically ill advised, harmful, or wrong, but because they may *appear* improper in court (Williams, 1997, 2000). Besides dual relationships, other practices considered high-risk and therefore not advisable by many attorneys and ethicists include scheduling clients at the end of the day, self-disclosure, leaving the office with a client, and giving a client a comforting hug (Austin, 1998; Pope & Vasquez, 1998; Woody, 1998). Fear of lawsuits and of hypervigilant regulatory and consumer protection agencies have created great dread and trepidation among therapists, particularly around the issue of dual relationships (Ebert, 1997). "Risk Management" may sound like practical or pragmatic advice, but in fact is a misnomer for a practice in which fear of licensing boards and attorneys, rather than clinical considerations and the needs of the client, determines the course of therapy.

10. *Promotion of a connection between nonsexual and sexual dual relationships: The supposition of a 'slippery slope.'* One of the main arguments against dual relationships is the snowball effect, described by Gabbard (1994) as follows: "... the crossing of one boundary without obvious catastrophic results (making) it easier to cross the next boundary" (p. 284). Kenneth Pope (1990), a prominent authority on ethical matters, asserts what has become a professional standard: "... nonsexual dual relationships, while not unethical and harmful per se, foster sexual dual relationships" (p. 688). Based on the same perspective, Strasburger et al. (1992) state, "Obviously, the best advice to therapists is not to start (down) the slippery slope, and to avoid boundary violations or dual relationships with patients" (pp. 547–548). Borys and Pope (1989), Evans, 1997 as well as Sonne (1994) also agree that nonsexual dual relationships are likely to lead to harm or sexual dual relationships. Sonne describes how a therapist and client who play tennis with each other can easily begin to carpool or drink together. Sonne goes on to declare that "With the blurring of the expected functions and responsibilities of the therapist and client comes the breakdown of the boundaries of the professional relationship itself" (p. 338). Clearly, the most distinguished scholars on dual relationships imply a direct causal link not only between dual relationships and harm, but also between sexual and nonsexual dual relationships. While the slippery slope claim has

been shown to be illogical, fear based, and syllogistic (Ebert, 1997; Lazarus, 1994; Zur, 2001a), it is nevertheless referred to extensively and presented as evidence based and factual rather than as a hypothetical speculation. It is reminiscent of those who fear and believe that one puff of marijuana will inevitably result in hard core drug addiction.

11. *Distribution of illusory research findings based on partisan inquiries and falsely representative samples.* Several surveys have been conducted on dual relationships in therapy, most of which have significantly low return rates that put the validity of the findings into question. The return rates reported by Baer and Murdock (1995); Borys and Pope (1989); Epstein, Simon, and Kay (1992); Lamb and Catanzaro (1998); Pope, Tabachnick, and Keith-Spiegel (1987); Ramsdell and Ramsdell (1993); and Sharkin and Birky (1992) were 38%, 49%, 21%, 60%, 45%, 26%, and 32%, respectively. Given the witch-hunt–like atmosphere around the issues of boundaries and dual relationships (Ebert, 1997; Herlihy & Corey, 1992; Lazarus, 1998; Williams, 1997), most therapist or client respondents who believe that crossing traditional boundaries can be curative are highly unlikely to respond to such surveys (Williams, 1992, 2001; Yalom, 1997). Researchers' promises of confidentiality and anonymity are not likely to help such practitioners to overcome their deep fear and trepidation of loss of license, public shame, and prosecution. In addition to sampling problems, many of the survey instruments suffer from a significantly biased wording of questions, which in turn affect the validity of the instruments. Consistent with the general perpetuation of the myth of the depravity of dual relationships, the criticism of existing research has been largely ignored by the researchers themselves and by those who back their conclusions on these questionably validated studies.

SUMMARY

All of the major professional associations unanimously acknowledge that nonsexual dual relationships are neither always unethical, nor always avoidable. Using very similar wording, all the codes (e.g., American Psychological Association, 1992) emphasize that therapists must avoid any form of sexual interaction with clients and that they must exclude only those nonsexual dual relationships that might impair their judgment and objectivity, or harm or exploit patients. Additionally, dual relationships are unavoidable in many settings, such as rural, military, deaf, church, ethnic minority, and other small communities. Dual relationships have also been shown to be beneficial clinically as they increase trust, familiarity, and therapeutic alliance between therapists and clients. Nevertheless, the faulty belief that nonsexual dual relationships are essentially unethical, inherently exploitative, and inevitably lead to sex and harm continues to dominate the field of psychotherapy. This chapter documents several ways by which consent has been manufactured in regard to the opposition to dual relationships.

Notably, there are a handful of journals and books that consistently have not been part of this movement to manufacture consent about the depravity of dual relationships. The few publications that repeatedly encourage critical thinking about the complexities of nonsexual dual relationships primarily include three journals: *Professional Psychology: Research and Practice* (e.g., Hansen & Goldberg, 1999; Schank & Skovholt, 1997), *Psychotherapy: Theory, Research, Practice, Training* (e.g., Rubin, 2000; Williams, 1997), and *The Independent Practitioner* (e.g., Saunders, 2001; Williams, 2001; Zur, 2001a). Similarly, the limited number of books that also support this line of critical thinking include Herlihy and Corey (1992), Heyward (1993), Howard (1986), and Lerman and Porter (1990).

To discard the option of healthy, productive nonsexual dual relationships in psychotherapy based on the inaccurate negative impression imposed by gatekeepers and others in opposition of dual relationships is not only unfair to clients, but an insult to the concept of critical thinking and inimical to the purpose of the profession. If the misinformation currently being disseminated is effective in curtailing the willingness of therapists to act according to the best interests of clients, then the patterns of blind compliance and fear-based avoidance behaviors will become even more entrenched.

The key for therapists' effectiveness is to be well informed and to think critically while keeping in mind the simple objective of best serving the client. Hansen and Goldberg (1999) reflect on the presentation of dual relationships as harmful and 'slippery': " . . . when a psychologist sees professional behavior contrary to his or her personal values, the observer may well cry 'unethical,' when a more apt response might be 'I disagree' " (p. 499).

REFERENCES

American Psychological Association. (1992). Ethical principles of psychologists and code of conduct. *American Psychologist, 47,* 1597–1611.

Austin, K. M. (1998). *Dangers for therapists*. Redlands, CA: California Selected Books.

Baer, B. E., & Murdock, N. L. (1995). Nonerotic dual relationships between therapist and clients: The effect of sex, theoretical orientation, and interpersonal boundaries. *Ethics & Behavior, 5* (2), 131–145.

Barnett, J. E. (1992). Dual relationships and the federal trade commission. *The Maryland Psychologist, 3,* 12–14.

Barnett, J. E. (1996). Boundary issues and dual relationships: Where to draw the line? *The Independent Practitioner, 16* (3), 138–140.

Barnett, J. E., & Yutrzenka, B. A. (1994). Nonsexual dual relationships in professional practice, with special applications to rural and military community. *The Independent Practitioner, 14* (5), 243–248.

Bersoff, D. N. (Ed.). (1996). *Ethical conflicts in psychology*. Washington, DC: American Psychological Association.

Bersoff, D. N. (Ed.). (1999). *Ethical conflicts in psychology*. Washington, DC: American Psychological Association.

Borys, D. S. (1992). Nonsexual dual relationships. In L. Vandecreek, S. Knapp, & T. L. Jackson (Eds.), *Innovations in clinical practice: A source book* (Vol. 11, pp. 443–454). Sarasota, FL: Professional Resource Exchange.

Borys, D. S. (1994). Maintaining therapeutic boundaries: The motive is therapeutic effectiveness, not defensive practice. *Ethics and Behavior, 4* (3), 267–273.

Borys, D. S., & Pope, K. S. (1989). Dual relationships between therapist and client: A national study of psychologists, psychiatrists, and social workers. *Professional Psychology: Research and Practice, 20,* 283–293.

Brown, L. S. (1989). Beyond thou shalt not: Thinking about ethics in the lesbian therapy community. *Women and Therapy, 8,* 13–25.

Brown, L. S. (1990). Ethical issues and the business of therapy. In H. Lerman & N. Porter (Eds.), *Feminist ethics in psychotherapy* (pp. 60–69). New York: Springer.

Brown, L. S. (1991). Ethical issues in feminist therapy. *Psychology of Women, 15,* 323–336.

Brown, L. S. (1994). Boundaries in feminist therapy: A conceptual formulation. *Women and Therapy, 15,* 29–38.

Bugental, J. F. (1986). Existential-humanistic psychotherapy. In I. L. Kutash & A. Wolf (Eds.), *Psychotherapist's casebook* (pp. 222–236). San Francisco: Jossey-Bass.

Chomsky, N. (1988). *Manufacturing consent*. New York: Pantheon.

Craig, J. D. (1991). Preventing dual relationships in pastoral counseling. *Counseling and Values, 36,* 49–55.

Ebert, B. W. (1997). Dual-relationship prohibitions: A concept whose time never should have come. *Applied & Preventive Psychology, 6,* 137–156.

Ellis, A. (1977). *How to master your fear of flying*. New York: Institute for Rational-Emotive Therapy.

Epstein, R. S., & Simon, R. I. (1990). The exploitation index: An early warning indicator of boundary violations in psychotherapy. *Bulletin of the Menninger Clinic, 54,* 450–465.

Epstein, R. S., Simon, R. I., & Kay, G. G. (1992). Assessing boundary violations in psychotherapy: Survey results with the Exploitation Index. *Bulletin of the Menninger Clinic, 56,* 150–166.

Evans, D. R. (1997). *The law, standards of practice, and ethics in the practice of psychology.* Toronto: Mond Montgomery.

Gabbard, G. O. (1994). Teetering on the precipice: A commentary on Lazarus's "How certain boundaries and ethics diminish therapeutic effectiveness." *Ethics & Behavior, 4* (3), 283–286.

Gabbard, G. O., & Nadelson, C. (1995). Professional boundaries in the physician-patient relationship. *Journal of the American Medical Association, 273* (18), 1445–1449.

Geyer, M. C. (1994). Dual role relationships and Christian counseling. *Journal of Psychology and Theology, 22* (3), 187–195.

Grosso, F. C. (1997). *Ethics for marriage, family, and child counselors.* Santa Barbara, CA: Author.

Gutheil, T. G. (1994). Discussion of Lazarus's "How certain boundaries and ethics diminish therapeutic effectiveness." *Ethics and Behavior, 4* (3), 295–298.

Gutheil, T. G., & Gabbard, G. O. (1993). The concept of boundaries in clinical practice: Theoretical and risk management dimensions. *American Journal of Psychiatry, 150,* 188–196.

Hansen, N. D., & Goldberg, S. G. (1999). Navigating the nuances: A matrix of considerations for ethical-legal dilemmas. *Professional Psychology: Research and Practice, 30* (5), 495–503.

Hargrove, D. S. (1986). Ethical issues in rural mental health practice. *Professional Psychology: Research and Practice, 17,* 20–23.

Hedges, L. E. (1993). In praise of the dual relationship. *The California Therapist, May/June,* 46–50.

Herlihy, B., & Corey, G. (1992). *Dual relationships in counseling.* Alexandria, VA: American Association for Counseling and Development.

Heyward, C. (1993). *When boundaries betray us: Beyond what is ethical in therapy and life.* New York: HarperCollins.

Howard, D. (1986). *The dynamics of feminist therapy.* New York: Haworth Press.

Jennings, F. L. (1992). Ethics of rural practice. *Psychotherapy in Private Practice (Special Issue: Psychological Practice in Small Towns and Rural Areas), 10* (3), 85–104.

Johnson, W. B. (1995). Perennial ethical quandaries in military psychology: Toward American Psychological Association and Department of Defense collaboration. *Professional Psychology: Research and Practice, 26,* 281–287.

Keith-Spiegel, P., & Koocher, G. P. (1985). *Ethics in psychology: Professional standards and cases.* New York: Random House.

Kitchener, K. S. (1988). Dual role relationships: What makes them so problematic? *Journal of Counseling and Development, 67,* 217–221.

Kitchener, K. S. (1996). Professional codes of ethics and ongoing moral problems in psychology. In W. O'Donohue & R. F. Kitchener (Eds.), *The philosophy of psychology* (pp. 361–370). London: Sage Publications.

Koocher, G. P., & Keith-Spiegel, P. (1998). *Ethics in psychology: Professional standards and cases*. New York: Oxford University Press.

Lakin, M. (1991). *Coping with ethical dilemmas in psychotherapy*. New York: Pergamon Press.

Lamb, D. H., & Catanzaro, S. J. (1998). Sexual and nonsexual boundary violations involving psychologists, clients, supervisors, and students: Implications for professional practice. *Professional Psychology: Research and Practice, 29* (5), 498–503.

Langs, R. J. (1974). The therapeutic relationship and deviations in technique. In R. J. Langs (Ed.), *International journal of psychoanalytic psychotherapy* (Vol. 4, pp. 106–141). New York: Jason Aronson.

Lazarus, A. A. (1989). *The practice of multimodal therapy*. Baltimore: The John Hopkins University Press.

Lazarus, A. A. (1994). How certain boundaries and ethics diminish therapeutic effectiveness. *Ethics & Behavior, 4,* 255–261.

Lazarus, A. A. (1997). *Brief but comprehensive psychotherapy: The multimodal way*. New York: Springer.

Lazarus, A. A. (1998). How do you like these boundaries? *The Clinical Psychologist, 51,* 22–25.

Lazarus, A. A. (2002). Something must be done about the totalitarian mentality of many ethics committees and licensing boards. In J. K. Zeig (Ed.), *The evolution of psychotherapy IV: A meeting of the minds*. Phoenix, AZ: Zeig, Tucker, & Theisen.

Lerman, H., & Porter, N. (Eds.). (1990). *Feminist ethics in psychotherapy*. New York: Springer.

Montgomery, M. J., & DeBell, C. (1997). Dual relationships and pastoral counseling asset or liability? *Counseling and Values, 42* (1), 30–41.

Nagy, T. F. (2000). *Ethics in plain English: An illustrative casebook for psychologists*. Washington, DC: American Psychological Association.

O'Connor-Slimp, P. A., & Burian, B. K. (1994). Multiple role relationships during internship: Consequences and recommendations. *Professional Psychology: Research and Practice, 25,* 39–45.

Pepper, R. S. (1991). The senior therapist's grandiosity: Clinical and ethical consequences of merging multiple roles. *Journal of Contemporary Psychotherapy, 21* (1), 63–70.

Pope, K. S. (1986). New trends in malpractice cases and changes in APA liability insurance. *Independent Practitioner, 6,* 23–26.

Pope, K. S. (1988). Dual relationships: A source of ethical, legal, and clinical problems. *Independent Practitioner, 8* (1), 17–25.

Pope, K. S. (1989). Therapist-patient sex syndrome: A guide to assessing damage. In G. O. Gabbard (Ed.), *Sexual exploitation in professional relationships* (pp. 39–55). Washington, DC: American Psychiatric Press.

Pope, K. S. (1990). Therapist-patient sex as sex abuse: Six scientific, professional, and practical dilemmas in addressing victimization and rehabilitation. *Professional Psychology: Research and Practice, 21,* 227–239.

Pope, K. S. (1991). Dual roles and sexual intimacy in psychotherapy. *Ethics and Behavior, 1* (1), 21–34.

Pope, K. S. (1994). *Sexual involvement with therapists: Patient assessment, subsequent therapy, forensics.* Washington, DC: American Psychological Association.

Pope, K. S., Tabachnick, B. G., & Keith-Spiegel, P. (1987). Ethics of practice: The beliefs and behaviors of psychologists as therapists. *American Psychologist, 42,* 993–1006.

Pope, K. S., & Vasquez, M. J. T. (1998). *Ethics in psychotherapy and counseling: A practical guide for psychologists.* San Francisco: Jossey-Bass.

Ramsdell, P. S., & Ramsdell, E. M. (1993). Dual relationships: Client perceptions of the effect of client-counselor relationship on the therapeutic process. *Clinical Social Work Journal, 21* (2), 195–212.

Rogers, C. R. (1942). *Counseling and psychotherapy.* Boston: Houghton Mifflin.

Rubin, S. S. (2000). Differentiating multiple relationships from multiple dimensions of involvement: Therapeutic space at the interface of client, therapist, and society. *Psychotherapy: Theory, Research, Practice, Training, 37* (4), 315–324.

Saunders, T. R. (2001). After all, this is Baltimore: Distinguished Psychologist of the Year address. *The Independent Practitioner, 21,* 15–18.

Schank, J. A. (1998). Ethical issues in rural counseling practice. *Canadian Journal of Counseling, 32* (4), 270–283.

Schank, J. A., & Skovholt, T. M. (1997). Dual relationship dilemmas of rural and small-community psychologists. *Professional Psychology: Research and Practice, 28,* 44–49.

Sears, V. L. (1990). On being an "only" one. In H. Lerman & N. Porter (Eds.), *Feminist ethics in psychotherapy* (pp. 102–105). New York: Springer.

Sharkin, B. S., & Birky, I. (1992). Incidental encounters between therapists and their clients. *Professional Psychology: Research and Practice, 23* (4), 326–328.

Simon, R. I. (1989). Sexual exploitation of patients: How it begins before it happens. *Contemporary Psychiatry: Psychiatric Annals, 19* (2), 104–187.

Simon, R. I. (1991). Psychological injury caused by boundary violation precursors to therapist-patient sex. *Psychiatric Annals, 21,* 614–619.

Simon, R. I. (1992). Treatment boundary violations: Clinical, ethical, and legal considerations. *Bulletin of the American Academy of Psychiatry and Law, 20,* 269–287.

Simon, R. I. (1995). The natural history of therapist sexual misconduct: Identification and prevention. *Psychiatric Annals, 25,* 90–94.

Smith, A. J. (1990). Working within the lesbian community: The dilemma of overlapping relationships. In H. Lerman & N. Porter (Eds.), *Feminist ethics in psychotherapy* (pp. 92–96). New York: Springer.

Sonne, J. L. (1994). Multiple relationships: Does the new ethics code answer the right questions? *Professional Psychology: Research and Practice, 25* (40), 336–343.

St. Germaine, J. (1996). Dual relationships and certified alcohol and drug counselors: A national study of ethical beliefs and behaviors. *Alcohol Treatment Quarterly, 14* (2), 29–45.

Staal, M. A., & King, R. E. (2000). Managing a multiple relationship environment: The ethics of military psychology. *Professional Psychology: Research and Practice, 31* (6), 698–705.

Stockman, A. F. (1990). Dual relationships in rural mental health practice: An ethical dilemma. *Journal of Rural Community Psychology, 11* (2), 31–45.

Strasburger, L. H., Jorgenson, L., & Sutherland, P. (1992). The prevention of psychotherapist sexual misconduct: Avoiding the slippery slope. *American Journal of Psychotherapy, 46* (4), 544–555.

Tomm, K. (1993). The ethics of dual relationships. *The California Therapist, January/February,* 7–19.

Williams, M. H. (1992). Exploitation and inference: Mapping the damage from therapist-patient sexual involvement. *American Psychologist, 47,* 412–421.

Williams, M. H. (1997). Boundary violations: Do some contended standards of care fail to encompass commonplace procedures of humanistic, behavioral and eclectic psychotherapies? *Psychotherapy, 34,* 239–249.

Williams, M. H. (2000). Victimized by "victims": A taxonomy of antecedents of false complaints against psychotherapists. *Professional Psychology Research & Practice, 31* (1), 75–81.

Williams, M. H. (2001). The question of psychologists' maltreatment by state licensing boards: Overcoming denial and seeking remedies. *Professional Psychology: Research and Practice, 32* (4), 341–344.

Woody, R. H. (1998). *Fifty ways to avoid malpractice.* Sarasota, FL: Professional Resource Exchange.

Yalom, I. D. (1980). *Existential psychotherapy.* New York: Basic Books.

Yalom, I. D. (1997). *Lying on the couch.* New York: Harper Perennial.

Zur, O. (2000). In celebration of dual relationships: How prohibition of nonsexual dual relationships increases the chance of exploitation and harm. *The Independent Practitioner, 20,* 97–100.

Zur, O. (2001a). Out-of-office experience: When crossing office boundaries and engaging in dual relationships are clinically beneficial and ethically sound. *The Independent Practitioner, 21* (2), 96–100.

Zur, O. (2001b). On analysis, transference, and dual relationships: A rejoinder to Dr. Pepper. *The Independent Practitioner, 21,* 202–204.

The Last Word

Nicholas A. Cummings, PhD, ScD

T he editors and chapter contributors to this volume, through a diverse series of approaches and considerations, have dispelled for all time the monolithic notion that dual relationships are always harmful and should be avoided. Dual relationships in therapy may be harmful or beneficial, to be avoided or unavoidable, inadvertent or inevitable; in short, they just are. In this sense dual relationships are like rain, which just is. Rain is usually beneficial, but it may be harmful (floods) or desperately needed (drought). No one would consider banishing rain; we do try to prohibit dual relationships.

For 9 years I sat on the APA Insurance Trust and also served as its chair. During this period several hundred malpractice cases, or threats of malpractice, were studied, and the conclusion was that approximately 90% could be attributed to dual relationships gone awry. Not satisfied with this simplistic explanation, I spent a lot of time studying the events and interviewing the perpetrators, and I found that in all but a few notable exceptions the therapist exercised poor judgment and disregarded what would be best for the client. Almost all had never read the APA Code of Ethics until they were sued. In my interviews with them it was apparent this was by far not the first instance of poor therapeutic judgment, although the event that brought them down was perhaps the poorest of their frequent poor judgments. The problem was not so much dual relationships, but the manner in which they conducted themselves in situations that would never have been a problem for most psychotherapists. But for a couple of notable exceptions, they were mediocre or worse therapists whose conduct would not have appreciably improved had they read the APA Code of Ethics. There is no substitute for a skilled, conscientious psychotherapist, and for those who lack good judgment, it cannot be mandated by a licensing board or code of ethics.

Very few psychologists practicing today remember that when their pioneering colleagues first began offering their services to the public through independent practice more than 50 years ago there was no licensing, professional liability insurance, third-party reimbursement, and, of course, no APA Code of Ethics. The practicing psychologist had no recognized standing in the eyes of the public, the government, or the courts. A malpractice suit could well mean going into debt the rest of the psychologist's life, as there was no insurance coverage to buffer the financial risk. No wonder that prior to World War II there were less than 200 psychologists in full-time private practice scattered about the country. This all changed shortly after the war, when psychologists, dissatisfied with the domination of psychiatry, entered private practice in droves. I was one of these and was typically both exhilarated and frightened. The APA at the time was solely a scientific and academic body. It ignored the trend of clinicians toward private practice, and not only did it have no guidance, assistance, or protection to offer, it strongly recommended that psychologists not enter independent practice.

Most of the psychologists in private practice before World War II were women who specialized in treating children. Their highest degree was the masters in psychology. An exception was Florence Mateer, PhD, who had a flourishing general psychological practice in Columbus, Ohio, for 2 1/2 decades beginning about 1920. She eventually retired from practice and moved to California where she taught at the Claremont Graduate School. I met her in 1949, the year I first began seeing private patients in a specially constructed office in the front part of my home. She was eager to see more psychologists enter independent practice, and she became a friend and mentor whose experience and encouragement were invaluable during those scary days.

At the time Columbus was a city large enough so that Florence Mateer did not expect to run into her patients (yes, in that era the designation was patient, not client), but small enough so that she invariably did. Being active in civic affairs, the possibility of what is now known as dual relationships was very real. She served on the governing bodies of a number of civic, community, and charitable groups, ranging from the school board, vice president of the local Red Cross chapter, the mayor's advisory council, through no less than a dozen others. She recalled that there were always at least one, and usually two or three of her patients or ex-patients serving with her in these groups. It became much more complicated during the Great Depression of the 1930s when emotional problems ran high and the need for psychotherapy and counseling increased dramatically; but because there was over 50% unemployment, no one had any money to pay for her services.

Dr. Mateer became animated whenever she discussed how her patients paid for her services: barter became the economy of the Great Depression in this hard-hit city. Her lawn was mowed and her garden was tended, several patients got together and painted her house, others cleaned her house, while an unemployed auto mechanic repaired and maintained her car. Dr. Mateer seldom bought food, because those of her patients that had farms brought everything from fresh produce and milk to meat and potatoes. I initially assumed that she kept an arm's length from this bartering, but she informed me that would have been an injustice to her patients who were so grateful and conscientious that left to their own devices, her patients would far overpay her in kind. So Dr. Mateer receipted each barter on its value and rendered statements showing payments in full. She acknowledged and encouraged self-respect and personal pride in her patients.

Being a prominent member of the relatively small community, did she attend weddings, funerals, bar mitzvahs, baptisms, graduations, and other such events? Unless there was an important and unique reason not to do so, Dr. Mateer invariably did, and she sent gifts as appropriate. The prevailing wisdom of the time was psychoanalytic anonymity, relatively easy because psychoanalysts were shielded by the nature of the metropolis where most practiced. How in the 1930s in economically depressed Columbus, Ohio, did she maintain her therapeutic neutrality and perspective? How did Dr. Mateer thread her way through a dual relationships minefield? Interestingly, she had never heard the term dual relationships until I used it to describe her practice of 25 years. Her answer was amazingly simple: "Hippocrates admonished us to first do no harm. Then just add to that the admonition to always do the right thing, no matter what the situation."

The rather simple Hippocratic Oath (circa 400 B.C.) was the primary, very effective ethical code in health care for almost two and a half millennia. It was overshadowed in the 20th century by a newly developed series of precise, legalistic codes promulgated first by medicine, then quickly followed by all the other professional societies. The first APA Code of Ethics adopted in the 1950s was a welcomed, workable document that proffered a wide range of ethical dilemmas followed by a discussion of possible solutions. With each revision that code became more and more detailed, rigid and mandatory. Eventually it came under severe criticism from those who saw it as stifling, inflexible, and lacking common sense on the one side, and those on the other side who saw it as insufficiently detailed and nonprecise and in need of greater sanctions. What happened in the latter half of the 20th century that seemed to so distort the doctor-patient relationship that the straight-jacketing of practice was viewed as a necessity?

It is a little known fact that the Hippocratic Oath, along with delineat-ing the obligations of the physician, also stated the obligations of the patient. Among these were the obligations to comply with the prescribed regimen and to pay the fee. This exquisite balance of doctor-patient obligations defined a workable relationship for almost 25 centuries. If the patient were displeased with the treatment, she or he would see their money wasted and would seek another practitioner. In turn, the physician had to be responsive to the needs of the patient or be replaced. What interfered with this pristine, delicate balance that we used to call the ideal doctor-patient relationship? For 2,000 years dual relationships abounded, for practitioners and their patients lived in close proximity in towns and villages. What changed? It was the advent of third-party payment that upset the delicate, workable balance of the doctor-patient relationship. I am not suggesting that we do away with third-party reim-bursement. Psychologists welcomed it and flourished, and the status of psychology as the preeminent psychotherapy profession would not have occurred without it. However, once a third party intruded into the doctor-patient relationship, it was never the same. Now the patient is beholden to the insurer, and the doctor works for the third-party payor. The patient, no longer paying for the service, is willing to accept pro-tracted, often ineffective treatment that would never be tolerated if payment were out of pocket. Insurance plans attempting to curtail unnecessary payments sought to eliminate the patient's choice of doc-tor, dictating rather one who would be more likely to follow insurance company guidelines. In a sense, the doctor was in the pay of the third-party payer, not the patient. Mandating behavior, especially when it is as specialized, esoteric, and personal as health care, is impossible, but it has not discouraged the lawmakers, the architects of ethics codes, licensing boards, and managed care organizations from trying to do just that. But once the true doctor-patient relationship was broken, everything other than the prescribed code of practice became a poten-tial dual relationship to be avoided.

Much of the prohibitions of dual relationships are attributed to Sigmund Freud, yet those who knew him describe him as amazingly pragmatic and flexible. A story related to me by Madame Suzanne Bernfeld, wife of Siegfried Bernfeld, PhD, pioneer and founder of the San Francisco Psychoanalytic Institute, demonstrates this. She and Siegfried met while both were in analysis with Freud in Vienna. They developed a relationship and eventually decided to marry. This was a taboo as it was regarded as "psychoanalytic incest," being in treatment with the same psychoanalyst. They shuddered as they anticipated telling Freud, and Siegfried finally admitted he lacked the courage and Suzanne would have to tell him. She recalled lying on the couch, her heart racing in fear as she blurted out that she and Siegfried were about to marry. After minutes of deafening silence, Freud arose, walked across the room to the bookcase, and picking up an artifact she had once admired, he handed it to her, saying, "My wedding present." Was this a dual relationship on the part of Sigmund Freud?

Erik H. Erikson, my training analyst, described to me his usual procedure when a child was referred to him for treatment. He immediately invited himself to dinner and spent the entire evening in the home of the family. He insisted that he learned more from this encounter than he would have through several sessions with the child and family, or from psychological testing. Is this a boundary crossing?

In the mid-1980s I pioneered the first and only clinically driven managed behavioral health care company. Rather than management by denial of services, we managed by expanding services, access, and penetration. We were determined to treat the patient early and effectively, and all of the psychological interventions excluded by third-party payers were eagerly offered (marital counseling, stress management, smoking cessation, assertiveness training, house calls for bedridden agoraphobics, etc.). Our mantra was that "the patient is entitled to relief from pain, anxiety, and depression in the shortest time possible and with the least intrusive intervention." In 7 years we grew to 14.5 million enrollees served by 10,000 psychotherapists in 39 states. In those 7 years there was not a single malpractice suit or patient complaint that had to be adjudicated. In everything we did we applied the rule of doing the right thing. Yet we often found our interventions skirting the edges of the APA Code of Ethics. We were not actually in violation; the code was simply irrelevant to what we were doing. How, for example, do you teach an agoraphobic how to buy a pair of socks without succumbing to panic, unless you go into the department store so as to desensitize her? And how do you teach a chronic schizophrenic in an independent living program how to order a meal in a restaurant without his collapsing into psychosis from fear, unless you have dinner with him?

In my half-century as a therapist, no matter whatever else I did, I averaged 40 to 50 45-minute therapy sessions per week. I was known in San Francisco as the psychotherapist of last resort, and colleagues sent to me their failures or their seemingly intractable clients. My weekly caseload abounded with Axis II, suicidal, borderline personality, psychotic, or severely addicted persons. Yet I never experienced a malpractice suit or the threat of one. Like Columbus, San Francisco is large enough so you do not expect to run into your patients, but small enough so you invariably do. The encounters are more often simple and inadvertent rather than complex, yet they threaten the so-called dual relationship. I recall a very pretty but thoroughly borderline woman who had eliminated all of her previous psychotherapists by seducing them, at least emotionally, but also sexually on two occasions. In therapy I had to place boundaries on Gena's exhibitionism and flagrant seductiveness. She accepted these, but always added, "Someday I'm going to catch you outside your office and you'd better watch out!" One morning I was driving to the office in a downpour, and while stopped at a red light, I saw Gena standing on the corner drenched. She was waiting for the bus, obviously going to our scheduled session. She saw me, but beyond her looking at me smiling, she made no other overture. What should I do? I could pretend I did not see her, but Florence Mateer would say not being genuine is not doing the right thing. I opened the door and called for her to get in. Gena jumped into the seat next to me and, as if to drain the rain off her soaked clothing, she coyly lifted her skirt, saying, "You're so sweet to give me a ride." I replied, "This gives us an extra 20 minutes to your therapy session today." Then I proceeded as if we were in my office, incorporating the chance encounter into her treatment. She not only cooperated, she later told me that was the turning point in her therapy. She realized lovers were a dime a dozen while a therapist who could cut through her defiance and hostility in order to help her was rare, indeed. I recall that night after I had concluded a strenuous and tiring day, I silently thanked the long-deceased Florence Mateer for teaching me how to do the right thing. Her admonition to first do no harm and always do the right thing had helped me navigate for decades potentially troublesome therapeutic waters far better than had a well-meaning, overideational ethics code.

I hope you have enjoyed reading this remarkable and refreshing array of chapters as much as I have.

Summary of Key Points

Nonsexual Dual Relationships in Psychotherapy and Counseling

1. Ethical guidelines of *all* major psychotherapists' professional associations [e.g., the American Psychological Association (APA), the National Association of Social Workers (NASW), the American Counseling Association (ACA), the American Association for Marriage and Family Therapists (AAMFT), the Canadian Psychological Association (CPA), and the California Association for Marriage and Family Therapists (CAMFT)] do *not* mandate a blanket avoidance of all dual relationships, but they all prohibit exploitation and harm of clients. All decree that:

   - Sexual dual relationships with ongoing or current clients are always unethical.
   - Nonsexual dual relationships are not always avoidable.
   - Nonsexual dual relationships are not always unethical.
   - Therapists must avoid *only* dual relationships that might impair their judgment and objectivity, interfere with performing therapy effectively, or harm, exploit, or undermine their patients.

2. Nonsexual dual relationships do not necessarily lead to exploitation, sex, or harm.
3. The "slippery slope" argument, which asserts that the crossing of small insignificant boundaries inevitably leads to sex and ex-

ploitation, is an unfortunate example of irrational and syllogistic reasoning.

4. Because dual relationships are more inclusive, increase familiarity, and reduce the power differential between therapists and clients, they are more likely to prevent exploitation and abuse rather than cause or lead to it.

5. Dual relationships are unavoidable in rural, military, and other small communities, such as the deaf, disabled, gay, universities, among members of the same church, and ethnic minorities.

6. Dual relationships are often a desirable, expected, essential and inherent aspect of interdependent rural and small communities, as they increase familiarity, build trust between therapists and clients, and therefore are likely to enhance therapeutic effectiveness.

7. The prohibition of dual relationships in therapy comes from four sources:

- Federal and state professional regulatory agencies. They instituted the prohibition in an attempt to protect consumers from harm by exploitative therapists.
- Traditional psychoanalysts. They embraced this prohibition primarily for the purpose of ensuring the degree of detachment and neutrality that is necessary for the "analysis of the transference."
- Our litigious culture. Several factions induce fear in therapists of courts, boards, ethics committees, and attorneys. This fear manifests itself through the blind application of strict risk-management guidelines and compels most therapists to employ defensive practices that include extreme measures, such as the absolute avoidance of all dual relationships.
- The mainstream, traditional, urban psychotherapeutic model versus the rural community model. Much like the analytic model in large urban areas, there is a strong emphasis on privacy, anonymity, separation, and strict boundaries in therapy.

8. "Risk Management" may sound like practical or pragmatic advice about avoiding dual relationships and other interventions, but in fact it is a misnomer for a practice in which fear of attorneys and boards, rather than clinical concerns, determines the course of therapy.

9. Therapists are trained, hired, and paid to provide the best care possible for their clients, and this may include engaging in dual relationships. They are not paid to act defensively. Thus, it could be argued that counselors and clinicians are professionally obligated to include dual relationships in their interventions when they assess that this might potentially benefit particular clients.

10. Predatory therapists will exploit with or without prohibitions on dual relationships.

11. Avoiding all dual relationships keeps therapists in unrealistic and inappropriate power positions, increasing the likelihood of exploitation. Underscoring the virtues of selected dual relationships may alter the power differential between therapists and clients in a manner that better facilitates health and healing.

12. Strict, unbending adherence to inflexible rules of boundary limitations may undermine rapport and damage the therapeutic alliance.

13. The absolute ban on dual relationships and the ensuing isolation decreases therapeutic effectiveness because clients' difficulties, many of which were caused by familial-childhood isolation, often cannot be healed by further therapeutic isolation.

14. Therapists are forced to rely on the client's report as the main source of knowledge. Dual relationships can provide additional clinically meaningful information, which can be of inestimable benefit. Therapeutic effectiveness can be diminished by exclusive reliance on a client's subjective perceptions.

15. Unlike the common myth, acquaintance between therapists and clients outside the consulting room does not detract, but in fact can enhance therapeutic effectiveness. (Even those who subscribe to notions of "transference analysis" will find that greater familiarity usually generates grist for the 'transference mill.')

16. Not all therapeutic approaches disparage dual relationships. Behavioral, Humanistic, Cognitive, Family Systems, Group and Existential therapy, at times view dual relationships as an important and integral part of the treatment plan.

17. In many cases, boundary crossings (vs. boundary violations, which inflict harm on clients) are confused with dual relationships. Boundary crossings are not unethical and often constitute the most caring, humane, and effective interventions. Examples of boundary crossings (which are not dual relationships) are:

hugging a grieving client, conducting a home visit with an ailing elderly client, flying with a client who has fear of flying, having a lunch with an anorexic client, going for a vigorous walk with a depressed client, or going to a show where the client is performing.

18. Dual relationships, such as having lunch or socializing with clients, asking a client for a ride to a nearby garage, playing recreational sports together, and bartering, can increase trust, familiarity, and therapeutic effectiveness and speed up the healing process if conducted with thought and care.

19. Dual relationships with seriously disturbed (psychotic) clients, and those with borderline, histrionic, narcissistic, violent, antisocial, or litigious proclivities, are often counterproductive and may lead to clinical, ethical, or even legal complications.

20. The prohibition of dual relationships may be unconstitutional as it is too vague and too broad and may also violate therapists' and clients' constitutional rights of privacy and freedom of association.

21. In a healthy society, unlike our modern culture, people cherish their reliance on one another. The more multiple the relationships, the richer and more profound the individual and cultural experience. Wise elders and practical neighbors all contribute advice and guidance, as well as physical and spiritual support. In ministering to the needs of members of the community, it is detrimental for healers, rabbis, priests, and therapists to shun dual relationships. It makes fundamental sense to depend on them for the insight and intimate knowledge that such relationships provide.

22. Graduate education too often instills a fear of licensing agencies and lawsuits, and it also delivers inadequate instruction about personal integrity, individual ethics, and how to navigate the complex issues of boundaries, duality, and intimacy in therapy. It may also help if graduate schools devoted more attention to screening out emotionally disturbed or mentally unhealthy students who are likely to become exploitative therapists.

In summary, dual relationships are neither always unethical nor do they necessarily lead to harm and exploitation, nor are they always avoidable. Dual relationships can be helpful and beneficial to clients if implemented intelligently, thoughtfully, and with integrity and care.

Guidelines to Nonsexual Dual Relationships in Psychotherapy

GENERAL ETHICAL-CLINICAL GUIDELINES FOR PSYCHOTHERAPY

- Always do whatever it takes to help clients.
- Make sure that you do no harm to clients in the process.
- Never exploit a client.
- Place the client's interest above your own. Avoid situations where there are conflicts of interest.
- Place clients' welfare above your fear of boards, courts, and attorneys.
- Show only respect for your clients and never humiliate them or assail their dignity.
- Provide a safe and trusting haven for healing and growth. Cold, distant, disconnected, and punitive relationships injure clients and do not promote healing.
- Protect and respect the client's privacy and confidentiality (unless by doing so you would fail to safeguard the client, society, etc., from harm).
- Remember you are paid to do a job, not to protect yourself. Clients do not pay you to employ risk management or defensive techniques.

- Develop clear treatment plans that are based on the client's problems, needs, gender, personality, situation, venue, environment, and culture.
- Whenever possible, develop an empirically based treatment plan.
- Intervene with your clients as outlined in each of their treatment plans, *not* according to any graduate school professor's or supervisor's dogma or even your own beloved theoretical orientation. Technical eclecticism is often the most helpful approach.
- Consult with colleagues for their input and assistance if necessary.

DUAL RELATIONSHIPS GUIDELINES

- Include dual relationships in your treatment plans when you assess them to be helpful to the client. In other situations, however, dual relationship should be ruled out. Make sure you know the difference and articulate it in the treatment plan.
- Before entering into a dual relationship, take into consideration the welfare of the client, personality, effectiveness of treatment, avoidance of harm, exploitation and conflict of interest, and the risk of impairment of clinical judgment. These are the paramount and appropriate concerns.
- Before entering into a dual relationship, carefully weigh the complexities, richness, potential benefits and drawbacks, and likely risks that may arise.
- Recognize the fact that dual relationships are not avoidable and are often part of the acceptable and expected norm in many communities, such as the military, rural, deaf, gay, church, colleges, minority, and other small close-knit and interdependent populations.
- When dual relationships are unavoidable proceed with caution. Discuss the complexities of such dual relationships with your clients before and throughout the treatment.
- Before entering into a dual relationship, discuss the risks and benefits with the client. Make sure the client fully understands them, and secure a written and signed agreement. Informed consent is the best way to treat clients with respect and to avoid misunderstandings or false accusations.
- Do not let fear of lawsuits, licensing boards, or attorneys determine your clinical interventions, including decisions about dual relationships. Do not let dogmatic thinking affect your critical thinking.

Act with competence and integrity while minimizing risk by consulting and following these guidelines.

- Do not enter into sexual relations with a current client because it is likely to impair your judgment, nullify your clinical effectiveness, and render you and your client vulnerable to emotional upheaval. It is always unethical and in many cases illegal.
- Remember that articulating the rationale for entering into dual relationships in the treatment planning is an essential and irreplaceable part of your clinical records and your first line of defense.
- Make sure your clinical records document clearly all aspects of dual relationship interventions, such as consultations, substantiation of your conclusions, potential risks, and benefits of significant interventions.
- Before entering into dual relationships, study the clinical, ethical, and legal complexities and potential ramifications of doing so.
- Consult with clinical, ethical, or legal experts in complex dual relationship cases, or whenever you feel confused or uncertain about your treatment trajectory, and incorporate the outcome of such consultations into the treatment plan.
- Minimize the extent of unavoidable dual relationships (such as those in small communities) if you assess that they may interfere with treatment or distress the client.
- Contemplate your own needs and biases before entering into a dual relationship.
- Sometimes dual relationships take an unexpected turn and you must change your treatment accordingly.
- If you have to disengage from dual relationships with a client, due to unforeseen problems, do it in such a way that the best interests of the client are served. You may be best advised to discuss the matter with a respected colleague for guidance and direction.
- It is probably best to avoid entering into a dual relationship, if there are ambiguous or complex issues involved, especially if you have some anticipatory misgivings.
- Avoid dual relationships with seriously disturbed (psychotic) clients, and those with borderline, histrionic, narcissistic, violent, antisocial, or litigious proclivities.
- Rather than operating out of fear and misinformation about dual relationships learn how to navigate the complex issues of boundaries, duality, power, and intimacy in therapy.

Author Index

Subject Index